THE HISTORY OF PUBLIC HEALTH AND THE MODERN STATE

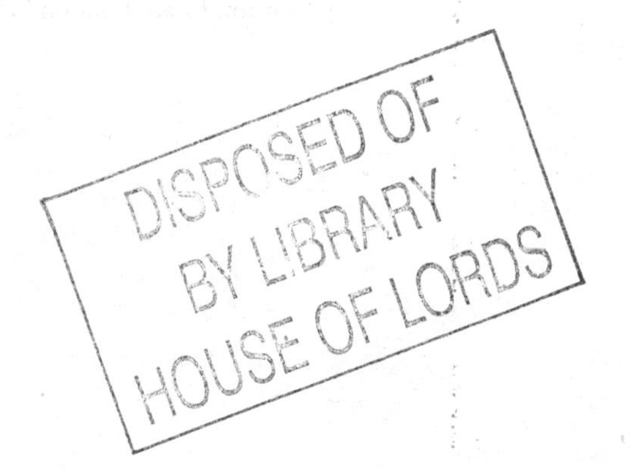

THE WELLCOME INSTITUTE SERIES IN THE HISTORY OF MEDICINE

Forthcoming Titles

The History of Medical Education in Britain
Edited by V. Nutton and Roy Porter

Medicine in the Enlightenment
Edited by Roy Porter

Academic inquiries regarding the series should be addressed to the editors W. F. Bynum and Roy Porter at the Wellcome Institute for the History of Medicine, 183 Euston Road, London NW1 2BE, UK

THE HISTORY OF PUBLIC HEALTH AND THE MODERN STATE

Edited by
Dorothy Porter

First published in 1994
by Editions Rodopi B. V., Amsterdam – Atlanta, GA 1994.

Design and Typesetting: Christine Lavery, the Wellcome Trust.
Printed and bound in the Netherlands by Editions Rodopi B. V.,
Amsterdam – Atlanta, GA 1994.

Front cover: Seven members of the French committee on
vaccination rail at Tapp, a health officer in the seventh
arrondissement of Paris, who resists the introduction of vaccination
into that part of the city. Coloured etching, *c.* 1800.
Wellcome Institute Library, London

British Library Cataloguing in Publication Data
A catalogue record for this book is available from the British Library
ISBN: 90-51 83–552-3 (geb)

CIP-GEGEVENS KONINKLIJKE BIBLIOTHEEK, DEN HAAG
The History of Public Health and the Modern State
Amsterdam – Atlanta, GA Rodopi. – ill.
(Clio Medica 26/The Wellcome Institute Series
in the History of Medicine, ISSN: 0045-7183)

Met index lit. opg.
ISBN: 90-51 83–552-3 (geb)
Trefw.: gezondheidszorg; geschiedenis.

Printed in The Netherlands

Contents

Acknowledgements

As editor my grateful thanks go to the authors of the essays in this collection. They have been faithfully cooperative, prompt and supportive throughout the entire production of the volume. I am deeply indebted to their superb scholarship, good humour and faith. I should also like to thank various unknown referees of both abstract and completed essays who have given valuable advice.

Notes on Contributors

Professor David Arnold, Department of History, School of African and Asian Studies, University of London, UK.

Professor Linda Bryder, Department of History, The University of Auckland, New Zealand.

Professor Jay Cassel, Department of History, York University, Canada.

Professor Elizabeth Fee, Johns Hopkins University School of Hygiene and Public Health, Department of Health Policy and Management, USA.

Professor Mahito H. Fukuda, Nagoya University Language Centre, Japan.

Professor Christopher Hamlin, Program in History and Philosophy of Science, University of Notre Dame, USA.

Professor Karin Johannisson, Uppsala University, Office for History of Science, Sweden.

Dr Maryinez Lyons, Institute of Commonwealth Studies, SOAS, University of London, UK.

Professor Matthew Ramsey, Department of History, Vanderbilt University, Nashville, Tennessee, USA.

Professor Milton I. Roemer, School of Public Health, University of California, Los Angeles, USA.

Susan Gross Solomon, Department of Political Science, University of Toronto, Canada.

Dr Paul Weindling, Wellcome Unit for the History of Medicine, Oxford, UK.

Introduction

Dorothy Porter

In his pioneering *History of Public Health,* published in 1958, George Rosen, the great medical historian and professor of public health at Yale University, suggested that 'The protection and promotion of the health and welfare of its citizens is considered to be one of the most important functions of the modern state.'[1] This book evaluates that assertion and explores the comparative history of health policy in numerous political states in the modern era. Rosen's survey was an exemplary work documenting health regulation in Western societies from the ancient Greek world to the modern United States. It was written at a time when public health appeared to be triumphant in achieving massive reductions in mortality in the West, when scientific medicine seemed to have almost eliminated the menace of pestilence. Our book comes at a time when the problems of world health seem to be far from resolved. Western mortality reduction was matched by ever rising levels of chronic morbidity. Despite the eradication of smallpox, announced by the World Health Organization in 1979 new unfathomable infections have appeared as major international health threats. This book is written at a time when the capabilities of scientific medicine and the ideology of prevention are being tested and cross-examined. Thus our book interrogates public health's past from a different angle of vision, posing new questions, seeking new understanding.

Rosen's story was a chronological account of social progress, arising from the technological advance of science and medicine, in combating endemic and epidemic disease. His history consisted of two components:[2]

> One is the development of medical science and technology. Understanding the nature and cause of disease provides a basis for preventive action and control. However, the effective application of such knowledge depends on a variety of nonscientific elements, basically on political, economic, and social factors. This is the other major strand in the fabric of public health.

For Rosen, the growth of public health paralleled the rise of centralized government, or, as he termed it, 'the great Leviathan, the modern state, whose outlines slowly appear out of the storm-sea of politics like a whale coming to the surface'.[3] He believed that as the modern state began to emerge from the late sixteenth century, so the incipient ideas of national health slowly gained ground in a process which he elsewhere described as a movement *From Medical Police to Social Medicine*.[4]

Rosen pointed out that the early modern state, supported by the political philosophy of mercantilism, was concerned with health. Mercantilism viewed the monarch's subjects as his paternalistic property and equated the entire well-being of society as coterminous with the well-being of the state. It was based, Rosen suggested, on a form of political bookkeeping which enabled the state to measure its strength in terms of the size of its healthy population and guided its administrative goals and objectives. Rosen then traced, from the eighteenth to the twentieth centuries, the steps taken towards social and cultural enlightenment which established health as a right of democratic citizenship long after it was first declared so by the revolutionaries in France in the 1790s. It was a process driven on and speeded up by the penalties of industrialization and urbanization and was radically stimulated by the development of laboratory based experimental science. The story of public health was, for Rosen, one of triumph of knowledge over ignorance, cultural enlightenment over barbarism and the emancipation of modern society from the primitive bondage of disease. In this way public health exemplified the political vision which Rosen and other like-minded intellectuals of his era shared of the historical march towards rational government. It was a political philosophy which reflected a mid-twentieth-century belief in the power of scientific logic to bring about the rational organization of society through comprehensive planning of economic, social and medical relations.[5]

Rosen's somewhat heroic vision was matched by other historians of public health in the 1950s and early 1960s such as the political biographers Samuel Finer, R. A. Lewis and Royston Lambert and the English public health officers who wrote outstanding administrative histories, William Fraser and Colin Fraser Brockington.[6] Their work stimulated a wealth of new research and has informed and influenced many later historians.[7] Subsequently, however, new historical problems appeared which began to challenge the heroic history of public health progress. To begin with, doubt about the role of medicine and public health in the reduction of mortality was aired in *The Rise of Modern Population* by Thomas McKeown in 1976. McKeown attributed it largely to improved nutritional status and standards of living.[8] He allowed that modern medicine had relieved suffering but accredited lengthened life expectancy to heightened immunity resulting from improved diet. McKeown agreed that public health had reduced infant mortality by preventing infantile diarrhoeas through clean water supplies and efficient drainage and sewage removal. But he claimed that the retreat of the great killers of the past, especially those affecting young adults and people in the prime of life, such as tuberculosis, resulted above all from reduced levels of malnutrition. McKeown's thesis spawned a growth industry in historical demography attempting to test, support or refute his hypothesis.[9] Although his arguments have been substantially challenged McKeown irrevocably cast a shadow of doubt over the heroic history of public health.

If Mckeown questioned the historical effectiveness of state medicine, the work of Michel Foucault suggested that it could be positively repressive. In his analysis of the characteristic relation ship between knowledge and power in modern society, Foucault identified a new form of authoritative 'gaze'. Foucault believed that from the time of the Enlightenment scientific categories of knowledge had come to dominate Western culture. But this 'rationalization' of society was constituted by the development of disciplinary knowledges and languages. In modern Western cultures power operated through new mechanisms of surveillance which achieved extensive behavioural discipline by turning the individual and his subjective experience into a subjugated body. Foucault picked out, medicine, psychiatry, criminology and the modern discourse surrounding sexuality amongst the new dialogues of repression. The rise of scientific medicine, Foucault suggested, had achieved a medicalization of social relations which turned sickness into a form of deviance. This enhanced the professional power of medicine to police health and illness. The 'body' had thus become the focus of a wide range of surveillance and disciplinary control in which the role of the medical profession was critical.[10] The birth of the clinic, the growth of the teaching hospital, institutionalized the medical gaze. This expanded into the bio-politics of populations and facilitated the regulation of the production and reproduction of life by the state.[11]

Following Foucault, some historians have identified the political regulation of health and the prevention of disease as based upon the power of disciplinary knowledge. This has led to the exploration of the conflict between increased distribution of the opportunities for health and the expansion of the regulatory power of the state, inevitably contrasting the civil liberties of the individual with the collective needs of the community.[12] These questions have been most acutely addressed in the analysis of the role of eugenics in the modern campaign for avoiding disease and planning a healthy society. Some historians have interpreted Francis Galton's creed for improving the human race through selective breeding as the ultimate technocratic nightmare.[13] Contemporary historians, such as Daniel Kevles, Paul Weindling, Greta Jones, Pauline Mazumder and others have deciphered the late nineteenth and early twentieth century discourse on biological degeneration in order to draw out the totalitarian implications of the eugenic solution to the health of populations. Such investigations contest the image of rational political planning which was advocated by Rosen's generation of historians. They hold up the eugenically inspired policies of compulsory sterilization and racial genocide as a warning about the way in which comprehensive planning can cross the line from emancipatory to murderously repressive public policy.[14]

Images of health bureaucracy becoming despotic technocracy have inspired investigation into the professionalization of public health. Older historical accounts concentrated on singularly important doctors in their role as administrators, such as John Simon, Britain's first chief medical officer from 1854 to 1876.[15] But more contemporary research has turned to a broader review of the various occupational groups who made up public health services. In the United States and in Britain Elizabeth Fee, Christopher Hamlin, Dorothy Porter and Jane Lewis have tried to discover who were public health workers, both medical and non-medical.[16] They have asked questions about their training and their professional ideologies. How did public health professionals consolidate their power to direct and implement public policy? To what extent did the professionalization of public health constitute a 'medicalization' and were some Victorians correct in equating the expansion of public health with the establishment of medical despotism?[17] Above all, does the analysis of the public health service confirm or refute Harold Perkin's assertions about the rise of professional society? Is the public health service an example of how the growth of the modern bureaucratic state is coterminous with the rise of the power of the professions? Do public health professionals feature in a new pattern of power and control in contemporary societies?[18]

Thus a new anti-heroic history of public health was inspired by Foucault and might equally be understood as a product of its times. It was formulated in the midst of late twentieth-century debates questioning the ambiguities of the Enlightenment, the rise of rational society, the expansion of the bureaucratic state and the normative basis of scientific rationality and its logic of domination.[19] The anti-heroic historiography interrogated the story of public health progress by attempting to deconstruct the dialectics of biology and culture. This has also been been reflected in the social history of disease. Studies on the black death, early-modern and modern plague, nineteenth century cholera, yellow fever, smallpox, typhus, tuberculosis and twentieth century polio and influenza have addressed the way in which disease is both framed and frames the processes of historical transition.[20] The arrival of AIDS as a world-wide pandemic has encouraged historians to cooperate with other social scientists to interpret how epidemics are constructed by and construct social relations.[21] The variety of responses to epidemics have been scrutinized, both religious and secular. Recent research has focused especially on the reciprocity of social dislocation and epidemic spread and the implications of the metaphoric meaning of disease in the semiotics of cultural representation.[22]

The essays here attempt to locate public health within the social history of biology and culture. But what emerges from them is that, above all, public health cannot be addressed as a monolithic march towards either inevitable progress or totalitarian repression. The variation between national contexts of power in which political responsibility for health developed, highlights its multiple and often contradictory dimensions. My aim in this Introduction is to draw out how, when the stories here are taken collectively, they challenge some of the main tenets of both the heroic and anti-heroic history of public health.

Mercantilism and Medical Police

The health of its population is a prerequisite for the survival of all human societies and since ancient times rules and protocols have been devised to promote it. The Hippocratic discourses on the effects of *Airs, Waters and Places* on local endemnicity, for example, provided crucial advice for colonization in Ancient Greece.[23] Health regulation has been greatly spurred by the impact of epidemic infectious diseases. Certain diseases were long held to be spread through human contact which led to the isolation of sufferers in colonies or lazarettos to protect the healthy. From the fourteenth century the role of civil authorities in instituting isolation greatly expanded in Europe when a number of Mediterranean city states introduced quarantines to protect themselves against the major epidemic of bubonic plague which began in 1346 – commonly known as the Black Death. The historians Richard Palmer and Carlo Cipolla have highlighted the way in which epidemic emergencies enhanced the power of Renaissance Italian city states to create strict civil regulation despite opposition from religious and mercantile interests.[24] Similarly, Paul Slack has pointed to the introduction of compulsory municipal quarantines against plague in sixteenth- and seventeenth-century England.[25]

From the fifteenth century the Western World rose to global dominance in wealth, trade, and military power. But as the West grew wealthier it did not grow healthier. Scholars such as William McNeill and Alfred Crosby have chronicled the devastation and sometimes decimation of the West's populations by endemic infections and waves of epidemics and pandemics.[26] The precise circumstances of early capitalism, with its inevitable accompaniments of crowded, cramped urban living, created the profoundest health problems. The contradiction between the health and wealth of nations was not lost, however, on mercantilist political and economic thought which developed the first systematic assessment of the health of the state. As mentioned above Rosen demonstrated how the philosophy which underpinned the political arithmetic of the late seventeenth-century English gentlemen-scholars William Petty and John Graunt also justified the creation of the late eighteenth-century schemes for medical police originated by the Austrian physicians Johann Peter Franck, Wolfgang Thomas Rau and Anton Mai. Rosen posited a model of medical police originating in the German context which withered away as state medicine emerged with the rise of industrial democracies in the nineteenth-century.[27]

Paul Weindling points out here in his chapter on 'Public Health in Germany', that although Austria continued to be the source of much innovation in the field of public health none of the German states translated mercantilist philosophies of health care into systematic state policies. Instead Karin Johannisson in her chapter 'The People's Health: Public Health Policies in Sweden' shows it was eighteenth-century Sweden which took them thoroughly to heart. She demonstrates how shockingly low levels of population in Sweden, discovered in an early eighteenth-century survey, galvanized the state into action on health and pronatalism. Sweden's homogenous society and universal episcopal bureaucracy enabled the state to institute the first comprehensive system of population registration and census taking. The promotion of fertility and personal hygiene education, the policing of sexually and socially transmitted diseases through policies of isolation and treatment, and the development of municipal hospitals were instituted in eighteenth-century Sweden in the name of strengthening the state through population growth. This comprehensive system was established through Sweden's effective local secular and episcopal bureaucracies long before Johann Peter Frank included such measures in his theoretical system of medical police. Throughout Europe, however, mercantilist concerns over healthy population levels promoted ever stricter enforcement of port quarantines, border *cordon sanitaires* and the policing of public nuisances and civil disorder.

Weindling discusses how the ideology of medical police justified dominance of public health administration in Germany by legally trained civil servants almost until the end of the nineteenth century. It took the triumphs of bacteriology to legitimate the medical take-over of the direction and control of health policy in unified Germany after 1871. But, he notes, the concept of medical police survived the medicalization of public health in Germany and provided legitimation of the policies of racial hygiene instituted under the Third Reich.

In his essay on 'Public Health in France' Matthew Ramsey says that the concept of medical police helped to found a primitive health administration under the *ancien régime* initiated by Louis XIV's minister of finance, Colbert. By the end of the eighteenth century this was administered through the Societé Royale du Médecine founded to police medical nostrums and quackery, distribute medicine chests to rural health authorities and to set up a network of reporting on local epidemics.[28] But Ramsey suggests that the fundamental principles of medical policing continued to fit well with a post-revolutionary strong centralized state in the early nineteenth century which had little regard for civil liberties but equally little enthusiasm for collective intervention. He demonstrates that political and economic individualism in France supported the policing of individual hygienic responsibility and avoided addressing the collective needs of the community.

But mercantilism and medical police were not the only impetus to public health innovation prior to the nineteenth century. Rosen pointed out how Enlightenment humanitarianism emphasized the role of philanthropy in facilitating self-help and civic improvement. As Christopher Hamlin in his essay here on 'State Medicine in Great Britain', and James Riley and John Pickstone elsewhere, have highlighted, town improvement commissioners in late eighteenth-century England sought to bring about the 'civilizing process' amongst the wretchedly squalid poor by inducing self-improvement through environmental improvement.[29] Furthermore, as Roy Porter has demonstrated, the largest expanding free-market economy in Europe made civic environmentalism a profitable trade, spawning new commercial enterprises in night soil collection, street widening, paving and lighting.[30] Christopher Hamlin suggests that when combined with the theories of political economy, sanitary reform and evangelical piety, this Enlightenment humanitarianism emerged as a sort of 'moral ecology' amongst nineteenth century public health enthusiasts such as Thomas Southwood Smith, the Unitarian doctor who was Chadwick's closest ally.[31] But, as Ramsey notes, the Parisian *parti d'hygiène* of the 1830s equally drew upon such ideological resources.

By far the most important ideological influence on late eighteenth-century rhetoric about health and the political state, however, was the Enlightenment philosophy of revolutionary democracy. Thomas Paine did not include health amongst the property rights to which all free men are innately entitled but, as George Rosen discovered, Thomas Jefferson declared that sick populations were the product of sick political systems.[32] According to Jefferson, despotism produced disease, democracy liberated health. Which is why, Matthew Ramsey tells us, the revolutionary committees on salubrity and public assistance under the French Constituent Assembly and the National Convention between 1790–2 declared health to be one of the rights of man. Thus the colours of health citizenship were pinned to the mast of political obligations of the modern democratic state. Elsewhere scholars such as Dora Weiner and Ludmilla Jordanova have pointed out, however, that health citizenship was two-sided because Idéologues, such as Constantine Volney, believed that the body of the democratic citizen was an economic unit of the free state.[33] Thus *Citizen Patient* had a duty to keep well, through temperance and healthy regimen.[34]

Democratic rhetoric on health citizenship failed to translate into reality in any late Enlightenment state. But, as Ramsey and Weindling show, it was still idealistically burning in the hearts of the German and French revolutionaries of 1848. The mantle of health reform was, however, inherited by utilitarian political economy. It was the economic value of preventing premature mortality to the expanding industrial state which was ultimately responsible for public health reform in early nineteenth-century Europe.

Industrialization and Centralization

Rosen and his contemporaries believed that the massive scale of health problems created by industrialization and urbanization provoked central government response.[35] As we have already noted from the example of Sweden, however, industrialization was not a prerequisite for state action on population health. In other national contexts discussed here, the discourses on state medicine often preceded industrialization.

The historical example which underlay the traditional model of the centralization of public health administration was Victorian Britain. In Britain massive and rapid industrialization and urbanization provoked advocates of utilitarian economic individualism to consider how state intervention might maximize the opportunities for free enterprize. Led by Jeremy Bentham's secretary and most ardent disciple, Edwin Chadwick, public health reform in England was a crusade to reduce the financial burden of destitution through a campaign against epidemic infections caused by 'filth'.[36] Hamlin shows here, however, that the public health movement was also influenced by philanthropic goals. It included individuals such as the great philanthropist and the first president of the Board of Health, the Seventh Earl of Shaftesbury and the author of famous sanitary surveys in Manchester and London and first secretary to the Department of Education at the Privy Council, Sir James Phillips Kay-Shuttleworth. Shaftesbury, Kay-Shuttleworth and the only medical inspector to the Board of Health, Thomas Southwood Smith, all aimed to reform the 'ragged' classes by educating them into the role of civically hygienic citizens.[37] Philanthropic reformers perceived public health as a campaign of humanitarian improvement of the poor by eliminating environmental filth and moral depravity with one stroke.

Charles Rosenberg and Barbara Rosenkrantz have extensively discussed how environmental hygiene as evangelical moral reform also underlaid the early public health movement in the United States.[38] President Zachary Taylor responded to the 1848 cholera epidemic by ordering a national day of fasting. He believed this was the way America could atone for the fact – as he saw it – that industriousness had turned into ambition and pious prudent profit-making and thrift into avarice and greedy accumulation. Early health reformers, such as Henry Griscom in New York and Lemuel Shattuck in Boston, believed that environmental improvement to prevent epidemic disease was a moral mission. While evangelical hygiene still identified the poor as the carriers of corruption it also admonished the wealthy for failing to act. Yet, as Elizabeth Fee discusses here in her essay on 'Public Health and the State: The United States', philanthropic paternalism was undermined by the increasingly ruggedly individualistic culture in America from the time of Andrew Jackson.[39] For most of the nineteenth century public health in the United States was limited to *ad hoc* measures and the efforts of voluntary agencies in response to emergencies, such as yellow fever and cholera epidemics. Long-term institutional development was sporadic and often ineffective until the last quarter of the nineteenth century.

The utilitarian solution to the health penalties of industrialization and urbanization involved the libertarian British Victorian state in a dilemma. This dilemma was an inherent feature of what George Kitson Clark and Oliver MacDonagh[40] long ago reappraised as the nineteenth-century revolution in government; i.e. the influence of utilitarianism upon the growth of bureaucratic government dominated by professional civil servants.[41] Hamlin discusses how tensions between the growth of central state intervention and the *laissez-faire* tenets of British politics remained unresolved throughout the nineteenth and early twentieth century up to the First World War. The champions of English liberalism and local democracy lashed out equally at paternalism and centralization slowing the pace of bureaucratic growth and ousting Chadwick from power (once called England's Prussian Minister by Lord John Russell).[42] Such tensions were expressed dramatically in the contradiction between state enforcement of health and the civil liberties of individuals in such measures as compulsory smallpox vaccination.

In Britain, compulsory health regulation stimulated popular resistance movements such as the Anti-vaccination League and Association to Repeal the Contagious Disease Acts.[43] These organizations succeeded in repealing the compulsory laws on infant vaccination and the inspection and detention of prostitutes.[44] Numerous authors here show, however, that many other nineteenth-century industrializing nations excluded such conflicts by simply avoiding the expansion of the central state altogether.[45] In France, Ramsey points out, the legacy of the revolution left a fundamental ideological contradiction between the supremacy of the rights of individual citizens and the paternalistic duties of the republic of virtue.[46] The post-Napoleonic state emerged strong at the centre, protecting property rights, but highly resistant to interventionist action. Thus, while France led the intellectual and practical development of public hygiene in the 1830s and 1840s the French state, Ramsey suggests, never translated this into policy innovation. The *parti d'hygiène* identified the social and economic aetiology of preventable mortality but relied on the remoralization of the poor to resolve the relationship between poverty and disease.[47]

In the United States, Fee stresses, the dominant *laissez-faire* political philosophy resisted paternalistic public policy reforms throughout the nineteenth century.[48] This was equally the case in the British colonies of Canada, Australia and New Zealand. In this context, paternalism was the key characteristic of the motherland which the new worlds wanted to leave behind.[49] Jay Cassel suggests in his chapter on 'Public Health in Canada' that cultural rivalries amongst the Canadian colonies ensured diversity. Yet in both British and French provinces public health was largely ignored because the high value placed upon unfettered market opportunity endorsed resistance to the adoption of metropolitan public health measures. Low taxation and opportunity for profit were always prized above the need for sanitary reform by both the British and French Canadian communities.

Linda Bryder shows in her chapter 'A New World? Two Hundred Years of Public Health in Australia and New Zealand', that European colonials were equally determined to resist old world paternalism in both of the Antipodean states. She demonstrates that it was the native indigenous populations which suffered most from this policy.[50] Economic growth and colonization in the nineteenth century had massive health consequences for Aborigine and Maori communities. Though often politically ignored or glossed over by the colonial governments, economic development also had high costs for the immigrant white urban poor within these increasingly affluent states. The much-vaunted environmental paradises of these new worlds could not mask ever-rising mortality rates from the 1860s from the classic epidemic infections which accompany economic growth and urbanization. No significant attention was paid to them, however, until, as Bryder suggests, a new language of social biology began to redefine the problem of population fitness in the early twentieth century.[51]

In colonies used by the European powers for the exploitation of their natural resources the role of centralized health administration in the nineteenth century varied. In his chapter on 'Crisis and Contradiction in India's Public Health', David Arnold shows that through apathy and neglect Victorian British rulers in India failed to build up the system of local administration required to implement central government initiatives. Instead the military became the main organ of administration.[52] This was effective, however, only in the context of preserving white British communities. By contrast, in her essay on 'Public Health in Colonial Africa: The Belgian Congo' Maryinez Lyons demonstrates that from the 1880s the rulers of the Belgian Congo universally enforced rigorous social hygiene. The goal of centralized disease prevention, however, was not the improvement of community health but eliminating shortages of native labour power.[53] In the context of imperial economic and political exploitation, therefore, the role of centralized control of population health varied widely from one colony to another.

Central state intervention was equally resisted in Europe and North America by the strength of local government and regional diversity. Weindling illustrates how, despite the image of Prussian domination, the federated German states retained high levels of local autonomy well beyond unification in 1871. This pattern of power resulted in a great deal of variation in health administration between states, so that while in Prussia it was most highly developed and routinized, numerous innovations were made by smaller states such as Saxony. In Germany all state-trained doctors who became health officers, *Kreisärzte,* remained subordinate to civil service control. Local diversity meant wide variety in the level of interventionist regulation, for example of infectious and sexually transmitted diseases. Thus, despite a degree of growing central regulation after 1871, Weindling suggests that German public health administration continued to be a diverse patchwork.[54] Even under Nazi totalitarianism local variations persisted.[55] In France also, Ramsey points out, until the end of the nineteenth century, local autonomy resulted in as much diversification. The Paris Health Council established the most comprehensive administration, but Rhineland provinces retained German-style systems of cantonal public health officers and local government health bureaucracies. French port quarantine authorities, such as Marseilles, maintained their traditional high degree of autonomy except in times of epidemic emergencies. Then the central state imposed unprecedented interventionist policies in sanitary cordoning and isolation.

In the United States, Fee points out that 'states' rights' have remained a barrier to the development of a Federal health department up to the present day.[56] In the first decade of the twentieth century a 'Committee of One Hundred' health reformers, officials and intellectuals forcefully lobbied for the creation of a Federal department but their attempt was blocked by political resistance to centralization. Public health administration spread slowly and unevenly from major east coast urban centres like Boston and New York to southern and mid-west and western territories. Wide varieties in local environments over the vast continental territory facilitated particular responses to public health necessities. And although, as John Duffy has emphasized,[57] coherence was first instituted through sanitary administration in the Civil War, Fee shows that *ad hoc* initiative resisted the professionalization of public health in the United States until the late nineteenth century. Coordinated public health response remained in the hands of a quasi-military agency, the Marine Hospital Service (transformed into the U.S. Public Health Service in 1912).[58]But national policy, Fee insists, eluded United States public health organization without the establishment of a Federal Government department and individual state authorities dominated a diverse agenda.

Centralization was thus resisted by both the forces of anti-paternalism and *laissez-faire* politics on the one hand and the issue of local diversity and autonomy on the other. The strongest representation of centralization in our collection is the story that Susan Gross Solomon tells in her chapter on 'The Expert and the State in Russian Public Health: Continuities and Changes Across the Revolutionary Divide'. She points out that in Russia the universal training and employment of doctors by the Tsarist state always ensured powerful central control of all health and medical services. Central control continued after the 1917 revolution. Russian physicians constantly sought greater influence in the central bureaucracy by trying to convert government policy on population health to their own professional goals and methods. Physicians did not gain such influence, however, until experts played a greater role in policy making in the Soviet system in the 1920s.[59]

Centralized administration in Russia, however, was long an inherent feature of its political history.[60] It was not the political consequence of the rise of industrial society. Even in modern corporatist Japan, later but rapid industrialization did not create the level of centralized bureaucracy that might be expected. In his essay on 'Public Health in Modern Japan: from Regimen to Hygiene', Mahito Fukuda tells us that under the Meiji Restoration, which replaced the Tokugawa Shogun military dictatorship from 1868, medical education and public health reforms became the responsibility of the Department of Medical affairs in the Ministry of Education. This was part of a major government initiative to increase production, promote industry, enrich the country and strengthen the army. But a separate government department of health did not emerge until after the Second World War, which still hesitates to implement highly interventionist public health policy. As a result, Fukuda points out the cause of preventive medicine remains underdeveloped in modern Japan. Our essay collection, therefore, suggests that the historical model of inevitable centralization of public health administration in industrial societies requires serious revision.

Medicalization and Professionalization of Public Health

If industrialization did not automatically produce centralization then did the medical 'gaze' induce the state regulation of the bio-politics of populations? Was the rationalization of public health a medicalization of power?[61]

Early public health reform was dominated by an idiosyncratic collection of political radicals, civil servants, philanthropists, and moral crusaders. From the mid-nineteenth-century in Europe, however, it became increasingly professionalized. The 1848 revolutions in France and Germany witnessed doctors demanding that medicine take a new spiritual lead in recasting the values of modern society.[62] Jules Guérin, the editor of the Paris *Gazette Médicale*, hailed the dawn of an epoch of 'social medicine'. Rudolf Virchow, the German founder of cellular pathology, urged doctors to become advocates for the poor.[63] In France and Germany, however, doctors did not begin to make a significant mark in public health until after Pasteur and Koch had achieved their great propaganda coups with the new science of bacteriology in the 1870s and 1880s.[64] Despite Virchow's medical reform movement and the demand of Germany's most famous public health campaigner, Max Von Pettenkofer, for the creation of academic hygiene as a university discipline, Weindling shows this was not established until the 1890s. The French academic medical élite were central in forming the *parti d'hygiène*, but Ramsey agrees with Bruno Latour, that not until after *The Pasteurization of France*[65] did the medical administration of public health become a national policy agenda.

From 1854 in England one of London's élite surgeons, John Simon, succeeded to Chadwick's public health throne. But as Hamlin argues, although the medical cavalry appeared to arrive in England with Simon's appointment as Britain's first Chief Medical Officer, the pace of public health legislation slackened.[66] It was rather the ever increasing number of doctors taking up state medical appointments in the localities that established a powerful medical influence within the system. But doctors, Hamlin shows, were only one amongst many professional groups vying for control of local health administrations. Furthermore, as the recent studies edited by Fee and Acheson have shown, by the last quarter of the century British medical men increasingly obtained post-graduate specialist qualifications in preventive medicine, which some took up as a full-time occupation and renounced therapeutics entirely.[67] And as Dorothy Porter has discussed elsewhere, by 1900 the Society of Medical Officers of

Health, self-consciously proclaimed preventive medicine to be a separate profession with its own agenda which would replace the need for therapeutics altogether.[68] Thus the British public health service was made up of medically trained men who had little in common, and were often hostile to, the clinical medical profession. Jane Lewis has shown that in the twentieth-century British public health officers lost their battle with the medical profession to dominate the nationalization of health care services. She points out that this resulted largely out of a failure to institutionalize a coherent professional ideology that moved with the times.[69]

Doctors were more successful at dominating the development of state medicine in the colonial context. As opportunities for public health employment expanded in the British colonies, specialized qualifications became a valuable exportable asset. Bryder shows how considerable numbers of Australian and New Zealand doctors took up the new opportunities for specialized training in Britain and went back to dominate the development of Antipodean public health administrations. Arnold and Lyons demonstrate that physicians were equally influential in the Indian and African colonies as the instruments of colonial rule; indeed this often extended beyond the field of health administration. The medical profession was not, however, the only agency involved in bringing western medicine and health regulation to indigenous communities. The Christian missionary movement also fulfilled this role.[70]

In her analysis of the American Public Health Association Barbara Rosenkrantz established that when it was formed in 1872[71] it brought together many public health-minded reformers. Physicians participated more as philanthropists rather than specialists in disease control. But Fee suggests here that even when specialist public health training was institutionalized in the United States in the 1890s the shortage of doctors meant that few medical men took it up. Thus public health schools in America began and continued to train social workers, civil engineers and community nurses to qualify as specialists in public health. In the United States, therefore, public health remains an eclectic discipline.[72] When doctors did enter the profession, however, they aimed to dominate it.[73] Thus, Fee concludes, medicine retained an ambiguous and somewhat contradictory relationship to public health in the United States. On the one hand the medical profession wanted to distance themselves from the degraded status of public health practice and on the other they sought to maintain a controlling influence upon it.[74]

In Germany and Russia medical education had always been

controlled by the state. As noted above, in Russia all medical appointments were made by the state and many doctors opted to work in the *zemstvo* system of community health centres, introduced by the Tsar in the 1860s, where they could maximize their medical autonomy. Solomon suggests that doctors eventually gained greater influence in state health policy in the 1920s. Then, however, they gained status only by becoming specialists in a new discipline called social hygiene which mixed political commitment with technical knowledge.

Without evidence of an unchallenged domination of public health administration by doctors it would be hard to sustain an argument for the expansion of the medical gaze to the bio-politics of populations. The professionalization of public health emerges here as the result of a more eclectic combination of expertise. But this is not to deny that professional ideology itself was not a powerful force in the regulation of population health. What the essays here show is that in the intricate dialectics of professional ideology, the influence of medical knowledge was differentiated and diffuse.[75]

Medical theory was one powerful influence on professionalization of public health. Yet even this was not straight forward.[76] The early nineteenth-century controversies over the causation of disease were interpreted by historians, such as Erwin Ackerknecht, as being responsible for the support and abandonment of quarantine and the support or resistance to the sanitary improvement of towns.[77] Elsewhere Margaret Pelling and Christopher Hamlin have reinterpreted the status of pre-bacteriological aetiology, however, recasting it as a story with mixed rather than mutually exclusive metaphors.[78] In her book on *Cholera, Fever and English Medicine 1825–1865*, Pelling pointed out that in England at least, rigid anti-contagionism was largely confined to the narrow but powerful official orthodoxy of the Chadwickian circle of policy makers. Among the English medical profession as a whole, however, 'contingent-contagionism' dominated. This was a mixture of aetiological theories, which held that some diseases were caused by contact others by atmospheric pollution with miasmas.[79] Christopher Hamlin both here and in other scholarly articles has reformulated the debate suggesting that it is more useful to understand early nineteenth-century disease theory in terms of the division between pre-disposing and exciting causes. This linked disease theory into older humoralist views of their action within the body and showed how diseases could be pre-disposed by atmospheric conditions while at the same time be directly caused by an active, if occult, agency.[80] Here both Hamlin and Ramsey show that in both Britain and France no clear division of opinion existed between miasmatism or contagionism and that public hygiene called upon both.

If historiographical battles rage over the epistemological status of mid-century 'contingent-contagionism' the social history of the impact of bacteriology upon public health ideology is equally fraught. Numerous historians have pointed out that bacteriology inaugurated an era of professionalized 'new public health' in the United States.[81] Elizabeth Fee suggests here, however, that the 'new public health' narrowed the sanitary programme towards a pursuit of individual 'carriers' of infectious microbes. Elsewhere David Armstrong and Dorothy Porter, have claimed that bacteriology had a negligible effect in changing the implementation of policy and it was more influential in preparing the way for a shift towards a sociological approach to the health of populations.[82]

Recently historians have suggested that other late nineteenth-century biomedical theories also had a deep influence on preventive medicine. Greta Jones has described this as a marriage between eugenics and public health in the rise of social hygiene.[83] Here Paul Weindling discusses how in Germany, this movement was led by the powerful intellectual Alfred Grotjahn who, at the end of the nineteenth century, believed that the way to health lay in the pursuit of social pathology. Obvious links existed between social and racial hygiene but the road from social pathology to the 'final solution' was not, Weindling insists, a simple or linear progression.

Eugenics had a mixed reception among public health officials in Britain. Leading medical officers of health opposed the eugenic agenda for state medicine but did co-opt the language of social Darwinism and imperialism into their struggle to establish health and social welfare provisions for infants and mothers.[84] Early twentieth-century anxieties over population[85] quantity and quality also stimulated the development of maternal and child welfare elsewhere. Cassel, Bryder and Johannisson discuss how anxiety over depopulation and declining birth rates focused attention upon the health of mothers, babies and schoolchildren in Canada, Australia, New Zealand and Sweden after 1900. Karin Johannisson tells us that in twentieth-century Sweden the state medical system was expanded into a comprehensive welfare plan out of fears about degeneration and diminished population growth. Bryder and Cassel suggest that in the British settlement colonies the first real moves toward state medicine began with the creation of infant and maternal welfare designed to ensure continued imperialist domination. Though both European and colonial eugenists feared that proletarian fecundity threatened to outstrip the reproductive rates of the middle classes, contraception and abortion were almost universally outlawed on the assumption that the prudent and thrifty would use it and the feckless and reckless would go on breeding like rabbits.[86]

Pronatalism and infant and maternal welfare were heavily promoted in France at the end of the First World War when a massive public education campaign encouraged its demobbed sons to procreate as fast and often as possible. The pronatalist campaign, Ramsey points out, followed a period of rapid expansion in public health and social welfare legislation.[87] In Germany during the Second World War positive eugenics stimulated a bizarre system of special ante-natal clinics and orphan homes for the progeny of S.S. officers with suitably Aryan women. The attempt to breed a blond haired, blue-eyed race was supported by a broad sweep of policies providing public financial and tax incentives for early marriage and the production of large families amongst 'Aryan types'.[88]

Positive eugenics, therefore, played a part in the development of ante-natal and baby clinics, school inspection services, free school meals and family allowances. It did not, however, set an agenda of its own, but served as a rhetorical resource to support preventive medical programmes which already had their own momentum. The reduction of infant mortality, for example, had been a major public health priority of the nineteenth-century sanitary idea. This priority became recast in the biologistic language of social Darwinism in the twentieth century even though the political goals of maternal and infant welfare programmes everywhere, with the exception of Germany, remained the same.

Negative eugenics, on the other hand, inaugurated a social policy agenda of its own. The compulsory sterilization of certain categories of incarcerated felons and the mentally handicapped was legally instituted in the United States, Germany and Sweden before the Second World War.[89] In Sweden, Karin Johannisson shows, compulsory sterilization was a feature of the demographic focus of its twentieth-century politics. Paul Weindling discusses how in Germany sterilization policy was extended into a plan for the comprehensive extermination of Jews, political dissidents, the mentally handicapped and others deemed undesirable by the Third Reich.[90] Apart from the legal sterilization of criminals and mentally handicapped, eugenics in the United States provided ideological justifications for immigration restriction and the development of IQ testing. In both the United States and Germany, however, negative eugenics can be seen to have accommodated rather than invented a set of political goals whose origins have a much broader cultural base.[91]

In Russia the field of social hygiene expanded in yet another direction.[92] Susan Gross Solomon describes how community physicians turned themselves into specialists in social hygiene based upon the interface between sociology and biology. Eugenics was only one component of Soviet social hygiene which incorporated a broad array of sociological disciplines into preventive medicine in the 1920s. The post-revolutionary social hygienists, however, claimed continuity with the *zemstvo* physicians' concerns about socio-economic influences on health and also with their dedication to fulfilling the political interests of the 'people'. After 1917, community physicians sought to consolidate their status and power in the new Soviet state by institutionalizing the political role of preventive medicine in socialist health care. Solomon suggests that the social hygienists straddled the boundaries between social medicine as purely technical expertise, and socialist medicine as political action on health.

The boundaries between the medical and social sciences were further explored by clinicians in the United States and Britain in the twentieth century. Arthur Viseltear has described the attempts at Yale in the 1930s to establish a new interdisciplinary medical curriculum[93] and Dorothy Porter has discussed the work of leading British doctors who set up social medicine in the 1940s.[94] As Fee and Hamlin state here, however, none of these attempts practically enhanced the power or influence of preventive medicine either before or after the Second World War. Yet it is clear from Solomon's account that social medicine in Western democracies was imbued with the socialist ethos of the Soviet health system, not least perhaps because many Western visitors to the Eastern block transported their observations back home.[95]

The essays here show that the professionalization of public health resulted from an eclectic mixture of expert knowledge from both the medical and the social sciences. Medicine was only one component of the specialism of disease prevention and health preservation. It is also clear that the power of professionals was constrained within the socio-political environment in which it operated. The political complexion of governments and their priorities determined the power of professionals to dominate the regulation of health. Those priorities varied in different national contexts at different historical moments and ranged from the needs of the free-market economy and fears of imperial decline, to the needs of economic colonial exploitation, or the equalization of health opportunities. These were political rather than professional goals. While the ideological power of specialist expertise is not denied, to suggest that in public health this represented the diffusion of a purely medical gaze would be myopic.

Imperialism and the Transfer of Health Technology

Neither the heroic or anti-heroic historiography has really addressed the complex historical connection between public health and imperialism.[96] The essays here show that national political context is crucial. In Europe imperialist rivalries fuelled anxieties over the biological quality of national population stocks. In colonies used for European settlement, public health bolstered white domination. In colonies used for Western exploitation of resources, white ruler 'enclaves' were preserved either through exclusive health reforms or through draconian policies imposed upon the indigenous populations.[97] The transfer of public health technology from the metropolitan to the colonial context, however, was often met with resistance and created cultural conflict.[98]

British interest in India began as a purely commercial enterprise but from the early nineteenth century the imperial rulers started to aspire to cultural as well as economic colonization. But if servants of the British Crown in India in the 1820s, such as James Mill and T. B. Macaulay, sought to integrate India into a Utilitarian dream of administrative government their successors were disillusioned by the 1850s.[99] After the events of 1857 British attitudes began to reinterpret Indian cultural resistance as indelibly flawed with oriental 'backwardness'.[100] British rule became increasingly conservative and coercive in the second half of the nineteenth century, making allies only with the indigenous ruling castes and perceiving the mission to Westernize as a largely futile task.[101] David Arnold shows how many British sanitary reforms were reproduced in India carried along by the ethos of the Utilitarian experiment in government. Sanitary reforms, however, were exclusively implemented for the white communities and administered largely through the military organization. Numerous explanations have been offered to explain British refusal to address the health and social deprivation of its dependent colony. One argument has suggested that British focus was narrowly geared to economic exploitation and that any 'mission' to modernize, educate, or develop India was largely empty rhetoric. Another interpretation has cited resistance to the imposition of European culture. Yet a further explanation involves the question of conflict between the metropolitan and colonial administrations. British rulers in India were dependent upon policies dictated by the metropolitan administration at home and any autonomy of action was thus extremely limited. In this sense, both David Arnold and Maryinez Lyons show that colonial rule is a special category of 'modern state', divided within itself and always wrestling with challenges to its authority and control from its occupied subjects.

However, even when an obligation to apply public health reforms to the entire Indian population was theoretically acknowledged by the British, neglect, parsimony and bigotry about oriental 'backwardness' prevented progress. Public health measures were taken with regard to the Indian population only when white colonial lives were believed to be threatened, for example by plague in the 1890s. Then strict isolation and sanitary cordons were imposed, without consultation with Indian representatives, in order to limit the spread of the disease. Such impositions naturally generated violent hostility and met resistance. Tropical medicine was developed in highly prestigious scientific research establishments but new knowledge was not translated into practical policy. Having failed to provide the basic infrastructure for comprehensive, universal public health reform, British colonial rule left an impossible legacy for the independent Indian state.[102]

In Africa Maryinez Lyons shows how native lives counted only as economic units.[103] Exploitation of labour power was the relentless priority of Belgian occupation of the vast territories delineated as the Congo. Disregarding indigenous medical belief systems the Belgian rulers imposed health regulations which appeared completely irrational to native Congolese. Communities were uprooted and moved according to the demands of labour shortage and for the purposes of reducing the spread of infectious diseases. Areas deemed to be health risks, such as river banks became forbidden territories and attempts to control population movement were made through the introduction of health passports.

While some sanitary reforms were introduced, they were ruthlessly imposed without any attention paid to the cultural conflicts which they induced. Furthermore, such action was only taken when it was considered necessary to prevent sickness and premature mortality reducing the supply of the African labour force. Then housing and domestic hygiene measures were enforced, which created confusion, distrust and, occasionally, rebellion. Despite the crude attempts at oppressive social hygiene, the Congolese mortality rates, especially the infant mortality rate, remained shockingly high throughout the period of colonial rule, and left an impossible challenge for the independent state of Zaire.

The transfer of Western public health technology without direct colonial occupation had rather different results, however, in later industrializing nations such as Japan. Mahito Fukuda discusses how, as Japan began to emerge from a feudal agrarian society into a modern industrial economy it embraced the system of Western medicine initially imported by the Dutch and the Portuguese in the sixteenth and seventeenth centuries. Western and Oriental medicine have some common ancient roots, but their conceptualizations differed dramatically by the modern period and an awkward symbiosis began to be institutionalized. The way was prepared, however, for the importation from the late eighteenth century, of public health measures such as smallpox vaccination.

An explosion of interest in modern medical science developed from the middle of the nineteenth century after the long period of Japanese isolation was ended and contacts with the West renewed. The initial mix of traditional Chinese and Western medical practice became overwhelmingly dominated by the latter by the early twentieth century. Environmental reform and infectious disease control was greatly stimulated by epidemics, such as typhoid, cholera and tuberculosis, common also to the Western industrial nations. By the end of the nineteenth century Western innovations in disease prevention, such as bacteriological diagnosis and testing and anti-toxin therapy, were rapidly absorbed into the Japanese system. As in its economic development, the initial assimilation of Western innovation in medicine and disease prevention was superseded by indigenous Japanese scientific initiatives. And these are necessary to address some of the unique features of Japan's disease profile. Japan's most prevalent cause of death is cerebral apoplexy rather than, by contrast in the West, cardiac disorders. But, as in the West, Japan's dazzling development of advanced therapeutic technology has not been matched by equal concern with the promotion of preventive medicine.

Provision of Health Care

If early industrialization stimulated nineteenth-century sanitary reform, by the twentieth century the public health agenda moved on to the provision of therapeutic services. As the Reich Chancellor of united Germany, Otto von Bismarck, fought off socialism and strengthened Germany's industrial potential with a programme of social insurance, the British and French panicked about losing the imperial race.[104] The British public health profession proposed the construction of a unified health service funded by the exchequer and administered through local health departments. They argued for promotion to the status of medical civil servants working directly for the cabinet minister of a new government Ministry of Health.[105] Lloyd George, however, chose the alternative scheme of funding general practice through national health insurance of all employed workers earning wages below a fixed amount.[106] The unified service had to wait until the reconstruction of Britain after the Second World War. Even then, the opportunity to rationalize the provision of health services was missed for the sake of nationalizing free access to medical treatment.[107] As Hamlin demonstrates, in the course of the protracted negotiations surrounding medical services the cause of preventive medicine and public health was relegated to a secondary concern.

In Britain, sanitary reform was succeeded by the politics of service provision;[108] but in economies where industrialization came slightly later, the establishment of public health infrastructures and the question of medical service provision sometimes ran together. Ramsey points out that cities in France were still waiting to receive pure water supplies while the Fifth Republic planned the mixed private and public sector medical service system that exists to the present day.[109] Fee shows how, in the United States, the campaigns to eliminate malaria were still going on while the medical profession battled with New Deal politicians to prevent the introduction of health insurance.[110] In Japan preventive and therapeutic medicine continued to compete in an economic and political culture which is at once dedicated to both free-enterprise and corporatism. Even in Weimar Germany, Weindling notes, neither the welfare state nor public health provision was established as a universal system.[111] Bryder and Cassel agree that in Australia, New Zealand and Canada the first systematic and effective public health legislation came after the turn of the century and was intertwined with questions of health insurance and national welfare. Only in Sweden and Britain was a nineteenth-century sanitary revolution succeeded by a comprehensive national health service in the twentieth century.[112] Where collective provision in both preventive and therapeutic medical services was needed most it faced its greatest challenges, as in India and many African states, often exacerbated by the legacy of colonial occupation.[113]

The outcome of all these negotiations was massive diversity between health care systems throughout the world.[114] Milton Roemer discusses, however, that while individual nation states struggled with the question of the health of their own populations a new consciousness concerning the international relations of health was beginning to take root.[115] As the World Health Organization began to emerge from the United Nations after the Second World War the health of the citizen of Planet Earth began to be placed on the agenda of international politics. But until the most recent times this agenda has been restricted to issues like world vaccination campaigns and the creation of basic sanitary infrastructures and health service provision in developing countries. Only recently has the concept of health in the global village begun to be linked with universal human rights, environmental politics and the interdependence of states. Within the last decade the AIDS pandemic has heightened awareness that 'Health for All' can be achieved only through international cooperation and coordination.

Conclusion

What are the fundamental lessons to be gained from the histories of public health in national context collected here? Firstly they illustrate that the dialectics of political power, knowledge and expertise is crucial to the historical analysis of public health.[116] Furthermore, that dialectic is culturally bound, so comparative analysis of national political histories is essential. Public health administrations were not created as an automatic response to devastation by pandemic diseases or industrialization. Rather, public health was an expression of the way different societies addressed questions of social order and nationhood. Neither did medical theories uniquely determine national responses to questions of population health. Medical knowledge was only one component of public health expertise. And while public health expertise may serve as example of the rise of what Harold Perkin has described as 'professional society', or of the influence of technocratic values upon the art of public policy formation, the regulation of health remained bound to the politics of pluralistic interests. Perhaps, above all, what these essays show is that both the heroic and anti-heroic histories of public health assumed a monolithic model of power of both the state and scientific knowledge which simply fails to withstand textured, comparative historical analysis.

Collectively these essays dismantle any Whig interpretation of the history of public health, either heroic or anti-heroic. In its place they present a new model for guiding research. That model stresses the fact that societies address the question of population health within various theatres of power; despotic absolutism, liberal democracy, authoritarian and totalitarian regimes and, more often than not, a pluralistic milieux containing elements of many of them.[117] Only by addressing the expression of power within the history of a national culture can it be fully explored. Thus the history of public health must be examined within the emergence of many modern states, taking into account their historical diversities and continuities, contrasts and convergences. The history of public health in the national contexts surveyed here is a beginning.

This book is intended to be a new work of reference for those who work in public health, teach it, are studying it or are engaged in the historical analysis of the complex interaction of biology, culture and society. It hopes to extend the scholarship of great past historians of the subject cited above, and attempts to do justice to their superb legacy.

Notes

1. George Rosen, *The History of Public Health* (New York: MD Publications, 1958), 17. George Rosen was one of a generation of pioneering historians who founded medical history as an authentic discipline. He, together with Henry Sigerist, initiated many of the historical inquiries which are still being pursued today in the field. He eventually was elected to the Chair of History of Medicine at Yale University but had spent most of his career as a public health educator. Although not a Marxist, Rosen shared many of the beliefs and values of his fellow left-wing intellectuals such as Sigerist. For further discussion see, Charles Rosenberg, 'Introduction', in *idem, Healing and History. Essays in Honor of George Rosen* (New York: Science History Publications, 1979).
2. *Ibid.*, 109.
3. *Ibid.*
4. George Rosen, *From Medical Police to Social Medicine. Essays on the History of Health Care* (New York: Science History Publications, 1974).
5. See E. Morman, 'Scholarship as Advocacy: George Rosen as Historian and Public Health Educator', in *Abstracts of American Association for the History of Medicine 65th Annual Meeting,* Seattle, Washington (Seattle: AAHM, 1992), 1 (paper delivered at 65th Annual Meeting of the Association, 30 May – 3 June, 1992). For discussion of left-wing intellectuals and the scientific management of society see, Gary Werskey, *The Visible College* (London: Allen Lane, 1978); Alan M. Wald, *The New York Intellectuals: the Rise of the Anti-Stalinist Left From the 1930s to the 1980s* (Chapel Hill: University of North Carolina Press, 1987).
6. S. Finer, *The Life and Times of Edwin Chadwick* (London: Methuen, 1952); R. A. Lewis, *Edwin Chadwick and the Public Health Movement* (London: Longmans and Green, 1952); Royston Lambert, *Sir John Simon 1816–1904 and English Sanitary Administration* (London: Macgibbon and Kee, 1963); William Fraser, *History of English Public Health 1834–1939* (London: Ballière, Tindall

and Cox, 1950); Colin Fraser Brockington, *A Short History of Public Health* (London: Churchill, 1956).

7. To list the works inspired directly by the work of these authors, especially the work of Rosen would go beyond the scope of this paper but their influence continues to the present day. A brief list to show the range of new work now being completed in the field of public health history is: Jane Lewis, *What Price Community Medicine?* (Brighton: Harvester, 1986); Charles Webster, *Problems of Health Care, The National Health Service Before 1957* (London: HMSO, 1988); F. B. Smith, *The Retreat of Tuberculosis, 1850–1950* (London: Croom Helm, 1988); Linda Bryder, *Below the Magic Mountain* (Oxford: Oxford University Press, 1988); Anne Summers, *Angels and Citizens. Military Nursing in Britain* (London: Routledge, 1988); Ruth Barrington, *Health, Medicine and Politics in Ireland 1900–1970* (Dublin: Institute of Public Administration, 1987); John Duffy, *The Sanitarians. A History of American Public Health* (Urbana and Chicago: University of Illinois Press, 1990); LaVerne Kuhnke, *Lives at Risk, Public Health in Nineteenth Century Egypt* (Berkeley: University of California Press, 1990); Nancy Elizabeth Gallagher, *Egypt's Other Wars. Epidemics and the Politics of Public Health* (New York: Syracuse University Press, 1990); Christopher Hamlin, *A Science of Impurity. Water Analysis in Nineteenth Century Britain* (Bristol: Adam Hilger, 1990); Jonathan Barry and Colin Jones (eds), *Medicine and Charity Before the Welfare State* (London: Routledge, 1991); and many other works cited throughout this volume.
8. T. McKeown, *The Role of Medicine – Dream, Mirage or Nemesis* (London: Nuffield Provincial Trust, 1976); *idem*, *The Rise of Modern Population* (London: Edward Arnold, 1976).
9. See, for example, J. M. Winter, 'The Decline of Mortality in Britain 1870–1950', in T. Barker and M. Drake (eds), *Population and Society in Britain 1850–1980* (London: Batsford Academic and Educational, 1982), 100–20; D. J. Oddy, 'The Health of the People', in *ibid.*, 121–39. Ann G. Carmichael, 'Infection, Hidden Hunger, and History', *Journal of Interdisciplinary History*, 14 (1983), 249–64; John B. McKinley and Sonja M. Mckinley, 'Medical Measures and the Decline of Mortality', in Peter Conrad and Rochelle Kern (eds), *The Sociology of Health and Illness. Critical Perspectives* (New York: St Martin's Press, 1981), 12–30; and many discussions over the last 15 years in the journals *Population Studies* and *Journal of Interdisciplinary History*, especially Vol. 14 (1983).
10. See also, Norbert Elias, *The Civilizing Process*, 3 vols (New York: Pantheon Books, 1982 [1939]); Brian Turner, *The Body and Society*.

Explorations in Social Theory, (London: Basil Blackwell, 1984); E. Scarry, *The Body in Pain* (Oxford: Oxford University Press, 1985); Thomas Laqueur, *Making Sex. Body and Gender from the Greeks to Freud* (Cambridge, Mass.: Harvard University Press, 1990); Ludmilla Jordanova, *Sexual Visions. Images of Gender in Science and Medicine Between the Eighteenth and Twentieth Centuries* (London: Harvester Wheatsheaf, 1989); Paul Valery, 'Some Simple Reflections on the Body', in Michel Feher, Ramona Naddaff and Nadia Tazi (eds), *Fragments for a History of the Human Body. Part Two* (New York: Zone, 1989), 395–401; Dorinda Outram, *The Body and the French Revolution. Sex, Class and Political Culture* (New Haven, Conn.: Yale University Press, 1989).

11. See M. Foucault, *The Order of Things* (London: Tavistock, 1974); *idem, Madness and Civilization* (London: Tavistock, 1971); *idem, The Birth of the Clinic* (London: Tavistock, 1971); *idem, Discipline and Punish, The Birth of the Prison* (London: Tavistock, 1977); *idem, The History of Sexuality* (London: Tavistock, 1979). See also, G. Gutting, *Michel Foucault's Archeology of Scientific Reason* (Cambridge: Cambridge University Press, 1989); M. Hewitt, *Social Policy and the Politics of Life: Foucault's Account of Welfare* (Hatfield: School of Social Sciences, the Hatfield Polytechnic, 1982).
12. See, for example, David Armstrong, *The Political Anatomy of the Body* (Cambridge: Cambridge University Press, 1983); Bryan S. Turner, *Medical Power and Social Knowledge* (London: Sage, 1987).
13. See, for example, Sander Gilman and J. E. Chamberlin (eds), *Degeneration: The Dark Side of Progress* (New York: Columbia University Press, 1985); Daniel Kevles, *In the Name of Eugenics. Genetics and the Uses of Human Heredity* (New York: Knopf, 1985); Geoffrey R. Searle, *Eugenics and Politics in Britain 1900–1914* (Leyden: Noordhoff, 1976); C. Webster (ed.), *Biology, Medicine and Society 1840–1940* (Cambridge: Cambridge University Press, 1981); Donald MacKenzie, *Statistics in Britain, 1865–1930* (Edinburgh: Edinburgh University Press, 1981); Greta Jones, *Social Darwinism and English Thought: the Interaction Between Biological and Social Theory* (Brighton: Harvester Press, 1980); *idem, Social Hygiene in Britain* (London: Croom Helm, 1986); Linda Clark, *Social Darwinism in France* (Alabama: University of Alabama Press, 1984); D. Gasman, *The Scientific Origins of National Socialism: Social Darwinism in Ernst Haeckel and the German Monist League* (London: Macdonald, 1971); S. Trombley, *The Right to Reproduce: A History of Coercive Sterilization* (London: Weidenfeld and Nicolson, 1988); Mark Haller, *Eugenics: Hereditarian Attitudes in American Thought*

(New Brunswick: Rutgers University Press, 1984); Robert Bannister, *Social Darwinism: Science and Myth in Anglo-American Thought* (Philadelphia: Temple University Press, 1979); A. Farrell, *The Origins and Growth of the English Eugenics Movement, 1865–1925* (Ann Arbor: University Microfilms, 1970); Paul Weindling, 'The Medical Profession, Social Welfare, and the Birth Rate in Germany, 1914–18', in J. Winter and R. Wall (eds), *The Upheaval of War: Family, Work and Welfare in Europe 1914–1918* (Cambridge: Cambridge University Press, 1988), 417–37; Robert Proctor, *Racial Hygiene: Medicine Under the Nazis* (Cambridge, Mass.: Harvard University Press, 1989); Sheila F. Weiss, *Race, Hygiene and the Rational Management of National Efficiency: Wilhelm Schallmayer and the Origins of German Eugenics, 1890–1920* (Ann Arbor: University Microfilms, 1983); Pauline M. H. Mazumdar, 'Eugenicists and the Residuum: the Problem of the Urban Poor', *Bulletin of the History of Medicine,* 54 (1980), 204–15; *idem, Eugenics, Human Genetics and Human Failings. The Eugenics Society, its Sources and its Critics in Britain* (London: Routledge, 1992); Nancy Stepan, *The Idea of Race in Science* (Hamden, Conn.: Archon Books, 1982).

14. See Paul Weindling, 'Theories of the Cell State in Imperial Germany', in C. Webster (ed.), *Biology, Medicine and Society 1840–1940,* 99–155; *idem, Health, Race and German Politics between National Unification and Nazism, 1870–1945* (Cambridge: Cambridge University Press, 1989); Benno Mueller-Hill, *Murderous Science: the Elimination by Scientific Selection of Jews, Gypsies and Others, Germany 1933–1945* (Oxford: Oxford University Press, 1988).
15. Lambert, *op. cit.* (note 6); William M. Fraser, *Duncan of Liverpool. Being an Account of the Work of Dr W. H. Duncan Medical Officer of Health of Liverpool 1847–63* (London: Hamish Hamilton Medical Books, 1947).
16. E. Fee, *Disease and Discovery: A History of the Johns Hopkins School of Hygiene and Public Health, 1916–1939* (Baltimore: The Johns Hopkins University Press, 1987); *idem* and Roy Acheson, *The History of Education in Public Health. Health that Mocks the Doctors' Rules* (Oxford: Oxford Medical Publications, 1991); Dorothy Porter, 'Stratification and its Discontents: Professionalization and Conflict in the British Public Health Service', in *ibid.*, 83–113; Hamlin, *op. cit.* (note 7); Lewis, *op. cit.* (note 7).
17. For medicalization thesis see Ivan Illich, *Limits to Medicine, Medical Nemesis: The Expropriation of Health* (Harmondsworth: Penguin Books, 1977).

18. Harold Perkin, *The Rise of Professional Society. England Since 1880* (London: Routledge, 1989).
19. See, for example, Theodore W. Adorno and Max Horkheimer, *Dialectics of the Enlightenment* (London: Verso, 1979 [1944]); Max Horkheimer, *The Eclipse of Reason* (London: Oxford University Press, 1947); Herbert Marcuse, *Reason and Revolution: Hegel and the Rise of Social Theory* (London: Routledge, 1986 [1941]); *idem, One Dimensional Man: Studies in the Ideology of Advanced Industrial Society* (London: Routledge, 1991 [1964]); *idem, An Essay on Liberation* (London: Routledge, 1964); Jürgen Habermas, *Toward a Rational Society* (London: Heinemann, 1972 [1968]); *idem, Legitimation Crisis* (London: Heinemann, 1979 [1973]); Georges Canguilhem, *The Normal and the Pathological* (Boston: D. Reidel, 1978).
20. See, for example, Charles Rosenberg, 'Disease in History. Frames and Framers', *Milbank Quarterly*, 67 (1989), 1–15; *idem* and Janet Golden (eds), *Framing Disease. Studies in Cultural History* (New Brunswick: N.J., Rutgers University Press, 1992); Terence Ranger and Paul Slack (eds), *Epidemics and Ideas. Essays on the Historical Perception of Pestilence* (Cambridge: Cambridge University Press, 1992); Paul Slack, 'The Disappearance of Plague: An Alternative View', *Economic History Review*, 34 (1981), 469–76; Andrew B. Appelby, 'The Disappearance of Plague: A Continuing Puzzle', *Economic History Review*, 33 (1980), 161–73; K. F. Kiple and V. H. Kiple 'The African Connection: Slavery, Disease and Racism', *Phylon*, 4 (1980), 211–22; J. A. Carrigan, 'Yellow fever: scourge of the South', in T. L. Savitt and J. H. Young (eds), *Disease and Distinctiveness in the American South* (Knoxville: University of Tennessee Press, 1988), 55–78; M. Warner, 'Hunting the Yellow Fever Germ, the Principle and Practice of Etiological Proof in Late Nineteenth Century America', *Bulletin of the History of Medicine*, 59, (1985), 361–82; Anne Hardy, 'Urban Famine or Urban Crisis? Typhus in the Victorian City', *Medical History*, 32 (1988), 401–25; Bill Luckin, 'Evaluating The Sanitary Revolution: Typhus and Typhoid in London', in R. Woods and J. Woodward (eds), *Urban Disease and Mortality in 19th Century England* (London: Batsford Academic, 1984), 111–16. Donald R. Hopkins, *Princes and Peasants: Smallpox in History* (Chicago: University of Chicago Press, 1983); Bryder, *op. cit.* (note 7); Smith, *op. cit.* (note 7); R. J. Evans, 'Epidemics and Revolutions: Cholera in Nineteenth–Century Europe', *Past and Present*, 120 (1988), 123–46; *idem, Death In Hamburg. Society and Politics in the Cholera Years 1830–1910*

(Oxford: Clarendon Press, 1987); R. J. Morris, *Cholera 1832. The Social Response to an Epidemic* (London: Croom Helm, 1976); David Arnold, 'Cholera and Colonialism in British India', *Past and Present*, 113 (1986), 118–51; Stuart Galishoff, 'Newark and the Great Influenza Pandemic of 1918', *Bulletin of the History of Medicine*, 43 (1969), 26–258; J. E. Osborn (ed.), *History Science and Politics. Influenza in America 1918–1976* (New York: Prodist, 1977); N. Rogers, 'Dirt, Flies and Immigrants: Explaining the Epidemiology of Poliomyelitis, 1900–1916', *Journal of the History of Medicine and Allied Sciences*, 44 (1980), 486–505; Tod L. Savitt, and J. H. Young (eds), *Disease and Distinctiveness in the American South* (Knoxville: University of Tennessee Press, 1988); C. Herzlich, J. Pierret, *Illness and Self in Society*, (Baltimore: Johns Hopkins University Press, 1987).

21. E. Fee and D. M. Fox (eds), *AIDS: The Burdens of History* (Berkeley: University of California Press, 1988).
22. S. L. Gilman, *Disease and Representation: Images of Illness from Madness to AIDS*, (Ithaca: Cornell University Press, 1988); S. Sontag, *Illness as a Metaphor* (London: Allen Lane, 1979); *idem*, *AIDS and its Metaphors* (London: Allen Lane, 1989).
23. Wesley D. Smith, *The Hippocratic Tradition* (Ithaca: Cornell University Press, 1979).
24. Richard John Palmer, 'The Control of Plague in Venice and Northern Italy 1348–1600' (Ph.D Thesis, University of Kent, 1978); Carlo M. Cipolla, *Miasmas and Disease. Public Health and the Environment in the Pre-Industrial Age* (New Haven and London: Yale University Press, 1992).
25. Paul Slack, *The Impact of Plague in Tudor and Stuart England* (London: Routledge & Kegan Paul, 1985).
26. W. H. McNeill, *Plagues and Peoples* (New York: Doubleday, 1976); A. W. Crosby, *The Columbian Exchange: Biological and Cultural Consequences of 1492* (Westport, Conn.: Greenwood, 1972); *idem*, *Ecological Imperialism: The Biological Expansion of Europe, 900–1900* (Cambridge: Cambridge University Press, 1986); *idem*, *Epidemic and Peace 1918: America's Deadliest Influenza Epidemic* (Wesport Conn.: Greenwood, 1976); *idem*, 'Virgin Soil. Epidemics as a Factor in the Aboriginal Depopulation in America', *William and Mary Quarterly*, 33 (1976), 289–99.
27. Rosen, *op. cit.* (note 4), 120–58.
28. See also M. Ramsey, *Professional and Popular Medicine in France, 1770–1830. The Social World of Medical Practice* (Cambridge: Cambridge University Press, 1988).

29. James C. Riley, *The Eighteenth Century Campaign to Avoid Disease* (Basingstoke: Macmillan, 1987); John Pickstone, 'Ferriar's Fever to Kay's Cholera: Disease and Social Structure in Cottonopolis', *History of Science*, 22 (1984), 401–19.
30. Roy Porter, 'Cleaning up the Great Wen: Public Health in Eighteenth-Century London', in W. F. Bynum and Roy Porter (eds), *Living and Dying in London. Medical History* Supplement No. 11 (London: Wellcome Institute, 1991), 61–75.
31. R. K. Webb, 'Thomas Southwood Smith. The Intellectual Sources for Public Services', in Dorothy Porter and Roy Porter (eds), *Doctors and Politics* (Amsterdam: Rodopi, 1993).
32. George Rosen, 'Political Order and Human Health in Jeffersonian Thought', *Bulletin of the History of Medicine*, 26 (1952), 32–44.
33. Dora Weiner, 'Le droit de l'homme à la santé: une belle idée devant l'Assemblée constituante: 1790–1791', *Clio Medica*, 5 (1970), 208–23; Dora Weiner, 'Public Health Under Napoleon: the Conseil de salubrité de Paris, 1802–1815', *Clio Medica*, 9 (1974), 271–84; L. J. Jordanova, 'Guarding the Body Politic: Volney's Catechism of 1793', in Francis Barker *et al.* (eds), *1789: Reading, Writing, Revolution. Proceedings of the Essex Conference on the Sociology of Literature, July 1981* (Colchester: University of Essex, 1982), 12–21.
34. Dora Weiner, *Citizen Patient* (Baltimore: Johns Hopkins University Press, 1993).
35. Rosen, *op.cit.* (note 1), 192–293; see also R. H. Shryock, *The Development of Modern Medicine. An Interpretation of the Social and Scientific Factors Involved* (Madison: The University of Wisconsin Press, 1979), 211–47.
36. See Finer, Fraser, Lewis, *op.cit.* (note 6); See also M. Flinn, 'Introduction', in *Edwin Chadwick, Report on the Sanitary Condition of the Labouring Classes of Great Britain, 1842* (Reprinted, Edinburgh: Edinburgh University Press, 1965), edited by M. Flinn; A. S. Wohl, *Endangered Lives. Public Health Reform in Victorian Britain* (London: Methuen, 1984), 142–65.
37. See also, Wohl, *op.cit.* (note 36), 6–7, 142–4.
38. C. Rosenberg, *The Cholera Years 1832, 1849 and 1866* (Chicago: University of Chicago Press, 1962), 121–50; *idem*, and Carol Smith-Rosenberg, 'Pietism and the Origins of the American Public Health Movement', *Journal of the History of Medicine and Allied Sciences*, 23 (1968), 6–34; B. G. Rosenkrantz, *Public Health and the State. Changing Views in Massachusetts, 1842–1936* (Cambridge, Mass.: Harvard University Press, 1972), 8–36.
39. See also, Alfred A. Cave, *Jacksonian Democracy and the Historians*

(Westport, Conn.: Greenwood Press, 1980).

40. Oliver MacDonagh, 'The Nineteenth Century Revolution in Government: A Reappraisal', *Historical Journal*, 1 (1958), 52–67; G. Kitson Clark, 'Statesmen in Disguise: Reflections on the History of the Neutrality of the Civil Service', *Historical Journal*, 2 (1959), 19–39.
41. For context of this debate see A. V. Dicey, *Lectures on the Relation Between Law and Public Opinion in England During the Nineteenth Century* (London: Macmillan & Co., 1905); J. Bartlett Brebner, 'Laissez-faire and State Intervention in Nineteenth-Century Britain', *Journal of Economic History*, 8 (1948), suppl., 59–73; Henry Parris, 'The Nineteenth-Century Revolution in Government: A Reappraisal Reappraised', *Historical Journal*, 3 (1960), 17–37; Robert M. Gutchen, 'Local Improvements and Centralization in Nineteenth Century England', *Historical Journal*, 4 (1961), 85–96; Jennifer Hart, 'Nineteenth Century Social Reform: A Tory Interpretation of History', *Past and Present*, 31 (July, 1965), 39–61; *idem*, 'Sir Charles Trevelyan at the Treasury', *English Historical Review*, 75 (1960), 92–110; L. J. Hume, 'Jeremy Bentham and the Nineteenth Century Revolution in Government', *Historical Journal*, 10 (1967), 361–75; William C. Lubenow, *The Politics of Government Growth: Early Victorian Attitude Toward State Intervention 1833–1848* (Newton Abbot: David and Charles, 1971); S. E. Finer, 'The Transmission of Benthamite Ideas 1820–50', in Gillian Sutherland (ed.), *Studies in the Growth of Nineteenth Century Government* (London, Routledge & Kegan Paul, 1972), 11–32; David Roberts, 'Jeremy Bentham and the Victorian Administrative State', *Victorian Studies*, 2 (1959), 159–78; *idem*, *Paternalism in Early Victorian England* (New Brunswick, N.J.: Rutgers University Press, 1979); D. G. Paz, 'The Limits of Bureaucratic Autonomy in Victorian Administration', *The Historian*, 49 (February 1987), 167–83.
42. Anthony Brundage, *England's 'Prussian Minister'. Edwin Chadwick and the Politics of Government Growth, 1832–1854* (University Park, Pa.: Penn State University Press, 1988).
43. D. E. Porter and R. Porter, 'The Politics of Prevention: Anti-Vaccinationism and Public Health in Nineteenth-Century England', *Medical History*, 32 (1988), 231–52; *idem*, 'The Enforcement of Health', in E. Fee and D. Fox, *AIDS: The Burdens of History* (Berkeley: University of California Press, 1988), 96–120.
44. P. Mchugh, *Prostitution and Victorian Social Reform* (London: Croom Helm, 1982); J. Walkowitz, *Prostitution and Victorian Society: Women, Class and the State* (Cambridge: Cambridge

University Press, 1980).

45. See also David Held, 'Central Perspectives on the Modern State', in David Held, *et al.* (eds), *States and Societies* (Oxford: Basil Blackwell, 1990), 1–55.
46. See also, Lynn Hunt, *Politics, Culture and Class in the French Revolution* (Berkeley: University of California Press, 1984); R. E. M. Irving, *Christian Democracy in France* (London: 1973).
47. See also William Coleman, *Death is a Social Disease. Public Health and Political Economy in Early Industrial France* (Wisconsin: University of Wisconsin Press, 1982), 277–306.
48. See also, Duffy, *op. cit.* (note 7), 52–78; 93–109; Stuart Galishoff, Newark, *The Nations Unhealthiest City 1832–1895* (New Brunswick: Rutgers University Press, 1988); John Ellis, 'Businessmen and Public Health in the Urban South During the Nineteenth Century: New Orleans, Memphis and Atlanta', *Bulletin of the History of Medicine*, 44 (1970), 197–212; 346–71; John Duffy, *A History of Public Health in New York City 1625–1866*, 2 vols (New York: Russell Sage Foundation, 1968).
49. Peter Burroughs, 'Colonial Self-government', in C. C. Eldridge, *British Imperialism in the Nineteenth Century* (London: Macmillan, 1984), 39–64; J. M. Ward, *Colonial Self-Government: The British Experience 1759–1856* (Toronto: University of Toronto Press, 1976).
50. See also, M. F. Christie, *Aborigines in Colonial Victoria, 1835–1886* (Sydney: Sydney University Press, 1979); Raymond Evans, Kay Saunders and Kathryn Cronin, *Exclusion, Exploitation and Extermination: Race Relations in Colonial Queensland* (St Lucia: University of Queensland Press, 1988 [1975]); Henry Reynolds, *Frontier: Aborigines, Settlers and Land* (London: 1987).
51. See also Geoffrey R. Searle, *The Quest for National Efficiency. A S tudy in British Politics and Political Thought, 1899–1914* (Berkeley: University of California Press, 1971); Paul Kennedy, 'Continuity and Discontinuity in British Imperialism', in C. C. Eldridge, *op. cit.* (note 49), 20–38.
52. See also, David Arnold, 'Medical Priorities and Practices in Nineteenth Century British India', *South Asia Research*, 5 (1985); G. J. Meulenbeld, D. Wujastyk (eds), *Studies on Indian Medical History* (Gronigen: Egbert Forsten, 1987); R. J. Moore, 'India and the British Empire', in C. C. Eldridge, *op. cit.* (note 49), 65–84; P. J. Marshall, *Bengal, The British Bridgehead: Eastern India 1740–1828* (Cambridge: Cambridge University Press, 1988); C. A. Bayly, *Indian Society and the Making of the British Empire* (Cambridge: Cambridge University Press, 1988); G. D. Bearce, *The Raj in Fiction: A Study of*

British Attitudes Toward India (Delhi: B. R. Publishing Corporation, 1987); C. H. Philips and Mary Wainwright (eds), *Indian Society and the Beginnings of Modernization 1830–50* (London: University of London School of Oriental and African Studies, 1976); S. Gopal, *British Policy in India 1858–1905* (Cambridge: Cambridge University Press, 1967).

53. See also M. Gelfand, *A Service to the Sick: A History of Health Services for Africans in Southern Rhodesia* (Gwelo: Mambo Press, 1976); G. W. Hartwig and K. D. Patterson, *Disease in African History: An Introductory Survey and Case Studies* (Durham: Duke University Press, 1979); J. Iliffe, *The African Poor* (Cambridge: Cambridge University Press, 1987); J. N. Lasker, 'The Role of Health Services in Colonial Rule: The Case of the Ivory Coast', *Culture, Medicine and Psychiatry*, 1\3 (1978), 277–97; M. Vaughan, *Curing Their Ills: Colonial Power and African Illness* (Cambridge: Cambridge University Press, 1991).
54. See also J. R. Gillis, *The Prussian Bureaucracy in Crisis, 1840–1860* (Stanford: Stanford University Press,1971); M. Walker, *German Home Towns. Community, State, General Estate* (Ithaca: Cornell University Press, 1971).
55. See also, Ian Kershaw, *Popular Opinion and Political Dissent in the Third Reich: Bavaria 1933–1945* (Oxford: Oxford University Press, 1983); Timothy W. Mason, *Sozialpolitik im Dritten Reich: Arbeiterklasse und Volksgemeinschaft* (Opladen: Westdeutscher Verlag, 1977).
56. See also Alan Marcus, 'Disease Prevention in America: From a Local to a National Outlook, 1880–1910', *Bulletin of the History of Medicine*, 53 (1979), 184–203; Manfred Wassermann, 'The Quest for a National Health Department in the Progressive Era', *Bulletin of the History of Medicine*, 49 (1975), 353–80.
57. Duffy, *op. cit.* (note 7), 93–109.
58. Fitzhugh Mullan MD, *Plagues and Politics. The Story of the United States Public Health Service* (New York: Basic Books, 1989).
59. See also, Alec Nove, 'Is There a Ruling Class in the USSR?', in Anthony Giddens and David Held (eds), *Classes, Power and Conflict. Classical and Contemporary Debates* (London: Macmillan, 1992), 588–604; Murray Yanowitch, 'Work, Hierarchy and Management "Participation" in the Soviet Union', in *ibid.*, 605–28; Elizabeth Garnsey, 'Competing Interests, and the Soviet Occupational System', in *ibid.*, 629–42.
60. See Perry Anderson, 'The Absolute States of Western Europe', in David Held (ed.), *States and Societies* (London: Basil Blackwell,

1990), 137–50; Theda Skocpol, 'States and Revolutions: France, Russia and China', in *ibid.*, 151–69; Boris Frankel, 'On the State of the State: Marxist Theories of the State after Leninism', in Giddens & Held (eds), *op. cit.* (note 59), 257–73.

61. See Armstrong, *op. cit.* (note 12).
62. See also Roger Price, *The Revolutions of 1848* (London: Macmillan Education, 1988).
63. See René Sand, *The Advance to Social Medicine* (London: Staples Press, 1952), 201–6. On the role of the medical profession as the new public health 'priests' of society see, D. Porter, 'How Soon is Now? Public Health and the BMJ', *British Medical Journal*, 301 (1990), 738–40; *idem*, *A Political History of Public Health* (London: Routledge, forthcoming), ch. 6.
64. William Bulloch, *A History of Bacteriology* (Oxford: Oxford University Press, 1938); Peter Baldry, *The Battle Against Bacteria: A Fresh Look* (Cambridge: Cambridge University Press, 1976).
65. Bruno Latour, *The Pasteurization of France* (Cambridge, Mass.: Harvard University Press, 1988).
66. For alternative interpretation see, Anthony Wohl, *op. cit.* (note 36), 151–65.
67. Fee and Acheson, *op. cit.* (note 16).
68. D. E. Porter, 'Biologism, Environmentalism and Public Health in Edwardian England', *Victorian Studies*, 34 (1991), 159–78.
69. Lewis, *op. cit.* (note 7), 15–56. See also Webster, *op. cit.* (note 7), 17–43; 94–102; 107–42; D. Fox, *Health Policies, Health Politics, The British and American Experiences* (Princeton: Princeton University Press, 1986), 94–114. Margot Jefferys, 'The Transition from Public Health to Community Medicine: The Evolution and Execution of a Policy', *Society for the Social History of Medicine Bulletin*, 39 (1986), 47–63.
70. See Norman Etherington, 'Missionary Doctors and African Healers in Mid-Victorian South Africa', *South African Historical Journal*, 19 (1987), 77–91; Brian Stanley, *The Bible and the Flag. Protestant Missions and British Imperialism in the Nineteenth and Twentieth Centuries* (London: Apollo, 1990); C. Peter Williams, *The Ideal of the Self-governing Church. A Study in Victorian Missionary Strategy* (Leiden: E. J. Brill, 1990); Michael Gelfand, *Christian Doctor and Nurse: The Study of Medical Missions in South Africa* (Sandton: Aitken Family and Friends, 1984); Rasbahadur Sharma, *Christian Missions in North India 1813–1913* (Delhi: Mittal Publications, 1988); Marvin D. Markowitz, *Cross and Sword: The Political Role of Christian Missions in the Belgian Congo 1908–1960* (Stanford:

Hoover Institution Press, 1973).

71. Barbara Rosenkrantz, 'Cart Before Horse: Theory, Practice and Professional Image in American Public Health', *Journal of the History of Medicine and Allied Sciences,* 29 (1974), 55–73.
72. See Fee, *op. cit.* (note 16).
73. See also Paul Starr, *The Social Transformation of American Medicine* (New York: Basic Books, 1982), 180–97; James H. Cassedy, *Medicine in America. A Short History* (Baltimore: The Johns Hopkins University Press, 1991).
74. James G. Burrow, *Organized Medicine in the Progressive Era: The Move Toward Monopoly* (Baltimore: The Johns Hopkins University Press, 1977); R. Stevens, *In Sickness and In Wealth. American Hospitals in the Twentieth Century* (New York: Basic Books, 1989); *idem, American Medicine and the Public Interest* (New Haven, Conn.: Yale University Press, 1971).
75. For broader discussion of professional ideology and power see, Emile Durkheim, *Professional Ethics and Civic Morals,* transl. by Cornelia Brookfield (London: Routledge & Kegan Paul, 1957); A. M. Carr-Saunders and P. A. Wilson, *The Professions* (Oxford: Oxford University Press, 1933); Terence J. Johnson, *Professions and Power* (London: Macmillan, 1972); W. J. Reader, *Professional Men: the Rise of the Professional Classes in Nineteenth-Century England* (London: Weidenfeld & Nicolson, 1966); E. Freidson, 'The Theory of Professions: State of the Art', in R. Dingwall and P. Lewis (eds), *The Sociology of the Professions* (London: Macmillan, 1983), 19–37; D. Rueschemeyer, 'Professional Autonomy and the Social Control of Expertise', *ibid.,* 38–58; Guy Benventiste, *The Politics of Expertise* (London: Croom Helm, 1973). For discussion specifically of professionalization and medicine see E. Hughes, 'The Making of the Physician', *Human Organization,* 14 (1956), 22–5; N. Parry and J. Parry, *The Rise of the Medical Profession: A Study of Collective Social Mobility* (London: Croom Helm, 1976); R. K. Merton, *Some Thoughts on the Professions in American Society* (Providence: Brown University Papers, 37, 1960); *idem,* 'Some Preliminaries to a Sociology of Medical Education', in R. K. Merton, G. Reader and P. L. Kendall (eds), *The Student Physician* (Cambridge, Mass.: Harvard University Press, 1957), 3–79; Barbara Rosenkrantz, 'The Search for Professional Order in Nineteenth Century American Medicine', in J. Leavitt and R. Numbers (eds), *Sickness and Health in America. Readings in the History of Medicine and Public Health* (Madison: University of Wisconsin Press, 1985), 219–32; John Burnham, 'American Medicine's Golden Age: What Happened to it?', *ibid.,* 248–58; Ivan Waddington, *The Medical Profession in the*

Industrial Revolution (Dublin: Gill & Macmillan, 1984), 53–95; Irvine Loudon, *Medical Care and the General Practitioner 1750–1850* (Oxford: Clarendon Press, 1986), 65–85; Starr, *op. cit.* (note 73), 3–29; R. M. Morantz, *et al.* (eds), *In Her Own Words. Oral Histories of Women Physicians* (New Haven, Conn.: Yale University Press, 1986), 3–43; Rosemary Stevens, *Medical Practice in Modern England. The Impact of Specialization and State Medicine* (New Haven, Conn.: Yale University Press, 1966); George Rosen, *The Structure of American Medical Practice 1875–1941* (Philadelphia: University of Pennsylvania Press, 1983), 38–108; Frank D. Campion, *The AMA and U.S. Health Policy Since 1940* (Chicago: Chicago Review Press for the AMA, 1984); M. Jeanne Peterson, *The Medical Profession in Mid-Victorian London* (Berkeley: University of California Press, 1978), 244–82.

76. See Turner, *op. cit.* (note 12).
77. E. H. Ackerknecht, 'Anti-Contagionism Between the Wars', *Bulletin of the History of Medicine*, 22 (1948), 562–93.
78. M. Pelling, *Cholera Fever and English Medicine 1825–1865*, (Oxford: Oxford University Press, 1978), 300–12; C. Hamlin, 'Predisposing Causes and Public Health in Early Nineteenth Century Medical Thought', *Social History of Medicine*, 5 (1992), 43–70.
79. Pelling, *op. cit.* (note 78).
80. Hamlin, *op. cit.* (note 78).
81. G. Rosen, *Preventive Medicine in the United States, 1900–1975 Trends and Interpretations* (New York: Science History Publications 1926), 20–54; James Cassedy, *Charles V. Chapin and the Public Health Movement* (Cambridge, Mass.: Harvard University Press, 1962), 126–42, 157–80; Duffy, *op. cit.* (note 7), 193–220; B. G. Rosenkrantz, *Public Health and the State. Changing Views in Massachusetts, 1842–1936* (Cambridge, Mass.: Harvard University Press, 1972), 128–75.
82. See Armstrong, *op. cit.* (note 12); Porter, *op. cit.* (note 68).
83. Jones, *op. cit.* (note 13), *Social Hygiene in Britain.*
84. Porter, *op. cit.* (note 68); Jane Lewis, *The Politics of Motherhood. Child and Maternal Welfare in England 1900–1939* (London: Croom Helm, 1980), 27–43, 61–113; *idem*, 'Motherhood Issues' in the *Late Nineteenth and Twentieth Centuries*, in Katherine Arnup, Andre Levesque and Ruth Roach Pierson (eds), *Delivering Motherhood. Maternal Ideologies and Practices in the Nineteenth and Twentieth Centuries* (London: Routledge, 1990), 1–19; Deborah Dwork, *War is Good for Babies and Other Young Children. A History of the Infant and Child Welfare Movement in England 1898–1918* (London: Tavistock, 1987), 3–21; 167–207; 208–20; Anna Davin, 'Imperialism and

Motherhood', *History Workshop*, 5 (1978), 9–65; F. B. Smith, *The People's Health 1830–1910* (London: Croom, Helm 1979), 13–64; 65–135; 178–94.

85. See Richard A. Soloway, *Birth Control and the Population Question in England 1877–1930* (Chapel Hill: University of North Carolina Press, 1982); *idem, Demography and Degeneration. Eugenics and the Declining Birthrate in Twentieth-Century Britain* (Chapel Hill: University of North Carolina Press, 1990); James Woycke, *Birth Control in Germany 1871–1933* (London: Routledge, 1988).
86. *Ibid.*
87. See also Jean-Pierre Dumont, *La sécurité sociale toujours en chantier: Histoire - bilan - perspectives* (Paris: Les éditions ouvrières, 1981); Sanford Elwitt, *The Third Republic Defended: Bourgeois Reform in France 1880–1914* (Baton Rouge: Louisiana State University Press, 1986); Kerry Davidson, 'The French Socialist Party and Parliamentary Efforts to Achieve Social Reform, 1906–1914', (Tulane University, Ph.D Dissertation, 1970).
88. David Glass, *The Struggle for Population* (Oxford: Clarendon Press, 1936).
89. See Kevles, *op. cit.* (note 13); Haller, *op. cit.* (note 13); Weindling, *op. cit.* (note 13). But for defeat of eugenic attempts to achieve legislation on sterilization in Britain see, John Macnicol, 'Eugenics and the Campaign for Voluntary Sterilization in Britain Between the Wars', *Social History of Medicine*, 2 (1989), 147–62.
90. See also, Proctor, *op. cit.* (note 13); Weiss, *op. cit.* (note 13); Paul Hoedeman, *Hitler or Hippocrates. Medical Experiment and Euthanasia in the Third Reich* (Lewes: Book Guild, 1991).
91. See Kevles, *op. cit.* (note 13); Haller, *op. cit.* (note 13).
92. See also Susan Gross Solomon and John F. Hutchinson (eds), *Health and Society in Revolutionary Russia* (Bloomington: Indiana University Press, 1990).
93. A. J. Viseltear, 'Milton C. Winternitz and the Yale Institute of Human Relations: a Brief Chapter in the History of Social Medicine', *Yale Journal of Biology and Medicine*, 57 (1984), 869–89.
94. Dorothy Porter, 'Changing Disciplines: John Ryle and the Making of Social Medicine in Twentieth Century Britain', *History of Science*, 30 (1992), 119–47.
95. Sir Arthur Newsholme and John Adams Kingsbury, *Red Medicine: Socialized Health in Soviet Russia* (Garden City, N.Y.: Doubleday, Doran & Co., 1933); Henry Sigerist, *Medicine and Health in the Soviet Union* (New York: Citadel Press, 1947); Sydney Webb and Beatrice Webb, *Is Soviet Communism a New Civilization?* (London:

Left Review, 1936).

96. The history of 'disease, health, medicine and empire', however, is now an expanding field, see for example: David Arnold (ed.), *Imperial Medicine and Indigenous Societies. Disease, Medicine and Empire in the Nineteenth and Twentieth Centuries* (New York: St. Martin's Press, 1988); Philip Curtin, *Death by Migration. Europe's Encounter with the Tropical World in the Nineteenth Century* (Cambridge: Cambridge University Press, 1989); R. M. Macleod and Milton Lewis (eds), *Disease, Medicine and Empire. Perspectives on Western Medicine and the Experience of European Expansion* (London: Routledge, 1988).
97. For contemporary debates upon imperialism see P. D. Curtin, *Disease and Imperialism Before the Nineteenth Century* (Minneapolis: University of Minnesota Press, 1972); R. A. Huttenback, *Racism and Empire: White Settlers and Colored Immigrants in the British Self-governing Colonies 1830–1900* (Ithaca: Cornell University Press, 1972); R. Hyam and Ged Martin, *Reappraisals in British Imperial History* (London: Macmillan, 1975); P. Mason, *Patterns of Dominance* (London: Oxford University Press, 1970); B. Porter, *The Lion's Share: A Short History of the British Empire* (London: Longman, 1975).
98. For further discussion sec Waltraud Ernst, *Mad Tales from the Raj. The European Insane in British India 1800–1858* (London: Routledge, 1991); Vaughan, *op. cit.* (note 53).
99. See P. Spear, *The Oxford History of Modern India 1740–1975* (Delhi: Oxford, Oxford University Press, 1985); E. Stokes, *The English Utilitarians in India* (Delhi: Oxford, Oxford University Press, 1982 [1959]).
100. A. T. Embree (ed.), *1857 in India: Mutiny or War of Independence* (Boston: D. C. Heath & Co. 1960); T. R. Metcalf, *The Aftermath of Revolt* (Princeton: N.J., Princeton University Press, 1964); J. Pemble, *The Raj, the Indian Mutiny and the Kingdom of Oudh* (Hassocks: Harvester Press, 1977).
101. Gopal, *op. cit.* (note 52); B. Tomlinson, *The Political Economy of the Raj, 1914–1947. The Economics of Decolonization* (London: Macmillan, 1979).
102. See Roger Jeffery, *The Politics of Health in India* (Berkeley: University of California Press, 1988).
103. For further discussion of disease, medicine and imperialism in Africa see Philip Curtin, '"The White Man's Grave": Image and Reality', *Journal of British Studies*, 1 (1961), 94–110; John Ford, *The Role of Trypanosomiasis in African Ecology* (Oxford: Oxford University Press,

1971); Nancy Hunt, '"Le Bébé en Brousse": European Women, African Birthspacing and Colonial Intervention in Breast Feeding in the Belgian Congo', *International Journal of African Historical Studies*, 21 (1988), 401–32; Randall Packard, *White Plague, Black Labour: Tuberculosis and the Political Economy of Health and Disease in South Africa* (Berkeley: University of California Press, 1989); Gwyn Prins, 'But What Was the Disease? The Present State of Health and Healing in African Studies', *Past and Present*, 124 (1989), 159–79; Terence Ranger, 'Godly Medicine: the Ambiguities of Medical Mission in Southeast Tanzania', *Social Science and Medicine*, 15 (1981), 261–77; Maynard Swanson, 'The Sanitation Syndrome: Bubonic Plague and Urban Native Policy in the Cape Colony, 1900–1909', *Journal of African History*, 18 (1977), 387–410.

104. See E. P. Hennock, *British Social Reform and German Precedents. The Case of Social Insurance 1880–1914* (Oxford: Clarendon Press, 1987); Wolfgang J. Mommsen (ed.), *The Emergence of the Welfare State in Britain and Germany, 1850–1958* (London: Croom Helm, 1981).
105. Porter, *op. cit.* (note 16).
106. For discussion of the rise of the insurance mentality in Britain and Europe see Peter A. Köhler and Hans F. Zacher (eds), *Ein Jahrhundert Sozialversicherung in der Bundersrepublik Deutschland, Frankreich, Grossbriannien, Österreich und der Schweiz* (Berlin: Duncker & Humblot, 1981); Eric J. Evans (ed.), *Social Policy 1830–1914: Individualism, Collectivism and the Origins of the Welfare State* (London: Routledge & Kegan Paul, 1978); Michael Freedon, *The New Liberalism: An Ideology of Social Reform* (Oxford: Clarendon Press, 1978); José Harris, *Unemployment and Politics: A Study in British Social Politics 1886–1914* (Oxford: Clarendon Press, 1972); J. R. Hay, *The Origins of the Liberal Welfare Reforms 1906–1914* (London: Macmillan, 1975). For discussion of resistance to the development of social insurance in the United States see Ronald Numbers, *Almost Persuaded: American Physicians and Compulsory Health Insurance* (Baltimore: Johns Hopkins University Press, 1978); *idem*, 'The Spector of Socialized Medicine: American Physicians and Compulsory Health Insurance', in *idem*, *Compulsory Health Insurance. The Continuing Debate* (Westport, Conn.: Greenwood, 1982, 3–24; James G. Burrow, *Organized Medicine in the Progressive Era: The Move Toward Monopoly* (Baltimore: The Johns Hopkins University Press, 1977), 133–53; D. Hirshfield, *The Lost Reform: The Campaign for Compulsory Health Insurance in the United States from 1932 to 1943* (Cambridge, Mass.: Harvard University Press, 1970).
107. Webster, *op. cit.* (note 7).

108. Charles Webster, 'Health Welfare and Unemployment During the Depression', *Past and Present*, 109 (1985), 104–30; Derek Fraser, *The Evolution of the British Welfare State. A History of Social Policy Since the Industrial Revolution* (London: Macmillan, 1973); Rudolf Klein, *The Politics of the National Health Service* (London: Longman, 1989), 1–30; F. Honigsbaum, *Health, Happiness and Security. The Creation of the National Health Service* (London: Routledge, 1989), 1–21, 187–210; Fox, *op. cit.* (note 69), 94–114.
109. Douglas E. Ashford, *Policy and Politics in France* (Philadelphia: Temple University Press, 1982); *idem, British Dogmatism and French Pragmatism: Central-Local Policy Making in the Welfare State* (London: Allen & Unwin, 1982); Jean-Michel Belorgey, *La politique sociale*, (Paris: Seghers 1976); Judith F. Stone, *The Search for Social Peace: Reform Legislation in France 1890–1914* (Albany: State University of New York Press, 1985); *idem.*, 'The Radicals and the Interventionist State: Attitudes, Ambiguities and Transformations, 1880–1910', *French History*, 2 (June, 1988); Davidson, *op. cit.* (note 87); Jacques Donzelot, *L'invention du social: Essai sur le déclin des passions politiques* (Paris: Fayard, 1984); Dumont, *op. cit.* (note 87); Henry C. Galant, *Histoire politique de la sécurité sociale française 1945–1952* (Paris: Cahiers de la foundation nationale des sciences politiques, 1955); Pierre Laroque, 'Social Security in France', in Shirley Jenkins (ed.), *Social Security in International Perspective. Essays in Honor of Elvine M. Burns* (New York: Social Work and Social Issues No.1, 1969); Louis Calisti, *La mutualité en mouvement* (Paris: Éditions Social, 1982); Allen Mitchell, 'The Function and Malfunction of Mutual Aid Societies in Nineteenth-Century France', in Jonathan Barry and Colin Jones (eds), *Medicine and Charity Before the Welfare State* (London: Routledge, 1991), 172–89; William Logue, *From Philosophy to Sociology: The Evolution of French Liberalism, 1870–1914* (DeKealb: Northern Illinois University Press, 1983).
110. See also E. Sydenstricker, 'Health in the New Deal', *Annals of the American Academy of Political and Social Science*, 176 (1934), 131–7; Forrest A. Walker, 'Americanism Versus Sovietism: A Study of the Reaction to the Committee on the Costs of Medical Care', *Bulletin of the History of Medicine*, 53 (1979), 489–504; Paul Starr, *op. cit.* (note 73); F. Mullan, *Plagues and Politics. The Story of the United States Public Health Service* (New York: Basic Books, 1989), 82–127; Odin W. Anderson, *Health Services in the United States. A Growth Enterprise Since 1875* (Ann Arbor: Health Administration Press, 1985), 41–103; *idem, The Uneasy Equilibrium. Private And Public Financing of Health Services 1875–1965* (New Haven, Conn.:

College University Press, 1968), 57–103, 104–29; Fox, *op. cit.* (note 69), 37–51, 71–93; Michael R. Grey, 'Poverty, Politics and Health: The Farm Security Administration Medical Care Program, 1935– 1945', *Journal of the History of Medicine and Allied Sciences*, 44 (1989), 320–50.

111. Paul Weindling, 'The Modernization of Charity in Nineteenth-Century France and Germany', in Jonathan Barry and Colin Jones (eds), *Medicine and Charity Before the Welfare State* (London: Routledge, 1991), 190–206; W. R. Lee and Eve Rosenhaft (eds), *The State and Social Change in Germany 1880–1980* (Munich: Berg, 1990); Kershaw, *op. cit.* (note 55); Vernon L. Lidtke, *The Outlawed Party: Social Democracy in Germany, 1878–1890* (Princeton: Princeton University Press, 1966); Mason, *op. cit.* (note 55); Ludwig Preller, *Sozialpolitik in der Weimarer Republick* (Kronberg: Athenaum, 1978); Michael Prinz, *Vom neuen Mittelstand zum Volksgenossen: Die Entwicklung des sozialen Status der Angestellten von der Weimarer Republick bis zum Ende der NS-Zeit* (Munich: R. Oldenbourg, 1986); Gerhard A. Ritter, *Social Welfare in Germany and Britain: Origins and Developments* (Leamington Spa: Berg, 1986); Walter Vogel, *Besmirch Arbeiterversicherung: Ihre Entstehung im Kräftespiel der Zeit* (Brunswick: Rutgers University Press, 1951); Wolfgan Braumandl, *Die Wirtschafts – und Sozialpolitik des Deutschen Reiches im Sudenland 1938–1945* (Würnberg: Preussler, 1985).

112. Arnold J. Heidenheimer and Nils Elvander, *The Shaping of the Swedish Health System* (London: Croom Helm, 1980); Erik Allardt, 'The Civic Conception of the Welfare State in Scandinavia', in Richard Rose and Rei Shiratori (eds), *The Welfare State East and West* (New York, Oxford: Oxford University Press, 1986); Bent Rold Andersen, 'Rationality and Irrationality of the Nordic Welfare State', in Stephen R. Graubard (ed.), *Norden: The Passion for Equality* (Oslo: Norwegian University Press, 1986); Francis G. Castles, *The Social Democratic Image of Society: A Study of the Achievements and Origins of Scandinavian Social Democracy in Comparative Perspective* (London: Routledge & Kegan Paul, 1978); John Fry (ed.), *Limits of the Welfare State: Critical Views on Post-War Sweden* (Farnborough: Saxon House, 1979); Leif Lewin, *Ideology and Strategy: A Century of Swedish Politics* (Cambridge: Cambridge University Press, 1988).

113. P. Gifford and W. R. Louis (eds), *The Transfer of Power in Africa: Decolonization 1940–60* (New Haven: Yale University Press, 1982); R. F. Holland, *European Decolonization 1918–81: An Introductory Survey* (Basingstoke: Macmillan, 1985).

114. Peter Flora and Arnold J. Heidenheimer (eds), *The Development of*

Welfare States in Europe and America (New Brunswick: Transaction Books, 1981); Peter Flora, *et al.* (eds), *State, Economy and Society in Western Europe, 1915–1975* (London: Macmillan, 1987); Douglas E. Ashford, *The Emergence of Welfare States* (Oxford: Blackwell, 1988); Peter Flora (ed.), *Growth to Limits: the Western European Welfare State Since World War II* (Berlin: de Gruyter, 1986); Roger Girod, *et al.* (eds), *Social Policy in Western Europe and the USA 1950–80* (Basingstoke: Macmillan in association with Institute for Labour Studies, 1985); Margaret Weir, *et al.*, *The Politics of Social Policy in the United States* (Princeton: Princeton University Press, 1988); Abram de Swaan, *In Care of the State: Health Care, Education and Welfare in Europe and the USA in the Modern Era*, (Cambridge: Polity, 1988); Harold L. Wilensky, *The New Corporatism, Centralization and the Welfare State* (London: Sage Publications, 1976); Raymond Plant, *et al.*, *Political Philosophy and Social Welfare: Essays on the Normative Basis of Welfare Provision* (London: Routledge & Kegan Paul, 1980); Amy Gutman (ed.), *Democracy and the Welfare State* (Princeton: Princeton University Press, 1988).

115. Milton Roemer is one of the world's greatest authorities on the comparative analysis of health care systems as his many publications testify. See for example: Milton Roemer, *National Health Systems and their Reorientation Towards Health for All, Vol. 1* (New York, Oxford: Oxford University Press, 1991); *idem, et al.*, *National Health Systems and their Reorientation Towards Health for All* (Geneva: World Health Organization, 1984); *idem, Rural Health* (St Louis: Kimpton, 1976); *idem* and Ruth Roemer, *Health Manpower Policies in the Belgian Health Care System* (Washington: DEWH, 1977); *idem* and *idem, Health Manpower Policies Under Five National Health Care Systems* (Washington: DEHW, 1978).

116. Elmar Altvater, 'Some Problems of State Interventionism: The 'Particularization of the State in Bourgeois Society', in John Holloway and Sol Piccotto (eds), *State and Capital: A Marxist Debate* (London: Edward Arnold, 1978); John H. Goldthorpe (ed.), *Order and Conflict in Contemporary Capitalism* (Oxford: 1984); Kathi V. Friedman, *Legitimation of Social Rights and the Western Welfare State: A Weberian Perspective*, (Chapel Hill: University of North Carolina Press, 1981); Neil Gilbert, *Capitalism and the Welfare State: Dilemmas of Social Benevolence* (New Haven, Conn.: Yale University Press, 1983); Norman Ginsburg, *Class, Capital and Social Policy* (London: Macmillan, 1979); Ulf Himmelstrand, *et al.*, *Beyond Welfare Capitalism* (London: Heinemann, 1981); Roland Huntford, *The New Totalitarians* (London: Allen Lane, 1975); Julia Parker, *Social Policy*

and Citizenship (London: Macmillan, 1975); Stein Ringen, *The Possibility of Politics: A Study in the Political Economy of the Welfare State* (Oxford: Clarendon, 1987); Tony Cutler *et al.*, *Keynes, Beveridge and Beyond* (London: Routledge & Kegan Paul, 1986).

117. For current debates on the power and state in society see, Michael Mann, *The Sources of Social Power. A History of Power from the Beginning to A.D. 1760*, 3 vols (Cambridge: Cambridge University Press, 1986), Vol. 1, 1–33; Anthony Giddens and David Held (eds), *Classes, Power and Conflict. Classical and Contemporary Debates* (London: Macmillan, 1992); *idem*, *Central Problems in Social Theory* (London: Macmillan, 1979); *idem*, *The Constitution of Society* (Cambridge: Polity Press, 1984); *idem*, *Profiles and Critiques in Social Theory* (Berkeley: University of California Press, 1982); John Holloway and Sol Piccotto (eds), *State and Capital: A Marxist Debate* (London: Edward Arnold, 1978); David Held, *States and Societies* (London: Basil Blackwell, 1990); Simon Clarke (ed.), *The State Debate* (London: Macmillan, 1991); T. Skocpol, *States and Social Revolutions: A Comparative Analysis of France, Russia and China* (Cambridge: Cambridge University Press, 1979); J. Hall, *Powers and Liberties* (New York: Oxford University Press, 1985); M. Zeitlin (ed.), *Political Power and Social Theory* (Greenwich, Conn.: JAI Press, 1980), Vol. 1; C. Tilly (ed.), *The Formation of National States in Western Europe* (Princeton: Princeton University Press, 1975); P. Anderson, *Lineages of the Absolute State* (London: New Left Books, 1974).

1

Public Health in France

Matthew Ramsey

In the history of modern public health, France figures prominently as a pioneer and as the source of a programme emphasizing enlightened intervention from above.[1] Two related paradoxes, however, characterize the actual French experience. The first is that a country which helped create the modern public hygiene movement and establish public health as a scientific discipline was slow to apply public health measures on a wide scale. The second is that in France, whose name is virtually synonymous with centralization and the strong state, the central government long played a surprisingly limited role in public health. Far from subordinating the individual relentlessly to the public interest, France was one of the countries in which classic liberalism was most pervasive and persisted the longest. Although this pattern changed greatly in the twentieth century, particularly under the Fifth Republic, aspects of it are still recognizable today.

The Background: Old Regime and Revolution

The development of public health in modern France reflected the contradictory legacy of the French Revolution; its deeper roots lay in the Old Regime, in the efforts of the Bourbon monarchy to inject the state into the business of promoting the health and welfare of the king's subjects. Tocqueville's classic thesis on the continuities between the ambitions of the new and the old orders applies to public hygiene.

Traditional Public Health

In late-medieval and early modern France, as elsewhere in Europe, public health constituted neither a coherent discipline nor a well-defined administrative domain; rather, it represented the place of intersection of several predominantly local concerns and agencies. Public assistance constituted one such field of activity. Based primarily in an extensive network of hospitals, typically staffed by religious or members of the lay nursing orders created during the Counter Reformation,[2] its object was to succor the needy, some of whom happened to be sick.[3] Medical assistance outside the hospital setting was very limited; the model of the salaried town or district physician, well established in the Germanies and some other parts of Europe, was less widely emulated in France.[4] The municipality had primary responsibility for administering public assistance, though the Church also played an active role, as did guilds, confraternities and individual notables.

Measures to combat the spread of disease came under the rubric of 'police', broadly concerned with administration and maintenance of order, primarily in urban settings. In times of plague, many towns, starting in the late fifteenth and sixteenth centuries, appointed health councils or captains of health on the Italian model, with emergency powers;[5] in some places, notably port cities vulnerable to ship-borne diseases (Marseilles is the most prominent example), the board became permanent. In addition to these defensive measures, routine municipal ordinances governed such essential services as water supply and the disposal of refuse and excreta, as well as the great range of economic activities affecting the health of the population.[6] Yet these numerous practices fell far short of constituting a coordinated system of public health and left the vast rural majority of the French population largely untouched. Moreover, it was only in the last decades of the Old Regime that public health was fully recognized as a sub-discipline of medicine as well as a branch of police; such terms as 'public hygiene' (and even the expression 'medical police', commonly used as a synonym) did not gain wide currency until the end of the century. Readers who consulted the article on hygiene in Diderot's *Encyclopédie*, published in the middle decades of the century, would have found only a discussion of private hygiene as a means of promoting personal health; for public health, they would have had to turn to the article on police, where it figured as one of 11 administrative concerns subsumed under that rubric. In contrast, the article on hygiene that Jean-Noël Hallé (1754–1822) wrote in the 1780s for the *Encyclopédie méthodique*, gave extended consideration to 'public hygiene'.[7]

State Intervention and the Origins of the New Public Health

At the end of the Old Regime, the network of local institutions was still clearly recognizable; yet there had grown up next to it the rudiments of a new public health system, sponsored by the Crown, implemented by a specialized bureaucracy, and increasingly grounded in medical science.[8] Under the mercantilist assumptions of the early-modern state builders, the strength of the kingdom depended on a thriving and numerous population,[9] and at least since the late seventeenth century, the government had committed itself to promoting the health of all the king's subjects. Consolidating public health functions under state control also contributed to the broader political programme of the absolute monarchy, which sought to reduce the independence and authority of competing institutions.

Louis XIV's minister of finance, Colbert, established the institutional framework: an office known as the Contrôle Général des Finances, broadly concerned with the social and economic life of the kingdom, including health and poor relief; a corps of royal intendants served as its agents in the provinces. Starting late in the reign of Louis XIV, the government began shipping boxes of remedies to the countryside when an intendant reported an epidemic; the intendants also dispatched physicians and surgeons to the most seriously affected sites.[10] In 1720, after what proved to be France's last plague epidemic had broken out at Marseilles, the government attempted to coordinate prophylactic measures on a national scale. But this was an *ad hoc* response to a major crisis. For most of the Old Regime, France lacked a permanent institution at the national level devoted exclusively to public health, with the minor exception of a series of commissions that regulated proprietary remedies, starting in 1728.[11]

The establishment of a Royal Society of Medicine, during the reign of Louis XVI, filled this lacuna.[12] The Society originated in a corresponding committee created in 1776 by Turgot, then Controller-General, to combat epidemics and epizootics; it received royal letters patent and its official title in 1778. Nominally headed by Joseph Lassone, physician to the queen and First Physician in reversion to the king, the Society was in practice governed by its permanent secretary, Lassone's younger colleague, the anatomist Félix Vicq d'Azyr (1748–94), arguably the most prominent spokesman for public health in the last years of the Old Regime and the first years of the Revolution. Epidemics and epizootics remained among its principal concerns, together with the regulation of secret remedies and mineral waters; strongly influenced by the neo-Hippocratic currents of the eighteenth century, the Society asked its members and correspondents to compile medical topographies and keep detailed meteorological records[13] and encouraged the elimination of environmental health hazards.[14]

By the last decades of the Old Regime, then, a medical bureaucracy with jurisdiction over public health had begun to emerge, distinct from the old localist system of medical police as well as from the corporate network of faculties, colleges, and guilds that governed the practice of medicine, pharmacy, and surgery. The bureaucracy's purview extended to the population of the entire kingdom, not merely urban centres; indeed, the health of the peasantry was perhaps its foremost preoccupation, in keeping with the physiocratic sympathies of many of its most influential members. Ambitious proponents of the statist programme were far from satisfied, however; they hoped to see a national system of hospitals, welfare and medical assistance – all controversial proposals.[15] Critics of the hospital denounced it both as a charitable and as a medical institution, calling instead for home care and voluntary local assistance; the medical profession's detractors preferred to emphasize self-help, especially hygiene.[16] This discourse can be read as a liberal counter-programme, expressing distrust of the power vested in large public institutions, monopolistic professions and the central government. Nevertheless, broad agreement existed on the need to reform public assistance and medical police.

The Revolution and its Aftermath

The Revolution of 1789, by bringing into question all existing political and social institutions, gave new urgency to these debates.[17] Where once only piecemeal reform had seemed practicable, there now opened the possibility of replacing the existing patchwork of institutions with a comprehensive and rationally designed system of social welfare and public health; it might be paid for in large part, as some reformers had suggested at the end of the Old Regime, by nationalizing the wealth of the Church. The revolutionaries agreed that the people enjoyed a right to health,[18] though they differed on how to attain this goal: some emphasized active medical intervention, while a smaller group shared the Rousseauist vision of a regenerated society in which people would lead healthier lives, and the need for medicine and all its attendant institutions would wither away.[19]

The charge of developing a revolutionary programme for public health fell to two committees established in 1790 within the National Constituent Assembly: a committee on poor relief chaired by the duc de La Rochefoucauld-Liancourt (1747–1827), and a committee on health, headed by the physician Joseph-Ignace Guillotin (1738–1814) and closely linked to the Royal Society of Medicine (which presented its views in a 'New Plan for the Constitution of Medicine in France'). Both committees favoured a national programme of medical assistance to the indigent, and the health committee presented an elaborate plan that would have created the first fully developed national public health system anywhere and made medical care accessible to the entire population, although it contained no provision for a central administration.[20]

Little of this vast project was subsequently realized or even pursued. The National Convention, which ruled France from the fall of the monarchy in 1792 to the inception of the Directory regime in 1795, did adopt a generous law in May 1794 on public assistance in rural areas.[21] It called, among other things, for three salaried 'health officers' (the revolutionary name for medical practitioners) in each administrative district to treat the indigent sick; the government would provide supplies of medicine and food for the patients, and they would receive a monetary allowance for themselves and their children. The law proved difficult to implement, however, since the need was great and funds in short supply. Two other actions by the Convention seriously undermined public health. In keeping with the earlier programme of nationalization and with revolutionary anticlericalism, the government confiscated the hospitals' endowments and expelled the nursing orders, but without putting anything in their place.[22] The Convention also completed the work of shutting down the privileged medical institutions of the Old Regime, including the faculties and surgical corporations as well as the no longer royal Society of Medicine; although at the end of 1794 the Convention authorized three new schools to teach medicine (including public hygiene), regulation of medical practice and the remedy trade remained suspended for a decade. The immediate consequences of the Revolution for public health, it could be argued, were chiefly negative.

Under the Directory and the Napoleonic Consulate and Empire, the hospitals returned to something like the *status quo ante,* with the nursing orders restored and endowments reconstituted; administration and funding were once more in the hands of the municipalities (though with state oversight), an arrangement that remained firmly in place into the years following the First World War.[23] Outdoor relief was placed in the hands of municipal *bureaux de bienfaisance* (welfare bureaus); some hired physicians to care for the indigent, though neither in practice nor in intent did this arrangement realize the scheme imagined by the Convention two years earlier. No national agency replaced the Royal Society of Medicine. The government turned for advice to the Paris medical school (renamed faculty of medicine under Napoleon); starting in 1800, this work was coordinated by a Society of the School (later Faculty) of Medicine, composed of a commission of professors and 32 associates from outside the faculty. Several independent medical societies also appeared, starting, in 1796, with the Medical Society of Paris, a conscious rival of the Paris faculty that advised the Paris administration on questions of public health.[24] But the state, abandoning the commitments envisaged in 1790–1, had largely withdrawn from the fields of welfare and public health.

The Revolution brought great hopes and even greater disappointments to the cause of public health. One need not share the nostalgia for the Old Regime evinced by traditional conservative scholarship and some of the more recent work of neo-conservatives and other disabused liberals[25] to recognize the gulf between revolutionary theory and practice, and the deterioration of both public assistance and medical police. Although the old system of charitable relief was in many places already in decline at the end of the Old Regime and arguably antiquated in its underlying conception and design,[26] it made more generous provision for the sick poor than the revolutionaries found possible, and the work of the Royal Society of Medicine on epidemics and the remedy trade was cut short in its most vigorous phase. The Revolution can be credited, at most, with a longer-term and less direct contribution: by levelling the old institutions, it created the space in which new ones could arise.

This was hardly the revolutionaries' intention. But confiscated Church property failed to provide the financial base that reformers had anticipated for their dauntingly expensive enterprise, and the wars and political turmoil that consumed France during the 1790s would in any case have overwhelmed the ambitious projects of the Constituent Assembly. The programme also lost momentum to internal friction arising from reformers' divergent views on how best to promote health and from contradictions among the Revolution's most basic ideals – conflicts that have their counterparts in debates on civic rights and responsibilities in any modern democratic polity. The right to health and assistance, taken together with the proposed mechanisms for state intervention, ran counter to the revolutionary principles of economic freedom and the sanctity of private property. At a deeper level, revolutionary individualism, proclaimed in the Declaration of the Rights of Man of 1789, conflicted with the communitarianism expressed in the radical Revolution's conception of republican virtue; and the federalism and local autonomy favoured in the early stages of the Revolution found their antithesis in Jacobin centralization and the authoritarian state embodied by the Committee of Public Safety.

So far as the Revolution resolved these tensions, which were arguably present from the beginning, the outcome did not favour ambitious national programmes in public health. Although the revolutionaries reluctantly adopted price controls and, with greater enthusiasm, confiscated property belonging to the Church and counter-revolutionary *émigrés,* even the radical Republic valued property over social welfare, and memories of the Terror reinforced distrust of far-reaching statist solutions after the fall of Robespierre. The post-revolutionary settlement, epitomized in the Napoleonic Code, preserved equality before the law but rejected the communitarian promises of the Revolution as utopian and subversive. Government would be centralized and not particularly respectful of civil liberties, but it would protect property and would not attempt to control French social and economic life from Paris; the state would in a sense be strong but also non-interventionist. The vision of the enlightened reformers was far from dead, but the painful legacy of the Revolution made it difficult to realize – more difficult, perhaps, than under the old Monarchy – and set limits to public health reform for several generations. Tocqueville's thesis applies, with a proviso: France inherited from the Old Regime and Revolution both a statist programme born under the absolute monarchy and powerful forces that resisted it.

The Nineteenth Century

The subsequent development of French public health expressed the Revolution's contradictory heritage.[27] A public hygiene movement emerged whose goals in some ways recalled the revolutionaries' original ambitions. The movement had close links to the state and was marked by a strong centralizing impulse; what reforms took place owed less to private initiatives than in England (where the proponents of centralization, such as Jeremy Bentham and Edwin Chadwick, took the French model as their point of reference).[28] The result was something more than an extension of the Old Regime patterns of assistance and police. Yet the new laws and institutions, even had they worked as intended, would not have matched the contemporaneous achievements of France's neighbours in Western Europe, much less fulfilled the hopes of the revolutionary committees; the public hygiene movement in the nineteenth century attained only limited success in its struggle with the post-revolutionary forces opposing state intervention.

Although Napoleon greatly reinforced the national bureaucracy, the French state long tended toward neutrality in the social and economic domains. In public assistance, commonly seen as a duty of society but not an absolute right of the individual, the state merely seconded private philanthropy and mutual aid, with higher levels of government intervening when lower levels had proved inadequate (a principle that continued to dominate until the 1930s). Nor was health a right of French citizens guaranteed by the state, as some revolutionaries had envisaged. Public health measures continued to depend to a large extent on the goodwill and resources of local authorities, who often failed to cooperate even when national legislation theoretically compelled them to act. Administrative centralization did to some extent shape public health programmes, but in negative as well as positive ways; it has been argued that the structure of French politics and administration allowed interest groups to block reforms at the centre, safe in the knowledge that a victory secured in Paris greatly diminished the chance of independent initiatives in the provinces.[29]

The story of public health in nineteenth-century France is exceptionally complex, reflecting not only the ideological debates and changes in medical theory and practice common to all Western nations but also the particular pattern of instability that characterized modern French political history: after the destruction of the old monarchy, no regime until recent times could claim full legitimacy for itself, and only one, the relatively long-lived Third Republic (1870–1940), lasted so long as two decades. For the sake of convenience, the period may be divided schematically into three phases. The first, roughly 1800–30 (spanning the Consulate created by Bonaparte's *coup d'état* of 1799, the Empire of 1804–14, and the Bourbon Restoration), saw the beginnings of an organized public health movement and the creation of a first generation of institutions. A second phase, running from 1830 to about 1870, encompasses the July Monarchy of Louis-Philippe of the house of Orléans (r. 1830–48), the short-lived Second Republic that issued from the Revolution of 1848, and the Second Empire of Napoleon III, whose rise to power began with his election, as Louis-Napoléon Bonaparte, to the presidency of the Republic in 1848. During these decades, France lost its leadership position in public health; *laissez-faire* liberalism reached its acme under the July Monarchy, and the subsequent regimes produced only tentative experiments with new institutions and forms of medical assistance. The third phase, corresponding roughly to the years from the founding of the Third Republic to the beginning of the First World War (1870–1914), marked a watershed. In France, as elsewhere, public health was consolidated as a profession and refounded as a discipline on the basis of the new microbiology. These international developments, in conjunction with political changes peculiar to France, made possible a series of legislative enactments that involved the state in public health to an extent unprecedented in French history – though still below the level attained in several of France's neighbours.

The Early Hygiene Movement: 1800–30

In the first decades of the nineteenth century, a vocal public health movement emerged in France. An earlier generation might have looked for inspiration to the central Europe of Johann Peter Frank (whom Napoleon tried to recruit to France in 1802), and a later one to Chadwick's England or Virchow's Prussia; for the generation that reached adulthood in the years following the French Revolution, France provided the clearest (and arguably the first) model of public health as a coherent discipline.[30] The French hygienists were the heirs to the statist programme of the Enlightenment, mediated through the progressive thinkers of the revolutionary and Napoleonic era known as the Ideologues, whose ranks included the physician-cum-philosopher Georges Cabanis (1757–1808). Ideologue thought linked the 'moral' to the material world, psychology to physiology, and medicine to politics and the social sciences; it also accorded extensive authority to experts in the design and execution of public policy. Throughout the nineteenth century, an ambitious French tradition of political medicine assigned physicians a prominent role as advisers to legislators and promised that medicine applied to the public sphere would make society both healthier and happier.

Physicians made up the core of the movement, joined by prominent pharmacists, scientists and interested administrators. The three schools of health (later medical faculties) authorized by the revolutionary Convention provided the institutional base for the first generation, who had reached adulthood under the Old Regime. Hallé was the first occupant of the Paris chair; François-Emmanuel Fodéré (1764–1835), who held the chair at Strasbourg from 1814 to 1835, published standard textbooks on public health and legal medicine.[31] The leaders of the next generation of hygienists, most prominently Louis Villermé (1782–1863) and A.-J.-B. Parent-Duchâtelet (1790–1836), were primarily public health investigators rather than teachers and textbook writers, and they typically worked outside the faculties. Although they were active in the medical societies and new public health institutions that had emerged since the Revolution, they had neither a professional organization of their own nor a single well-defined institutional forum for promoting their goals. The movement's spiritual centre, indeed, was not an institution but a periodical, the *Annales d'hygiène publique et de médecine légale*, launched in 1829, the first journal of public health in any language and long the leader in its field.[32]

In France, then, the development of public health in the early nineteenth century depended chiefly on a specialized and committed group of activists within the medical élite. *L'hygiènisme* should not be identified with a larger social movement or even with the medical profession as a whole; few public health programmes involved more than a small minority of physicians, and many practitioners remained distrustful of a cause which, if it attained its goals, might deprive them of fee-paying patients and tend to transform them into functionaries. Nor could public health at this time be considered a profession. The salaried full-time public health officer was virtually unknown; the great majority of physicians who held posts in the field of public hygiene maintained a normal private practice, and many of their offices were unpaid.[33]

Both the public health movement and its allies among public officials found themselves constrained by the limits of the administrative machinery with which they had to work. The Ministry of the Interior, corresponding to the office of the Controller-General under the Old Regime, had primary responsibility for the health of the population on French territory; its statistical bureau, established in 1800, provided strong support to the hygienists' epidemiological and demographic investigations. But jurisdiction over health-related questions was dispersed among several ministries, including the Ministry of Agriculture and Commerce, which regulated economic activities. At lower levels, overseeing public health was one of many duties of prefects, sub-prefects and mayors, and rarely among their highest priorities.

Napoleon, though well aware of the potential benefits of public health measures (as his celebrated enthusiasm for vaccination attests), made only a limited contribution to developing the administrative apparatus to implement them. Even the vaccination campaign, though sponsored and supported by the government, was directed by an independent agency, the Central Vaccination Committee (1800), which owed its existence to the joint efforts of the medical élite (including Philippe Pinel and Michel-Augustin Thouret, director of the Paris medical school) and socially prominent philanthropists, the duc de La Rochefoucauld-Liancourt chief among them.[34] As an example of a more clearly bureaucratic institution, one could point to the departmental 'medical juries' established under the medical practice law of 1803 to examine and certify candidates in medicine and midwifery and also charged with inspecting pharmacies; not all *départements* had a regularly functioning jury, and the institution was ultimately abolished in 1854, but the more activist juries regularly investigated threats to public health, especially illegal medical practice and the sale of harmful drugs. In 1810 the imperial government appointed a special commission on secret remedies, in an effort to revive the systematic regulation provided by the Royal Society under the Old Regime, but after an initial burst of activity it lost momentum, and by 1813 it had ceased to function.[35]

The major institutional innovation of the Napoleonic years was not, indeed, the direct creation of the central government: it was the Paris prefect of police, Dubois, who established the Health Council (Conseil de Salubrité) of the *département* of the Seine in 1802.[36] France had had municipal health boards before, and the model survived in port cities exposed to ship-borne epidemics (indeed, a measure of 1802 called for similar agencies in all ports); the most powerful of the boards, the Intendancy of Health at Marseilles, controlled the application of quarantines to merchant shipping in the Mediterranean, a monopoly dating from the Old Regime.[37] The Paris council's activities can also be seen as a revival of the work carried out under the jurisdiction of the Paris lieutenant of police at the end of the Old Regime. In several important respects, however, the institution was a novelty. Unlike many of the Old Regime health boards, it functioned permanently; its personnel, drawn from among the leading lights of the public hygiene movement, enjoyed salaried lifetime appointments. More important, it devoted itself to perennial problems of public health in the life of a great city and not just epidemic emergencies: noxious industries (which were to be the single most important demand on its time), quacks, garbage, sewage and adulterated food, among many others. The Council, it is true, remained an advisory body without powers of enforcement, and it never took on the direct national role to which it aspired. Its influence, however, was truly national and even international, and it served as the model for other municipal and departmental health boards in the provinces.

It was the Restoration that created the first major national public health institutions of the new century. In 1820 it filled the lacuna left by the suppression of the old Royal Society by establishing a Royal Academy of Medicine; and in the early 1820s, in response to the threat posed by outbreaks of yellow fever in Spain, it created first an *ad hoc* commission and then a permanent national council to coordinate the defence of French frontiers against epidemic disease.

The Academy brought veterans of Old Regime medical institutions together with the leaders of the societies that had emerged under the Republic, effectively creating a single institutional base for the medical élite.[38] The Academy was to promote research, adjudicate questions of legal medicine and advise the government on all matters medical; above all, though, it was given explicit responsibility for all questions relating to public health. Like the Royal Society before it, the Academy dealt with epidemics, epizootics, secret remedies (including the larger problem of quackery), and mineral waters; it also took over coordination of the vaccination campaign from the Central Committee.

The government formed the Central Sanitary Commission in 1820 to design and oversee the system of cordons sanitaires, quarantines, and lazarettos intended to contain the spread of yellow fever, which had appeared in Cadiz the previous year, raising fears of the worst epidemic to invade French territory since the plague of 1720; the Commission's model was the Marseilles Intendancy of Health.[39] This temporary arrangement prepared the way for new legislation in 1822, following the reappearance of yellow fever closer to French borders, in Barcelona. The law established a permanent High Council of Health under the Ministry of the Interior and charged it with implementing a new code designed to guard against the transmission of epidemic disease from abroad; a network of subordinate sanitary commissions in the provinces would direct the actual work of enforcement.[40] In part because the threat of yellow fever subsequently abated, the provincial network did not fully materialize; the High Council, which was not closely connected to the public hygiene movement and was committed to a traditional model of medical police that emphasized containing the spread of contagion, exercised far less influence than the Academy and played only a marginal role in the development of public health as a discipline. Nevertheless, the legislation of 1822 did reorganize and effectively nationalize the system for sanitary protection of the frontiers; as one indication, the Minister of the Interior now had sole power of appointment to the once proudly autonomous Intendancy of Health at Marseilles.

Public health institutions and their programmes are shaped by the intersecting and sometimes mutually reinforcing influences of the political and medical cultures in which they operate. In early nineteenth-century France, the legal framework inherited from the Revolution held that citizens enjoyed certain fundamental rights, as the returning Bourbons were compelled to recognize in the Charter of 1814, the constitutional document of the Restoration. The most firmly established was that of property, but it was not absolute: like other rights it might be abridged to protect the rights of others or to serve an overriding public interest. The extent of the limits that the state might legitimately impose was a matter of debate. The school of political economy exemplified by Jean-Baptiste Say, the French disciple of Adam Smith, argued for minimal interference; *laissez-faire* not only respected individual rights but also promoted public prosperity. Say's critics, most prominently J.-C.-L. Simonde de Sismondi in his *New Principles of Political Economy* of 1819, emphasized the costs of *laissez-faire* in an era of emerging industrial capitalism and its tendency to promote the well-being of some classes over others (though few would have argued for state intervention to redress the balance).[41] The hygienists, though recruited from the ranks of the professional bourgeoisie and closely allied with the state, mostly embraced liberal political economy; Villermé saw the prosperity created by unfettered economic activity as essential to the well-being of the nation, since a poor population would not be healthy.[42] In practice, they used state institutions to control the most serious public nuisances, without trying to regulate industrial activities or work conditions more generally; above all, they avoided any suggestion that the state, in the name of promoting health, should raise the standard of living of the least advantaged members of society.

As in politics, so in medicine a flawed consensus provided an unsteady platform for the hygienists' programme. The broad outlines of aetiological thinking in the early nineteenth-century remained close to the neo-Hippocratic environmentalism of the Old Regime: hence the hygienists' emphasis on sanitary measures. But this was not quite the eighteenth-century world of medical topographies and epidemic constitutions. The Hippocratic preoccupation with climate and soil was giving way to an emphasis on social factors affecting health, the central concern in the work of Villermé. Many correspondents of the Royal Society had sought to understand disease in its social context, but where they had concentrated on what they saw as the unhealthful behaviour of an ignorant and superstitious peasantry, the hygienists increasingly focused on the characteristic pathologies of the industrial working class in urban settings.

The explanatory powers of environmentalism, however, were widely recognized to have certain limits. Much has been written about the early nineteenth-century debates on this question and the possible connections between 'contagionist' and 'anti-contagionist' positions, on the one hand, and political reaction and liberalism on the other.[43] It is important to recognize both the strengths and the weaknesses of this interpretation. A rigid distinction between contagionists and anti-contagionists will not work satisfactorily. Virtually all authorities recognized the influence of environmental factors (particularly airborne miasmas)[44] while also acknowledging that certain diseases, such as smallpox and syphilis, were transmitted directly from individual to individual through some process of contagion. They did differ noisily, however, on which diseases to assign to the latter category. The case of yellow fever was particularly problematic. The commission that the Restoration government initially sent to Spain, under the direction of Étienne Pariset (1770–1847), described yellow fever as contagious; the government accepted that interpretation, but other physicians, notably Nicolas Chervin (1783–1843), argued strongly against it. In 1828, the Academy of Medicine, parting company with the High Council of Health, endorsed the anti-contagionist position.

A similar point applies to politics. It is too facile simply to identify contagionism and quarantines with the Bourbons and reaction, and anti-contagionism with modern medicine and liberal politics; critics of contagionism based their arguments on what they saw as sound medical reasoning. Yet public health measures unquestionably carried political implications. The exponents of political economy (and mercantile interests) deplored the restraints on trade created by quarantines and cordons sanitaires; liberals unsuccessfully fought the legislation of 1822 because it imposed what seemed to them excessively harsh penalties and called for destroying contaminated articles without compensation. (It is sometimes forgotten that they would have protested even more loudly against the environmental medicine favoured by the public hygiene movement, had its programmes been rigorously compulsory rather than largely voluntary.)

The government responded to the shifting currents of these debates, though its general policy, broadly continuous with that of the Old Regime, was as much the product of inertia. Assistance remained primarily local, relying heavily on the network of hospitals – still catch-all asylums for the unfortunate, with only limited medical functions.[45] Outdoor relief was similarly organized at the local level, through the welfare bureaus (*bureaux de bienfaisance*) established by the Directory in 1796; as before, some had physicians attached to their staffs, who provided an increasing but still modest amount of medical care. The only nationally coordinated system of medical services took the form of a revived network of epidemic doctors and remedy boxes required by a decree of 1805.[46] Beyond this, most medical assistance was purely local and often voluntary. Apart from the welfare bureaus, some cities appointed neighbourhood doctors to serve the indigent. The Philanthropic Society of Paris, founded in 1780, established five dispensaries in 1803 with a salaried medical staff to treat the deserving poor; their patients numbered in the thousands but constituted only a small fraction of the population in need of assistance.[47] Private insurance schemes were still in their infancy; mutual aid and provident societies (technically illegal under the

Criminal Code of 1810, which banned associations of more than 20 persons) were not numerous and made only limited provision for medical care. The most remarkable innovation came at the regional level: in the Alsatian *département* of the Bas-Rhin, Adrien Lezay-Marnésia, a prefect who had served previously in annexed territory in the Rhineland, where he came to admire the German model of the district physician, issued a decree in 1810 establishing a network of public physicians in each canton, who were to serve both as public health officers and physicians to the poor. The doctors who held these posts also maintained their private practice; their annual stipend was set initially at 500 francs and, despite subsequent increases, remained well below the income that a successful university-trained physician could expect.[48] Two additional *départements* in the north-east emulated this model under the Restoration, and others adopted similar programmes in the decades that followed, leading many private practitioners to fear the development of a state medical service that would either absorb them or drive them out of business.

The dreaded 'medical functionocracy' did not materialize, however. Indeed, one of the characteristic features of French public health throughout the nineteenth century and beyond was the limited number of full-time salaried state medical personnel, outside the military services; the concept of the 'state physician' barely applies. The great majority of public medical appointments were part-time, and many were paid badly or not at all, although doctors attached to prisons, schools, the customs and the gendarmerie generally received better compensation than those on the staffs of hospitals or dispensaries, epidemic doctors, forensic experts and the rest. The élite regularly monopolized most appointments; there are even some indications that officials favoured prosperous practitioners whose wealth made them local notables (particularly during the Restoration and July Monarchy, when suffrage was limited to citizens whose payment on a property tax known as *le cens* exceeded a certain level). *Le cumul* – the accumulation of multiple appointments – was common. Less favoured colleagues might work as vaccinators and perform a few other modestly rewarded services, but this was not a reliable or substantial source of income. Public medicine, then, did not constitute an occupation in itself and was less readily available later in the century than in some other parts of Western Europe as an alternative to private practice for members of a medical proletariat.

Police measures, like public assistance, embodied a mixture of old and new. The most important national regulatory legislation, adopted in 1803, applied to the medical professions themselves. The state would now certify doctors of medicine and surgery, 'health officers' (a new second tier of medical practitioners, corresponding roughly to the lower-level surgeons of the Old Regime, and not to be confused with public health officials), pharmacists, and midwives, thus ending the period of deregulation that began when the Revolution dismantled the corporate institutions of the Old Regime.[49] The legislation on pharmacy contained restrictions on the sale of secret remedies, and an imperial decree of 1810 called for the wholesale examination of all such remedies, but both measures were subsequently undercut by decisions protecting the interests of established remedy owners: here property rights overrode concern for public health.[50] More sustained results followed from another imperial decree of 1810, which regulated potentially dangerous industrial establishments. This measure protected the neighbours of a factory, rather than the workers inside it, and neighbours' property rights as much as the broader interest of public health, but it gave the authorities a useful weapon against polluting enterprises. New plants were subject to inspection; industries classed as dangerous required the approval of the Council of State and had to be located away from residential areas. Implementation of this decree, which occupied much of the time of the Paris Health Council and its provincial emulators, required continual compromises between the interests of property and of public health; the hygienists, Villermé foremost among them, did not see industry in itself as a major cause of ill health, and the councils hesitated to discourage economic development.

In most other areas of medical police, regulation continued exclusively at the local level, as under the Old Regime. This was true, for example, of prostitution. Paris adopted a programme of surveillance and medical control at the beginning of the century: medical examinations were required in 1802, and a special dispensary was established three years later. Similar programmes appeared in provincial cities, but France remained without national legislation on this subject throughout the nineteenth-century, despite the best efforts of advocates such as Parent-Duchâtelet.[51]

Most sanitary legislation and measures to remove or control possible sources of infection were similarly local in scope. At the national level, two programmes designed to protect against epidemic disease stand out: the vaccination campaign launched at the beginning of the century, and the system of protection against imported epidemics, initially centered in seaports and then expanded and reinforced by the legislation of 1822.

The French received Jenner's discovery with the same enthusiasm that greeted it world-wide; the central government informally sponsored and supported the campaign but neither required vaccination nor introduced any other formal legislation on the subject.[52] (In contrast, one of the major objectives of the regional system of cantonal physicians in the Bas-Rhin was to vaccinate all children.) The keenest advocates of the procedure wished to make it obligatory; the opposing view prevailed, however, in large part on the grounds that the state, in deciding to vaccinate a child, would be usurping the position of the paterfamilias, whose commanding position in the family the Napoleonic Code repeatedly affirmed. This outcome was hardly unusual (in the early nineteenth century, only a few small kingdoms – Bavaria in 1807, Denmark in 1810 – attempted to introduce mandatory vaccination); the French response, however, contributed to a particularly tenacious pattern of resistance to the principle of obligation.

The defensive anti-epidemic legislation of 1822, in contrast, was thoroughly compulsory in spirit.[53] It gave the monarchy virtually dictatorial powers in times of epidemic emergency and effectively suspended the rights of citizens under the Charter of 1814. Physicians and officials were required to report epidemic diseases; quarantines and cordons sanitaires would protect France's ports and borders from the invasion of foreign scourges; and those who violated the regulations would be subject to drastic penalties, including fines as high as 20,000 francs, long terms at hard labour and even death. (The law's severity had the unintended effect of making the authorities reluctant to invoke it, and in part for this reason the number of cases prosecuted under it remained quite small throughout the century – a dozen in the cholera year of 1832, for example, and only 14 in 1903, following a major revamping of public health institutions, though in some years the numbers rose to several times that level.)[54] The powers assumed by the government recall those of the captains of health appointed in early modern cities to defend against plague; the whole scheme was a rationalized version of the monarchy's response to the outbreak of plague in 1720. The spirit of the legislation, it has been suggested, bespeaks the Old Regime paternalism and authoritarianism of the restored Bourbon monarchy – though it should be recalled that the procedures envisaged in the 1822 legislation were in every sense emergency measures, comparable to wartime restrictions on the activities of civilian populations. The steps taken by the central government in this period to reduce 'normal' morbidity and mortality were few and faltering.

Slow Maturation: 1830–70

The middle decades of the nineteenth century saw the full efflorescence of the hygiene movement. Parent-Duchâtelet and Villermé set the standard for careful empirical investigations and statistical analysis, the former in his work on sewers and prostitution, among many other subjects, the latter in his studies of cholera (which revealed striking divergences in the mortality rate for different classes) and above all in his report on the health of workers in the textile industry, whose afflictions he blamed more on living conditions and faulty regimen than on the factory itself.[55] The July Monarchy (1830–48) brought no major institutional innovations at the national level. The Academy of Medicine remained the chief advisory body, seconded by the Academy of Sciences and the Academy of Moral and Political Sciences, which the minister Guizot revived in 1832 (Napoleon had suppressed the corresponding section of the French Institute as a potential source of dissidence); this new assembly counted Villermé among its members and sponsored his study of textile workers. The liveliest institutions were the departmental and municipal health councils, whose number steadily increased.

The continued importance of local institutions was evident in 1832, when the first European cholera epidemic reached France. As the disease advanced across Europe in 1831, the government had sent commissions to investigate and had mounted a national defence of French ports and frontiers under the direction of the High Council of Health. Once the epidemic appeared on French soil, however, local and often *ad hoc* councils and commissions coordinated the response; Paris established a particularly elaborate hierarchy of special commissions and a network of medical stations to provide first aid to cholera victims in each neighbourhood.[56] The local agencies sought to dispatch victims to hospitals, thereby isolating them, but also called for cleaning up possible sources of infection; it has been argued that the Paris Health Council, rather than the Intendancy of Health at Marseilles, provided the model,[57] although in practice few sanitary improvements were actually made.

Reorganization of public health institutions had to await the Revolution of 1848, which, like the great revolution of 1789, occasioned a re-examination of existing institutions and practices, though much more briefly and on a far more limited scale. The Second Republic abolished the High Council of Health and replaced it with a Consultative Committee on Public Hygiene (CCHP), under the Ministry of Commerce and Agriculture (which, as the government department most directly concerned with the economic life of the nation, retained jurisdiction over key aspects of sanitary police); it continued to function, albeit with many modifications, into the next century. The CCHP was to supervise a network of advisory councils of public hygiene and health at the level of the *département* and arrondissement; the 65 existing councils, including the one in Paris, were incorporated into this system. The councils later took over responsibility for coordinating the work of epidemic doctors (1851) and inspecting pharmacies (1859). But the network was slow to develop, particularly at the arrondissement level. By 1861, only about a quarter of the *départements* had active councils; two decades later the proportion was closer to three-quarters.[58] The Second Republic also reorganized the system of sanitary protection of the frontiers and placed it under even tighter state control, eliminating the last vestiges of autonomy of the Marseilles Intendancy of Health. In 1850, when the Intendancy refused to accept limits on quarantines, the goverment, swayed by the anti-contagionist sentiments of the day, suppressed it and dispatched the physician François Mélier (1798– 1866) to Marseilles with the title of commissioner extraordinary. In 1853 Mélier was appointed the first French inspector general of sanitary services, with primary responsibility for shipping, lazarettos and quarantine ports. Maritime sanitation was henceforth a state service staffed by medical professionals, putting an end to the Old Regime tradition of lay municipal control.

Other new elements in the public health administration included corps of inspectors to implement regulations governing foundlings (1839), housing (1850) and other matters. But it would still be premature to speak of a public health profession and national bureaucracy. Many key appointees (such as housing inspectors) answered only to municipal authorities; and it is a measure of the weakness of the public health establishment that the institutions required by law, such as the health councils, served only as advisory bodies, whereas those institutions that did have powers of enforcement at the local level (such as a health inspectorate) remained optional.[59] In the first decade of the enabling legislation on housing, less than two per cent of *communes* (municipalities) chose to create an inspectorate. Britain established what was arguably a more effective bureaucracy under the General Board of Health (1848–58) and then the medical department of the Privy Council (to 1871), as well as a more specialized body of public health officials (medical officers of health), who founded a professional organization in London in 1856 and at the national level in 1873.

The fortunes of France's public health institutions reflect the larger transformation of French political life. It is a commonplace that the July Monarchy's sympathies for the capitalist bourgeoisie discouraged restraints on economic activity, but it is important not to exaggerate the contrast between a paternalist Restoration and a liberal July Monarchy, or the radicalism of French conceptions of political economy. Many industrialists themselves were more sympathetic to a Christian conception of a moral economy than to the hard version of utilitarianism represented by the new English poor law, and they displayed a certain paternalism in the treatment of their own workers.[60] Nor should we overstate the commitment of the hygienists to political economy. They recognized and deplored widespread poverty among the industrial working class (in this respect they were closer to Sismondi than to Adam Smith); and even though most advocated only limited government intervention, urging voluntary efforts and moral improvement among workers, they agreed that their condition demanded reform. Villermé, though a convinced liberal, made a significant exception to the principle of non-intervention: the state should protect children, since they could not be expected to help themselves.

Liberalism, moreover, faced challenges both from the Right and from the Left that carried implications for public health policy. Many on the Right, particularly among Legitimists who never accepted the Orléans dynasty of Louis-Philippe on the French throne, adopted a social Christian perspective that attributed to the government and élites the moral duty to succor the unfortunate, including those they saw as the victims of rapacious capitalism. Their outlook was typified by Alban de Villeneuve-Bargemont (1784–1850), author of a treatise on 'Christian political economy' (1834), who, as a prefect under the Restoration, had created the first departmental health council.[61] (Under the Second Empire, however, the generation of social Catholics represented by Frédéric Le Play [1806–82] embraced a different sort of paternalist social ethic, calling for the moral regeneration of the lower orders but without a substantial role for the government.) On the Left, radical republicans and socialists criticized the existing political and social order even more sharply; France in the 1830s and 1840s was the seedbed of modern socialism, and its exponents dilated on the theme that bad health resulted from social evils. Eugène Buret's study of the working classes in France and England, published in the same year as Villermé's report on the textile workers, offered a savage indictment of raw capitalism and called for state intervention.[62] The Saint-Simonians shared their founding father's longing for a new industrial order based on brotherhood and added an even more radical critique of economic individualism. They found a following among physicians, who agitated for sanitary reforms and volunteered their services at the public medical stations during cholera epidemics. Another strand of radical populist thought, represented by the chemist Raspail (1794–1878), indicted the medical profession itself and promoted a democratic vision of the people's health based on universal self-help.[63] All these figures remained outside or at most on the margins of the public health movement, but they briefly assumed much greater prominence in the first months following the February revolution of 1848, when hopes briefly flourished for a truly 'democratic and social' republic. The radical physicians Philippe Buchez and Ulysse Trélat were elected president and vice-president, respectively, of the Constituent Assembly; physicians made up four per cent of the membership, and many were sympathetic to the notion that the universal suffrage introduced by the revolution had as its natural counterpart a thoroughly democratic programme of 'social medicine' – a term first given currency in that year by the orthopaedist Jules Guérin (1801–86), editor of the *Gazette médicale de Paris*. In the heady days of that Paris spring, a group of progressive medical journalists, including Guérin, organized a junto to promote the 'brotherhood of physicians'; he used this platform to demand the creation of a Ministry of Progress or Public Health.

The public health project of 1848 failed even more rapidly than its counterpart of 1789, as power passed into the hands of men unsympathetic to socialism, democracy and even republicanism, though the reemergence of Catholic conservatives, who had suffered an eclipse under Louis-Philippe, opened the way to a small number of reforms. Bonaparte systematically repressed the Left after the coup of 1851. The future emperor, however, was a contradictory figure, who followed his uncle in basing an authoritarian regime on universal suffrage and, at the end of his reign, accepted a significant liberalization of the Empire; his economic policies encompassed both *laissez-faire* and state intervention. The treaty signed by France and England in 1860 marked the high point of free trade in the nineteenth century, and the regime substantially liberalized the regulations governing business enterprises; but Napoleon III saw himself as the protector of the poor (as a young man he had published a work on ending poverty), and he leaned toward a Saint-Simonian view of a partnership between state and industry. The consistent underlying strategy sought to promote economic and technological modernization, using competitive pressures where necessary. Helped by favourable economic circumstances (his reign coincided in part with a European boom),

Napoleon encouraged new programmes of assistance and undertook major public works projects; although public health was not among his government's primary commitments, the hygienists found the regime more congenial to their enterprise than any they had previously encountered.

The development of French medical thinking very roughly paralleled the fortunes of liberal political economy, though it would be misleading to suggest a direct causal relationship. The appearance of cholera in 1832 offered a new field for aetiological debates. A special commission appointed to investigate its effects, whose members included Villermé and Parent-Duchâtelet, attributed the disease to infection rather than contagion, although it heavily emphasized the social factors that made some elements of the population far more susceptible than others. The Academy of Medicine in 1846 declared plague non-contagious. The use of quarantines, which had proved particularly ineffective against cholera, was substantially curtailed in the late 1830s and 1840s. The sanitary code adopted in 1853 attenuated some of the repressive features of the 1822 law, though it was still much more restrictive than the British quarantine law of 1825, which left decisions in the hands of local authorities; it took no clear position on the question of contagion but empowered the inspector general of sanitary services to impose quarantines at his own discretion.

French medicine was slow to acknowledge the accumulating evidence of the transmissibility of specific diseases (Bretonneau on diphtheria, Semmelweis on puerperal fever, Snow on cholera, Budd on typhoid fever), which preceded the bacteriological discoveries of a later generation; once persuaded, medical authorities hesitated to pronounce diseases contagious for fear of alarming the public. But the implications had begun to sink in by the late 1850s, and by the time of the 1869 cholera epidemic, the public health community generally accepted that the disease spread through its victims' excreta. In the case of yellow fever, Mélier's own epidemiological work on the Saint-Nazaire outbreak of 1861 clearly established that it was an imported disease, though its exact cause remained unidentified. Mélier, however, remained sympathetic to the requirements of commerce, and the result was a compromise: a more rigorous programme of quarantine, but only where a threat clearly existed, and then only as long as absolutely necessary (yellow fever has a short incubation period).[64]

The question of the transmissibility of specific diseases should not obscure the larger debate on the sources of health and illness with which it was connected. The strictly environmentalist view of hygiene represented in England by Chadwick demanded sanitary intervention to remove sources of infection. The French from the outset placed as much or more emphasis on social factors – poverty and individual behaviour – that increased the individual's susceptibility to disease; some of Villermé's studies suggested that living surrounded by filth would not necessarily make one sick. The French also paid increasing attention to hereditary transmission of morbid tendencies, particularly the 'degeneration' induced by alcohol abuse and other vices, even before Morel's widely influential treatise of 1857.[65] This last approach attributed much illness to individual behaviour, which the family and local community were in the best position to influence.

Neither politics nor medical theory, then, supported a major transformation of the state's role in public health in the middle decades of the nineteenth century; the cautious innovations of this period tended to avoid compulsory measures dictated from the centre and relied instead on local agencies for implementation and enforcement. Welfare policy provides one illustration. Although a failed project in 1848 sought to organize the sort of national system of assistance envisaged by the revolutionaries of 1789, public relief continued to depend chiefly on the network of local welfare bureaus and hospitals, the latter only slowly assuming a more specialized medical role. (One key national measure, the legislation of 1838 governing the confinement of the mentally ill, had already separated and medicalized an important function of the old hospital by requiring each *département* to establish a special insane asylum headed by a doctor; funding, however, depended on the goodwill of the general council of each *département*.) In a gesture toward voluntarism, the revolutionaries of 1848 also freed mutual aid societies from criminal prohibitions; although the government subjected them to restrictions again in 1850 and 1852, Napoleon III strongly promoted (and in some cases subsidized) friendly societies and insurance programmes.

Medical assistance presents a similar picture. In 1854 and 1855 the government encouraged (but did not require) the *départements* to create programmes of free medical care for the rural poor.[66] Some had previously operated rural dispensaries or adopted the model of the cantonal physician. The idea of the medical functionary, however, remained controversial among physicians, who feared government controls and argued that the poor should be able to choose their own doctors. The great medical congress that met in Paris in 1845 rejected the idea,[67] as did the legislators of the Second Republic. Left to their own devices under the Second Empire, the *départements* set up a variety of programmes, generally somewhere between the cantonal physician system, in which a single salaried practitioner provided whatever services were needed to indigents on an official list, and, at the other extreme, the system adopted in the *département* of the Landes in 1856, in which indigent patients enrolled in the programme could consult the physician of their choice, who would be reimbursed on a fee-for-service basis. (In practice, by the 1880s, doctors were appointed to participate in the Landais plan, and not all *communes* paid them for each visit.) At the high point of this regime in 1868, 800,000 indigents living in 15,000 *communes* were enrolled in the medical assistance programmes of 52 *départements*. Urban residents, however, were still generally better provided for through dispensaries, physicians attached to welfare bureaus, and municipal medical services in some of the largest cities. Baron Haussmann (1809–91), as prefect of the Seine, established a system in 1853 that provided complete medical care for Paris's needy,[68] and Lyons adopted a similar programme in 1856. The post of municipal ward physician (*médecin de quartier*) brought a worker's salary and little prestige (hospital staff despised these neighbourhood drudges), but it represented a further step towards the creation of a public health service. The *médecins de quartier* were more closely linked to the municipal administration than the physicians attached to the welfare bureaus and typically performed functions beyond medical service to the poor (in Paris, for example, they sat on the housing inspection commissions). A similar trend could be seen in the provinces, where practitioners with titles such as physician of the poor, public assistance physician, and sanitary service physician combined medical assistance to the indigent with vaccination, forensic services and other public health functions.

Two major regulatory measures affecting health stand out in this period, one from the July Monarchy and the other from the Second Republic. Villermé's report of 1840 on textile workers helped inspire legislation the following year on child labour. This was neither the first such measure in Europe (legislation had appeared earlier in England, Prussia, Austria and the Italian peninsula) nor the most effective. The law, which applied to factories employing 20 or more workers, banned the employment of children younger than eight and limited the hours that children might work; but it imposed only modest penalties (light fines), and the inspectors appointed to enforce it were unpaid and mostly drawn from the manufacturing class. Even in this weakened form the measure drew strong opposition from legislators anxious to protect property rights; its passage marked the first significant state intervention on a social question.[69] Similar difficulties of enforcement limited the impact of the Melun housing law of 1850, named for its legislative sponsor in the National Assembly, Anatole de Melun, and inspired in large part by the reformist efforts of his brother Armand (1807–77), a prominent social Catholic.[70] This measure, which applied only to rented dwellings, empowered *communes* to appoint inspection commissions to investigate unhealthful lodgings; where appropriate, they could compel the landlord to take corrective action. Few municipal authorities followed through, and those that did faced unsympathetic courts, highly solicitous of property owners' rights (they refused, for example, to let the authorities force a proprietor to take specific steps to correct an unsanitary condition). But this was a symbolic foot in the door: the first legislation allowing government inspectors to violate the sanctity of a private dwelling.

The middle decades of the nineteenth century produced even less national legislation directed specifically towards fighting infectious disease; the experience of cholera provoked only short-term responses. In the continuing campaign to improve public sanitation and clean up public spaces, Paris led the way, thanks in large part to two activist prefects of the Seine, Rambuteau, under the July Monarchy, and his more celebrated successor, Baron Haussmann, under the Second Empire. The city became a less noisome place with the establishment of a municipal knacker's yard on the outskirts at Aubervilliers in 1839, and the closing in 1841 of the Montfaucon dump, which was located in the centre of the city and collected solid human waste, among other refuse. Thanks to Haussmann and the work of the engineer Eugène Belgrand (1810–78), champion of *le tout-à-l'égout* (a system that drained sewage, rain, and all forms of waste water into a common conduit), Paris received a greatly increased supply of clean water and a greatly expanded sewer system, although the water was not yet very widely distributed: half the capital's houses still did not have running water in 1870, and a large number of those that did had a supply on the ground floor only.[71] By the end of the century, though, when the city celebrated its modernity in a world's fair, it boasted a water supply of 249 litres per capita per day and a sewer system extending 1,113 kilometres, or 1 kilometre for every 2,240 inhabitants.[72] Sanitary reforms in Paris and some provincial cities stimulated hopes for improvements in personal hygiene, but national legislation of 1851 intended to encourage model public baths and wash-houses yielded only modest results.[73] The middle decades of the nineteenth-century, then, saw some local achievements, but little substantive progress toward the creation of a coherent national public health system.

The Critical Years: 1870–1914

In France as elsewhere, the late nineteenth and early twentieth centuries marked an epoch in the development of public health. The conjunction of a new public hygiene based on bacteriology with new conceptions of social welfare that challenged the *laissez-faire* assumptions of an earlier era was an international phenomenon. But the French experience was a distinctive one, in part because of the extraordinary prestige of Pasteur, in part because of the exceptional character of French politics. France in 1870 received its third republican regime in the space of less than a century and long remained the only republic among the major states of Europe. Promoting the people's health formed an integral part of republican ideology, even if France's parliamentary institutions proved singularly ineffective in putting that programme into practice. Liberal traditions and respect for property rights remained strong but yielded some ground to the claims of the collectivity, as voiced not by the growing ranks of the socialists but by moderate and progressive republicans who hoped to preserve social harmony by following a middle path between *laissez-faire* and socialism. Their success was unprecedented in the French context, but much less impressive when France was compared with several neighbours, particularly the new German Reich. Leaders of the French public health movement liked to argue, indeed, that France lagged farther behind than ever, and they referred repeatedly to English and German accomplishments.[74]

The French public health movement was reborn in the late nineteenth century. As in the early part of the century, it brought together an alliance of the medical élite (most prominently Paul Brouardel [1837–1906], dean of the Paris medical faculty), scientists (above all Pasteur), politicians (such as Léon Bourgeois [1851–1925] and Paul Strauss), and career administrators (notably Henri Monod [1843–1911]); but for the implementation of its programmes it depended on the participation of an expanding body of lower-level medical personnel dedicated primarily to work in the public sector. It should be stressed once more that this was not a full-fledged national public health service; apart from the maritime sanitation corps, which was staffed by state functionaries, the public health 'bureaucracy' consisted of a congeries of departmental and local health council members, epidemic doctors, participants in medical assistance programmes, inspectors enforcing the housing law of 1850, and the rest. Many physicians, however, combined several of these roles, functioning in effect as medical officers of health, and one can see several other early indications, starting in the 1870s, of the development of public health as a distinct profession. The year 1877 saw the creation of the first national organizations concerned with public health, the Société Française d'Hygiène and the Société de Médecine Publique et d'Hygiène Professionnelle. (The latter, however, contrary to what its name might suggest, was more a learned society than a professional organization; its 120 members, in addition to hygienists, included scientists, engineers and architects – Viollet-le-Duc, among others.) Three new specialized journals joined the *Annales d'hygiène*, the *Journal d'hygiène* (1875), the *Bulletin de la Société de Médecine Publique* (1877) and the *Revue d'hygiène et de police sanitaire* (1879). In addition, a new auxiliary occupation, the public health nurse, emerged at the turn of the century, as part of a more general transformation of the nursing field; the nurses' role was to conduct home visits, principally as part of the anti-tuberculosis campaign. The late 1800s saw the beginnings of the laicization of the hospital staffs (though this process was slow and very limited outside Paris) and the development of educational programmes for nurses in private schools and public hospitals.[75] The moving force behind the training of the *infirmières visiteuses* was Léonie Chaptal (1873–1937), great-niece of Napoleon's Minister of the Interior, the medically trained chemist Jean Chaptal. Faced with a shortage of adequately prepared personnel for the tuberculosis clinic that she ran in a working-class district of Paris, she opened a nursing school there in 1905 and actively promoted the use of the visiting nurse in the anti-tuberculosis campaign, in close collaboration with the sanitary service for Paris housing established in 1893 by the prefect of the Seine. By 1914, the public health nurses had become numerous enough to found their own national professional association.

In addition, starting in the 1870s, a series of voluntary associations and pressure groups were formed, some primarily professional, some mainly lay, some mixed, to fight smoking, alcoholism, tuberculosis, syphilis and prostitution; to protect the welfare and interests of children, pregnant women and the disabled; and to promote breastfeeding, 'puericulture', physical education and 'regeneration' of the population. (Puericulture, championed by Adolphe Pinard [1844–1934], professor of obstetrics at the Paris medical faculty, called for using scientific pre- and postnatal care to raise healthy children.)[76] Widening participation in such movements reflected the dissemination of the hygienists' themes in the general culture. To a far larger extent than its early nineteenth-century predecessor, the public health movement of the late nineteenth and early twentieth centuries relied on popular publicity to spread its message;[77] in the primary schools, which the Third Republic made free and compulsory, hygiene received some attention in classes on morality and civics, and it was added as a curricular subject in its own right at the beginning of the new century.

The eugenics movement also found its first French exponents, though not yet a large following. A eugenics society, which counted a majority of physicians among the founding members, appeared on the eve of the First World War, with Léon Bourgeois as its honorary president. Its president was Edmond Perrier (1844–1921), director of the Museum of Natural History and a specialist on invertebrate zoology, but also a writer on human evolution; other active participants included Pinard and Charles Richet, professor of physiology at the Paris faculty, whose catholic interests ranged from parapsychology to pacifism and evolution (he published a volume on 'human selection').[78] The French eugenists' generally positive approach, informed by a Lamarckian faith that improving the health of the current generation would benefit its posterity (as opposed to a negative eugenics that emphasized preventing the unfit from reproducing) resonated in public health circles and particularly influenced the social hygiene movement. The term 'social hygiene' could be used very loosely in the broad sense of preventive medicine applied to the population as a whole (it was not, as a rule, so narrowly associated with venereal disease as in English-speaking countries). But self-conscious social hygienists, who formed an Alliance of Social Hygiene and held a national congress in 1904, though in many respects a disparate lot, tended as a group to approach alcoholism, tuberculosis, venereal disease and other public health problems as symptoms of 'degeneration' and national decline; their expansive vision of science, which they believed would not just reduce morbidity and mortality but actively improve and 'perfect' the species, carried them outside the mainstream of public health.

The public health leadership, although sometimes echoing the pronouncements of earlier generations on hygiene as a social and political science,[79] focused on specific areas where medical treatment and prophylaxis could reduce morbidity and mortality; the old hygiene movement, which would have continued its campaigns with or without the development of microbiology, was nonetheless profoundly transformed by Pasteurianism, whose adherents dominated the Society for Public Medicine. To implement its programme, the public health lobby demanded a ministry of health, new coercive legislation (on vaccination, for example), and new institutions, such as tuberculosis sanatoriums. They looked with a mixture of envy and alarm across the Rhine to Germany, which by the end of the 1880s had a national public health office, national social insurance, and a series of public health measures based on the twin principles of state intervention and obligatory compliance. To their fellow citizens, demoralized by the Germans' easy victory in the Franco-Prussian war of 1870–1 and the subequent creation of a unified German Empire, and disturbed by the great disparity between the rates of population growth in the two countries, the reformers preached the importance of public health programmes for national security.

The headway that the public health movement made at the end of the nineteenth century was due in part to the creation of a new central health bureaucracy, which it helped inspire; here it was able to exercise an influence comparable to that of the hygienists on the Paris Health Council, but on a national scale.[80] France still had no ministry of health, but in the second half of the 1880s the government consolidated the bulk of the services connected with assistance and public health in the Ministry of the Interior; only unhealthful workshops and factories (the province of Commerce and Industry) and epizootics (Agriculture) lay outside its purview. In 1886 a Bureau of Public Health and Hygiene, which Monod was to head for two decades, was created in the ministry; it actively promoted expanding government intervention. In 1888, Bourgeois, a convinced Pasteurian, assumed the Interior portfolio, and a presidential decree established a High Council for Public Assistance (CSAP), under the ministry's jurisdiction, to make policy recommendations. In addition, the CCHP, headed by Brouardel since 1884, was moved from Commerce and Industry to the Ministry of the Interior.

This administrative reorganization reflected pressures within parliament to reform the administration of public health, but also the lack of a clear consensus on the model to adopt. In 1886, a group of physician legislators, joined by two prominent non-physician supporters of the cause of public health – the retired industrialist Jules Siegfried (1837–1922) and Charles Chamberland (1851–1908), the bacteriologist and collaborator of Pasteur – sponsored a bill to establish a ministry of health, a body of public health officials and a National Health Council to replace the CCHP. The following year, a government bill originating in the Ministry of Commerce and Industry, advised by the CCHP, naturally called for retaining the CCHP; it made no provision for an inspectorate or other major innovations, proposing instead to encourage better use of existing laws and institutions. The same committee of the Chamber of Deputies considered both bills; its reporter, Chamberland, dwelt on the gravity of France's public health problems and the need to reinforce the government's powers to correct them. As an alternative to an independent ministry of health, he put forward a compromise: a central health service within the Ministry of the Interior, advised by a higher council of public health, that would oversee a network of inspectors at the departmental level, charged, in turn, with guiding the activities of the local health councils.

Although no legislation resulted, and Chamberland's report was not even discussed in the Chamber, the government's decision to fashion a public health apparatus within the Ministry of the Interior represented a modest accommodation of the demand for reform. The transfer of the CCHP confirmed the growing influence of Pasteurian public health and symbolized a renewed emphasis on demography, health care and disease prevention (long among the concerns of the Minister of the Interior) as against the economic interests represented at Commerce and Industry. Monod now took the title of Director of Assistance and Public Health; he and Brouardel together constituted the nucleus of an activist public health lobby within the government. The CCHP remained only an advisory body, but it tirelessly promoted institutional reform (including the creation of a national public health service under a special ministry), new national legislation on public health, and Pasteurian ideas (Pasteur himself served as a member from 1881 until his death in 1895). It called for making disinfection services and supplies of pure water generally available; rejecting liberal objections, it favoured compulsory vaccination and mandatory reporting of contagious diseases and the cause of deaths.

Although the government subsequently established a few other mechanisms to address specific public health problems, such as an extra-parliamentary committee on tuberculosis, the services within the Ministry of the Interior remained the primary engine of reform at the national level. France lacked a public health system comparable to the one established in England under the Local Government Board by the Public Health Act of 1875. Monod, indeed, liked to call attention to the disparity between the English service, with its large central administration and network of health officers, and his own tiny staff.

At the regional and local level, the basic structure established in 1848 remained in place to the end of the century; by 1882 about three-quarters of the *départements* had active health councils, their role still largely confined to advising the prefect. Legislation of 1871 (on the departmental general councils) and 1884 (on municipal councils) clarified the powers of the *département* and *commune* in public health – and confirmed that jurisdiction was essentially regional and local – but did not require them to vote funds or mandate action by the authorities, although the prefect could intervene at the local level when a municipality had failed to act. Starting in 1888, a corps of regional inspectors of hygiene services, composed of professors from the medical faculties, supervised operations in the provinces. In the last two decades of the century, some 20 large cities organized municipal hygiene bureaus, with laboratories, disinfection services and the like. To this list one could add the Pasteur Institute in Paris (1888), private but 'recognized as publicly useful' (in the classic French formula), and its provincial offshoots in Le Havre, Lille, Nancy, Lyons, Grenoble, Marseilles, Montpellier and Bordeaux. These institutes and laboratories carried out research but also contributed directly to fighting infectious diseases, a practice that at times aroused opposition from local physicians, who feared unfair competition. Under Albert Calmette (1863–1933), the Pasteur Institute of Lille produced smallpox and rabies vaccine, analysed water samples, set up a model purification plant for treating industrial waste water, promoted industrial hygiene and occupational health (it diagnosed a parasitical infestation producing anaemia among miners, for example), and maintained a tuberculosis dispensary, among other projects, in addition to pursuing research on the causes and treatment of tuberculosis. Across the Mediterranean, at the Pasteur Institute of Tunis, Charles Nicolle (1866–1936) identified lice as the vectors of typhus.

Despite its institutional gains, the public health movement experienced repeated frustrations in its efforts to write its programmes into law. The political system of the Third Republic was both inherently inefficient and subject to multiple pressures from competing interest groups that often slowed or paralysed reform. The instability of governments and lack of continuity in legislative committees made it difficult to sustain the momentum of a legislative proposal, as did the cumbersome procedure for dealing with differences between the Chamber of Deputies (where most reform bills originated) and the much more conservative Senate. It helped to some extent that doctors made up more than 10 per cent of legislators and over 40 per cent of the Chamber's committee on public hygiene, which became a standing committee in 1898.[81] Outside parliament, the medical profession was far better organized than earlier in the century and constituted an increasingly effective pressure group. Not all medical men, though, were sympathetic to the programmes of the CCHP.

The General Association of French Physicians (1858), essentially a federation of mutual aid organizations, found itself displaced in the 1880s as a representative of professional interests by more militant *syndicats* (unions), closely identified with ordinary private practitioners, who feared increased state intervention and distrusted the medical élites who dominated the public health movement.[82]

The reform programme benefited, however, from larger transformations within French political culture. In France, as elsewhere, the late nineteenth century saw the waning of *laissez-faire* and growing support for government regulation and what might broadly be called protectionism (of which the Méline Tariff of 1892 is the best-known example). In social policy, the political majority proved increasingly receptive to welfare measures once favoured primarily by the Left and elements of the Catholic Right. For the first time since the Revolution of 1789, the notion that the state had a duty to solve social problems and, in particular, to provide for the least fortunate, gained wide acceptance: here was born, or reborn the idea of the welfare state (*l'État-Providence*, as its detractors called it).[83] The success of these principles owed something to nationalist fears of the consequences of demographic stagnation for French power and influence, and something, too, to the emergence of the political programme known as solidarism, whose most prominent spokesman was Léon Bourgeois. Solidarism had its strongest base in the Radical Party but drew adherents from across the spectrum of republican ideology; it sought to balance the rights emphasized by classical liberalism with obligations, and the claims of the individual with the claims of society. Individual rights did not include the right to put the health and lives of others at risk; social obligations included guaranteeing the bare necessities of life to all. This was neither socialism (respect for private property remained a central value), nor paternalist Christian corporatism, since the agency of assistance would be democratically elected governments; indeed, solidarism can be seen as a conscious attempt to arrive at an alternative to those programmes, which would help ease the adjustment of workers and peasants to modern society.

This endeavour met with predictable resistance from traditional liberals who distrusted state intervention, as well as from property owners and representatives of other private interests, who consistently rejected any expansion of government regulation of economic life.[84] One particularly difficult sticking point was the French tax structure, which relied heavily on indirect levies; they included a lucrative excise on alcohol, which created a serious conflict of interest for the government when it addressed alcoholism as a public health problem. The most promising potential source of revenue to pay for new welfare and health programmes was an income tax, which had been successfully used in Prussia and enjoyed strong support from the Left, but until the First World War, a majority successfully resisted it as an unacceptable intrusion into private affairs. Where medical personnel were involved, the physicians' *syndicats* fought hard to protect the 'liberal' model of medical practice, in which the relationship between patient and doctor was a freely chosen direct contract, and the physician retained complete autonomy in prescribing treatments. Most physicians also resisted obligatory reporting of contagious diseases and cause of death as a violation of the confidentiality of the doctor–patient relationship *(le secret professionnel).*

The solidarists, however, drew strength from Pasteur's triumphs in the 1880s. Apart from its sheer publicity value, Pasteurianism transformed the public health movement and the practice of public hygiene in ways that tended to disarm their adversaries.[85] Stopping the spread of microbes demanded certain costly projects, such as the public works needed to ensure pure water supplies and the safe removal of human wastes, but the traditional programmes of quarantine and massive clean-ups, which interfered with commerce and property rights, would be superseded by more focused measures of isolation, disinfection, and extermination of parasites and vermin (as animal vectors were discovered). The shift in approach was apparent, for example, in the measures adopted to counter the cholera outbreak of 1892, which entailed quarantining individual patients, decontaminating their immediate surroundings, and having the general population drink boiled or bottled water; in contrast, the programme adopted to combat the epidemic of 1884 had emphasized a general cleaning of public and private spaces and the elimination of suspected sources of infection (by closing certain food markets, for example). The new procedures were formalized in a decree of 1896, the seventh and last of a series implementing the legislation of 1822 on the sanitary protection of France's frontiers.

The changed political and medical context made possible a series of new enactments at the national level, mainly in the 1890s and the first half-decade of the new century. One law greatly expanded medical assistance, adumbrating the transition from older conceptions of subsidized health care as an aspect of poor relief to the principles of national insurance and general entitlement; another established France's first true national health code, which, although it still assigned responsibility for implementation chiefly to institutions at the departmental and local level, imposed an unprecedented set of uniform standards; and various other measures extended government regulation of economic activities that affected health.

The new programme of medical assistance markedly expanded support for treatment outside the hospital setting, typically in the patient's home. Even in the late 1880s, around the time of the creation of the High Council for Public Assistance, both general welfare programmes and programmes of medical assistance remained highly decentralized and barely functioned in many *départements*. One or more welfare bureaus, some with physicians attached to their staff, existed in 42 per cent of French *communes*, comprising 68 per cent of the population; the state provided less than 5 per cent of the total welfare budget, mainly for foundlings and mental patients. The network of medical services set up under the Second Empire was actually declining. In 1874 it continued to function in 44 *départements*, while 42 others did without; by 1887 the number of programmes had fallen to 38. The majority of *départements* relied on some version of the district physician; only a minority offered patients any choice or compensated the physician for each visit. Recognizing that France lagged behind other industrialized nations in the provision of medical services to the indigent, legislators sympathetic to the public health movement offered reform proposals starting in the early years of the Third Republic; it took until 1893, however, for an act to win passage. This bill was the first major project of the High Council for Public Assistance; the decision to focus on health care rather than housing or other needs reflects the Council's links to medicine and the emerging public health establishment.

The medical assistance act of 1893, which was first implemented in 1895 and remained in force until 1953, when the social security system completely displaced it, made medical assistance to the indigent an obligation for the *commune*, *département* and state. The scheme as a whole was highly decentralized. Each departmental general council voted a budget, which might be supplemented by state subsidies; in practice, the state had to augment its contribution substantially as the cost of the programme expanded far beyond initial expectations. *Communes* with existing programmes could opt out of the system; the legislators, who saw the bill as a device to bring modern medicine to the countryside and perhaps help slow the troubling 'rural exodus', had large urban centres in mind, but many rural *communes* applied for the exemption, reducing their own costs but also forfeiting outside funding. Home care would be preferred over hospitalization, but otherwise the precise design of the programmes was left to the *départements*; under heavy pressure from the medical *syndicats*, most opted for the Landais model, in which patients freely chose a doctor and the latter was reimbursed for services provided. The *syndicats* had strongly opposed both rural dispensaries and cantonal physicians, which they saw as a threat to private practice, although both reached more patients and cost less than the Landais system; the 1893 law, it has been argued, was as much a victory for private practitioners as for public health.[86] The law's proponents had estimated that 3–6 per cent of the population would be eligible for benefits; they failed to anticipate the extent to which the programme would stimulate demand. In 1895, 1.3 million citizens were enrolled, and 360,000 received treatment under the plan; by 1904, the number of participants had increased by about 50 per cent and the proportion claiming benefits by about 60 per cent. By 1914 expenditures had risen to 100 million francs.

The 1880s and 1890s also saw the growth of private insurance and the still more rapid expansion of mutual aid societies.[87] The membership of the societies doubled between 1870 and 1896 and more than doubled again by 1913, when over 20,000 societies enrolled 3.7 million members. From 1881 on, the state provided regular subsidies to supplement contributions from the *départements*, *communes* and participants. In early twentieth-century debates on providing medical coverage for the French population, many legislators were attracted to the model adopted in Belgium in 1899, which relied on state subventions to mutual aid societies, in contrast to the German model of compulsory insurance. Such programmes appealed to moderate republicans distressed by the limits of liberal medicine but reluctant to take away freedom of choice, although they had to recognize that the societies, which recruited heavily from the working-class élite and lower middle class, did not cover many workers too poor to join but not poor enough to qualify for government assistance. The medical profession remained wary, however, even though mutualism expanded the effective demand for professional services and offered the least favoured members of the profession, desperate for financial security, a useful alternative to the limited number of salaried posts available in the public sector. Since the societies typically signed contracts with physicians to provide services to their members for a fixed sum, the medical *syndicats* reacted to them with much the same distaste they showed for state programmes that did not conform to the liberal model of medical practice; some threatened to stage strikes and boycotts.

Both commercial insurance plans and mutualism benefited from a workmen's compensation law of 1898, which required proprietors of transportation companies, mines and factories using power machinery to pay for medical treatment for employees injured in work-related accidents, unless they belonged to a mutual aid society. The law applied to some 5 million workers; it was extended in 1899 to agricultural, and in 1906 to commercial, employees. These provisions represented the first attempt to provide general medical coverage to large groups of the population regardless of income. Medical *syndicats* and workers made common cause against employers who forced accident victims to be treated by a company doctor; the former established a professional pressure group, the National Union (*syndicat*) for Social Medicine, which, with labour support, won a law in 1905 that guaranteed free choice of physician and fee-for-service.

Another measure, adopted the same year, paid for home or hospital care for elderly invalids (70 years and older) and younger persons who were wholly incapacitated.[88] Thus by 1905, the year in which the long-standing struggles between Catholics and republican anti-clericals culminated in the formal separation of Church and State, the government had emerged as a serious rival to Catholic charities in providing for the health care needs of vulnerable social groups.

Just as medical assistance programmes had to accommodate the physicians, so most of the regulatory legislation adopted during the first decades of the Third Republic bore the marks of the perennial tension between economic interests and the concern for public health. The most prominent measure, a law of 1892 on medical practice, was also the most easily passed; by strengthening the existing provisions against illegal practice, it promoted the physicians' economic interests in the name of public health. This legislation, together with the law of 1893 on medical assistance, can be seen as a package in which physicians won a stronger professional monopoly and subsidies for private practice as the quid pro quo for expanding government health programmes.[89] Several other legislative measures extended special protection to children: the Roussel Law of 1874, which provided for national regulation to safeguard babies farmed out to paid wet nurses;[90] new legislation of the same year on child labour, which created the first inspectorate in this area; and a law of 1899 on 'morally abandoned' children, which empowered the authorities to declare the children of criminal, alcoholic and otherwise unfit parents wards of the state. Subsequent enactments regulated work by women and, on the eve of the First World War, provided for maternity leaves. In contrast, sponsors of new legislation on alcoholism and the trade in alcoholic beverages fought an uphill battle all the way.[91] A legislature dominated by liberal republicans deregulated the liquor business in 1880, leading to a rapid growth in bars and other outlets; a law of 1873 on alcoholism, passed by a more conservative and paternalist legislature before republicans consolidated their hold on the institutions of the Third Republic, applied only to gross public intoxication. After many skirmishes, in which physicians and solidarists joined forces in such organizations as the French Society Against the Abuse of Alcoholic Beverages, the temperance forces won a modest victory at the beginning of the First World War; they achieved a ban on the sale of absinthe, which was considered a particularly dangerous concoction – as opposed to wine, a patriotic beverage whose virtues even the physicians extolled (in 1900 wine, beer, cider, perry and mead had been officially classified as 'hygienic drinks', on which consumers paid lower taxes than on distilled alcohol). Yet the industry as a whole and the larger problem of alcoholism, a more serious threat to public health in France than anywhere else in Western Europe, remained untouched.

In the fight against infectious disease, the first three decades of the Third Republic brought only limited progress. Bacteriology had laid the foundations for a campaign against the most serious waterborne diseases, typhoid fever and cholera. A major outbreak of typhoid in 1882 led the Paris Municipal Council to press for connecting all outlets for waste water to the sewer system. The cholera epidemic of 1884 coincided with the adoption of the new municipal government legislation that enabled (but did not compel) mayors to force sanitary improvements. But reducing mortality from waterborne disease required major efforts, city by city, to improve water supplies and sewerage. The former was accomplished through a mixture of public and private enterprise (notably the General Water Company, founded in 1853), the latter by municipal governments; Paris adopted *le tout-à-l'égout* in 1894, but it became effective only around 1905, and it was not until the mid twentieth-century that pure water supplies and flush toilets connected to a sewer system became generally available to the French population.[92]

Still less progress was made against tuberculosis, a disease that by the end of the nineteenth-century claimed the lives of more French citizens than all other infectious diseases combined; France long had the worst mortality rates from tuberculosis in Western Europe. This dismal record cannot be attributed to lack of interest on the part of the public health leadership in the medical profession, administration and legislature. The Academy of Medicine expressed interest in sanatoriums on the American, German, and Swiss models; national congresses on tuberculosis met, starting in 1888, and reformers organized an anti-tuberculosis league. Pasteur's collaborator Jacques-Joseph Grancher (1843–1907) created a foundation in 1903 to help protect children at risk of infection; at the Pasteur Institute of Lille, Calmette and Camille Guérin (1872–1961) made important contributions to understanding the epidemiology of the disease and later developed the BCG vaccine (1921), which seemed at first to promise generalized immunity for the population. This was an affliction, moreover, that challenged all the liberal prejudices against compulsory measures, state financing and mandatory reporting of contagious diseases. Yet the obstacles remained, and positive action (building of sanatoriums, slum clearance) remained very limited.[93] The response to smallpox displayed similar vacillations through the end of the century. Despite the devastation wrought by the epidemic associated with the Franco-Prussian War and the manifest benefits conferred by obligatory vaccination in the Prussian army (and, after 1874, among the German civilian population), despite the strong endorsement of the Academy of Medicine (1881), the French continued for a generation to resist the principle of compulsion. The government did decide to vaccinate members of the armed forces (1876), to exclude unvaccinated children from public schools (1887), and to make vaccine available gratis to children in towns with 5,000 or more inhabitants; children were entitled to more protection, and soldiers to fewer rights, than other citizens.

The CCHP, since its inception, had urged adoption of a strong, coherent national health code, and a bill incorporating some of its desiderata passed the Chamber of Deputies in 1893, the same year as the law on medical assistance; it encountered serious opposition, however, in the Senate, the champion of property rights. A modified version finally received the approval of the upper chamber in 1901; the bill that passed into law the following year bore the marks of the Senate's efforts to guard against what some saw as the 'tyranny of hygiene'.[94] The public health law of 15 February, 1902, implemented one year later, incorporated a wide-ranging series of measures whose general thrust was to make the reduction of morbidity the permanent concern of French administrators; it did not replace (though it somewhat altered) the provisions for the sanitary protection of France's frontiers contained in the law of 1822, as modified by subsequent decrees. The new legislation made vaccination compulsory at the ages of 1, 11 and 21 required physicians and midwives to report certain contagious diseases to their mayor or sub-prefect (reinforcing a weaker clause in the medical practice law of 1892); and called on local authorities to deal with unhealthful sites and buildings. The 1850 legislation on unhealthful rented dwellings, now repealed, had been merely permissive; henceforth, administrators were required to intervene, and they receive expanded powers to discharge this responsibility. *Communes* were also to take action to stop epidemics and to make pure water supplies available. In any *commune* where mortality exceeded the French average for three consecutive years, the prefect would be obliged to investigate, and sanitary measures might be imposed at the expense of the *commune.* The law also provided for a major overhaul of the fragmentary public health bureaucracy dating from the Second Republic. Every *département* was required to have a health council, and every *commune* with 20,000 or more inhabitants (or as few as 2,000, if it possessed a hydropathic establishment) was to have a public health office; all *communes* were to adopt sanitary regulations. District commissions within each *département* would oversee the municipal health offices and, together with the departmental councils, would report annually to the CCHP on health conditions and sanitary activities. Whereas the legislation of 1848 had merely authorized health councils to offer advice to government officials on a series of questions related to public hygiene, such consultations were now mandatory. When a case of a reportable contagious disease was declared, the municipal health office, where one existed, or else an 'epidemics doctor', would insure the application of appropriate measures. To sweeten the pill, the law guaranteed proprietors full compensation for condemned property and provided that doors and windows created for reasons of health would not be taxed for five years (France's idiosyncratic tax code assessed apertures in buildings as external signs of wealth).

Resistance in the Senate and from the medical profession weakened several key provisions of the original bill. The public health bureaucracy would not be able to force sanitary improvements; only prefects and mayors would have coercive powers. Health council members would not be paid, and there would be no salaried inspectorate, though individual prefects might organize a service at the department level, using funds voted by the departmental general council; only three such agencies were created in 1903, and they were not made mandatory until 1935. Parliament, in other words, forwent the opportunity to create a national, professional public health service. It is revealing that the legislators chose to use the epidemic doctors, not so very different from their predecessors a century earlier, to respond to outbreaks of contagious disease.

As it was, many medical practitioners objected both to

mandatory reporting and to an article that authorized the CCHP to discuss questions relating to medical practice (even though the CCHP remained a consultative body without powers of initiative). On the former point, the defenders of professional confidentiality won a compromise in the form of a two-tiered list of reportable diseases, adopted in 1903 on the recommendation of the Academy of Medicine and the CCHP, which named 13 for which a declaration was required, but another nine (notably tuberculosis) for which it was merely suggested. The first group included typhoid fever, typhus, smallpox and varioloid, scarlet fever, measles, diphtheria, miliary fever, cholera and choleroid diseases, plague, yellow fever, dysentery, puerperal infections and neonatal ophthalmia (when the birth was not a secret), and epidemic cerebrospinal meningitis. The second class, in addition to tuberculosis, comprised whooping cough, influenza, pneumonia and bronchopneumonia, erysipelas, mumps, leprosy, tinea, and purulent conjunctivitis and granulomatous ophthalmia. There was a very rough medical logic at work here, since most of the common acute infections with high mortality rates were on the first list, but the deference shown *le secret professionnel* leaps from the page. Diseases associated with childbirth need not be reported when the mother wished to keep the birth concealed; tuberculosis, still widely considered shameful, was on the second list, even though it constituted the single greatest threat to public health; venereal diseases, which physicians hesitated to report even to the spouse of an infected patient, were omitted entirely (as, indeed, were all conditions believed to be hereditary and therefore ignominious, in the view of many). This was not, in short, the regulation that a social hygienist would have drawn up.

The limits of the new legislation are clear; but it is equally clear that it marked a watershed in the history of French public health.[95] It was the first true national health code, and it was conceived in a Pasteurian spirit; it established a national public health bureaucracy overseen by the CCHP (renamed the High Council of Public Hygiene and given increased powers in 1906); and it made obligatory several measures that had previously been voluntary or left to the discretion of local authorities (vaccination, disinfection). The momentum created in 1902 also led to additional legislation, notably a law of 1905 regulating the food industry; the new standards required food to be free of both toxic substances and harmful bacteriological contamination.

On the eve of the First World War, French public health was still characterized by the long-prevailing tension between *étatism* and centralization, on the one hand, and localism, voluntarism and the defence of individual rights on the other. Solidarism had found a way to tip the balance away from *laissez-faire;* new legislation introduced compulsory measures based on the contributions of bacteriology, as well as the beginnings of a system of social insurance distinguished from public assistance (though here the principle of compulsion was much less evident). In practice, however, resistance from property owners and from local authorities reluctant to commit funds remained strong. For partisans of public health, France lagged a generation behind several other Western European countries, particularly Britain and Germany. As scientists and theoreticians, French hygienists considered themselves the equal of any, but France's practical achievements fell far short of its contributions to the realm of ideas; certain health problems (alcoholism, tuberculosis) were more severe in France than elsewhere in Western Europe, and the government had done little to ameliorate them.

In earlier generations, many in France had sought a middle course between what they saw as the extremes of 'Anglo-Saxon' *laissez-faire* and Prussian statism; by the early twentieth century, this way of looking at the world seemed increasingly meaningless. Imperial Germany was in many ways more federal than the Third Republic; the *Länder* enjoyed considerable autonomy in public health matters, and the formal structure of the social insurance system was decentralized and corporatist. Britain developed a centralized public health bureaucracy significantly earlier than France and was in several areas likelier to use coercive measures (such as acquiring substandard housing through eminent domain for slum clearance); Lloyd George's act of 1911 on health and unemployment insurance was based on the compulsory German model.[96]

Had France itself become the extreme in the world of public health, a redoubt of liberty surrounded by more disciplined and less proudly individualist societies? In some respects this image would be misleading. France should not be compared to the isolated pockets of uncompromising *laissez-faire* found in some Swiss cantons or in Hamburg, where the government's reluctance to intervene led to disaster in the cholera epidemic of 1892.[97] Nor did France develop large and lively medical libertarian movements, such as the ones that fought compulsory vaccination in the United States, Britain and Switzerland (though the French did produce their own, more modest National League Against Obligatory Vaccination and participated in the international league, whose first meeting they hosted at Paris in 1880). Yet France unquestionably faced serious political constraints that hampered implementation of the resolutely statist programmes promoted by its public hygiene movement.

The record of the Third Republic in the field of public health would seem to exemplify Stanley Hoffmann's classic model of the stalemate society and republican synthesis that emerged in the last decades of the nineteenth century.[98] The post-revolutionary state was neither truly democratic nor truly authoritarian but non-interventionist – simultaneously centralized and limited, in a political culture that feared both revolutionary disorder and despotism. The relative stability finally achieved by the Third Republic, the fit between social structure and political institutions, depended on a consensus of interest groups maintained by shifting coalitions in the centre of the political spectrum; such an arrangement militated against the movement produced by a genuine alternation of Left and Right. Hygienists favouring drastic intervention ran up against a traditionally influential interest (property owners) and a newly influential one (the medical profession). They half succeeded in imposing their view that public health was a matter of life and death transcending normal politics, but they were compelled in the end to work within a political system in which they represented yet another interest group whose claims needed to be balanced against those of all the rest.

The Twentieth Century

Two decisive developments have shaped public health in contemporary France. The first it shares with the rest of the industrialized world: rightly or wrongly, attention has shifted from collective prophylactic measures to the costly business of making individual medical treatment available to the general population. The second, the changing role of the state, has parallels elsewhere but is in some respects peculiar to France. Routine politics can rarely transform entrenched institutions and practices in any society, but in the French system, more than most, crisis or change of regime has been the precondition for significant reform. In the twentieth century, both world wars opened the way to greater state involvement in public health; so did a third major upheaval – the Algerian crisis and the return of General de Gaulle in 1958, in a quasi-coup, as the last premier of the Fourth Republic and first president of the Fifth. The Second World War marked the critical watershed, because the Vichy regime of 1940–4 broke decisively with France's heritage of classical liberalism, and because the victorious forces of the Resistance repudiated the perceived weaknesses of the defeated Third Republic as much as Vichy's collaborationism; the widely shared sense of new possibilities in 1944–5 in some ways recalled the enthusiasms of 1789–90. The French restored the democratic republic but borrowed something from Vichy. The government of Marshal Pétain had attracted not only traditional conservatives and a smaller number of Nazi sympathizers, but also technocrats impatient with the internecine conflicts of the parliamentary system; some of the latter, with their vision of central planning, continued to influence policy after the war.[99]

Public Hygiene after the First World War

For the French public health system, struggling to implement the legislation of 1902, the crisis of 1914–18, which raised the incidence of disease among combatants and non-combatants alike, represented an unprecedented opportunity to demonstrate the principles of the new Pasteurian hygiene. The war effort also imposed an involuntary experiment in centralized organization and planning, which gave extraordinary powers to hygienists and allowed them to make their point: the hygiene services claimed credit for reversing the traditional ratio between deaths of soldiers due to enemy action and those due to disease, while also limiting morbidity and mortality among the civilian population.[100]

The French found a model for focused intervention against infectious disease in the anti-tuberculosis campaign of the special health commission sent to France in 1917 by the Rockefeller Foundation.[101] Tuberculosis was the logical target for such an undertaking: the disease accounted for about a sixth of deaths in France and perhaps a quarter in the large urban centres. The war had exacerbated an already difficult situation; many *poilus* contracted tuberculosis in the trenches, received medical discharges without the pensions to which wounded veterans were entitled, and returned home, where they infected their families. The basic approach to managing the disease, which had been thoroughly tested in Germany, entailed using dispensaries to track down cases, assist victims' families, carry out disinfection, and educate the public, in conjunction with sanatoriums to isolate patients and promote recovery. The wartime emergency had already facilitated passage in 1916 of a law that required each *département* to establish a tuberculosis dispensary; it was sponsored by Léon Bourgeois, a veteran of the anti-tuberculosis campaign (he had been named president of the tuberculosis commission within the Ministry of the Interior in 1903). This legislation, however, provided no additional state funding, relied heavily on voluntary efforts, and failed to add tuberculosis to the list of reportable communicable diseases; in 1917 France still had only 23 departmental dispensaries.

In collaboration with the American Red Cross, the Rockefeller workers established model programmes, emphasizing education and prevention, in areas where tuberculosis rates were high, notably the nineteenth arrondissement of Paris and the *département* of Eure-et-Loir; visiting nurses played a major role, and the Foundation encouraged the creation of schools to train them. Thanks in part to the impetus provided by the Rockefeller mission, parliament in 1919 passed a law based on a bill sponsored in 1917 by André Honnorat (1868–1925), a former journalist and founder of the National Alliance for French Population Growth, launching a project to build sanatoriums in all *départements*. By the time the Rockefeller commission completed its work in 1923 and transferred its responsibilities to a new French National Committee for Defence against Tuberculosis (headed by Honnorat until his death in 1925), the great majority of *départements* had permanent anti-tuberculosis programmes; 61 of the 79 had been sponsored by the Rockefeller team. In 1924, state expenditures in the anti-tuberculosis campaign exceeded 20 million francs, with more than double that amount coming from other sources, mostly the *départements*. Although the French death rate from tuberculosis remained the highest in Western Europe throughout the inter-war period, the government could no longer be accused of ignoring the problem.[102] A series of supplementary decrees in 1920, 1924 and 1932 extended implementation of the Honnorat law, and a decree of 1935 and a law of 1936 brought even private sanatoriums under government supervision and instituted a general state programme for placing tuberculosis patients in approved facilities.

The example of the anti-tuberculosis campaign and the perceived importance of public health to post-war recovery also contributed to the professionalization of the public health service. The staff physicians of tuberculosis dispensaries and sanatoriums were state functionaries, like the psychiatrists who ran the public insane asylums. In 1921, Léonie Chaptal presented a report on nursing to the High Council for Public Assistance, of which she had been a member since 1913, drawing in part on her own experience in the tuberculosis field; it inspired a decree the following year that formally recognized the nursing profession and established curricula and certificates for both hospital and visiting nurses (the latter could specialize in work with either tuberculosis patients or children). A year of special training would follow a common one-year introductory programme. State-certified nurses did not as yet enjoy a professional monopoly (they did not gain a rigorous one until after the Second World War), but they did, after 1925, have a national professional association, thanks largely to the efforts of Chaptal. The visiting nurses were agents of social welfare as much as medical auxiliaries, helping their clients, for example, to deal with insurance and public assistance programmes, and when a reform of 1938 effectively subsumed them into the new category of social worker (*assistante sociale*), it gave legal recognition to a situation that already existed *de facto*.[103]

Drawing on the momentum generated by the experience of 1914–18, the hygienists consolidated their institutional position in the years immediately following the war. The government finally elevated public health to ministerial status in 1920, when it created a Ministry of Hygiene, [Public] Assistance, and National Insurance [*Prévoyance Sociale*], built around the nucleus of the wartime military health service. A separate portfolio for public health was established in 1930, a practice followed by many, though not all, subsequent governments. In 1924, the legislature, following a proposal from the Paris office of the Rockefeller Foundation, established a National Social Hygiene Office, which was to concentrate at the outset on venereal disease and prostitution (French failings in this area had greatly exercised the American public health community since the arrival of US troops in 1917),[104] while also taking up the Rockefeller commission's struggle against tuberculosis; Foundation funding continued through the 1920s. Part propaganda office, part statistical bureau, the Office developed a variety of programmes, against cancer, diphtheria, typhoid fever, mental illness and infant mortality, as well as the more traditional 'social diseases'; a central nursing bureau was attached to it in 1925. The inter-war period was to prove the heyday of the social hygiene movement, led by figures such as the physician Just Sicard de Plauzoles, general secretary of the governmental Commission on Venereal Diseases (1920) and later of a High Council of Social Hygiene established in 1938. It continued, by and large, to promote its earlier vision of positive eugenics, though among French eugenists the emphasis gradually shifted toward controlling reproduction among the unfit; in the years immediately following the hard-won victory of 1918, *nataliste* sentiment remained strong, but by the early 1930s, when France's recovering birth-rate surpassed the slowing natality of England and Germany, and the rigours of the Depression revived Malthusian concerns over limited resources, it seemed reasonable to many to try to restrict the quantity but improve the 'quality' of the French population.

The advance of public hygiene remained a source of controversy for several groups: liberals and some physician allies who worried about creeping *fonctionnarisme* and the threat of tyranny through social hygiene;[105] elements farther to the Left on the political spectrum, who denounced it for distracting attention from the needed transformation of French society and for invading working-class households;[106] and eugenists, who criticized it for favouring the survival of the unfit. The existence of a national public health programme was never seriously in question, however; nor were its major efforts against infectious disease. They gained new strength from the Popular Front of 1936–8, which, true to the Left's vision of social medicine, promoted the concept of public health as a basic right; it brought the anti-tuberculosis campaign to a climax, thanks in major part to the efforts of the socialist Minister of Health and Physical Education, Henri Sellier (1883–1943) who had worked long and hard as mayor of Suresnes in the Paris suburbs and as head of the Public Office of Social Hygiene of the Seine to develop a programme of visiting nurses. Still, the system could not break entirely free of French traditions of economic and personal liberty and of privacy – expressed in a particularly strong conception of *le secret professionnel*, but also in widespread evasion of the income tax, to which a reluctant legislature had finally acceded during the First World War.

The government's regulatory activities bore the marks of these constraints, with a few exceptions. One notable curtailment of personal liberty, the 1920 law that forbade the advertising and sale of contraceptives, together with abortion and even public advocacy of the procedure, is attributable to the continuing fear of demographic stagnation after wartime losses. (These bans were not lifted until 1967 and 1974 respectively, when the first cohorts of the post-Second World War baby boom were themselves reaching child-bearing age.) The Third Republic resisted the eugenists' calls for a pre-marital medical examination and other mandatory investigations of the health of individual citizens. Regulation of alcoholic beverages weakened after the war; a High Committee on Population proposed new measures against alcoholism on the eve of the Second World War but did not win parliamentary approval. The Vichyites, who saw alcoholism as a major factor in the 'decadence' leading to France's collapse in the spring of 1940, used the decree powers of the new French State to enact the regulations, which restricted the number of bars but spared the still sacrosanct wine trade. In 1942 Vichy also adopted the requirement for a pre-marital medical examination, retained in subsequent versions of

French marriage law. After the war, the new republic showed less appetite for regulation than for other forms of state intervention in matters of public health, particularly where powerful economic interests were at stake. (With a certain consistency, the state itself retained its monopoly on the distribution of tobacco long after the physiological effects of smoking were well understood and public expenditures for the treatment of lung cancer were mounting.) Despite the promises of de Gaulle's provisional government, alcohol regulation faltered after 1944, under pressure from the producers' lobby. The efforts of the few political figures of the Fourth and Fifth Republics strongly committed to the anti-alcoholism campaign (notably Pierre Mendès-France, who as premier from June 1954 to February 1955 established an executive committee on alcoholism) met with the usual stiff opposition and sometimes ridicule; public tolerance of drinking and the perception that wine is a healthful beverage have only recently begun to decline among educated younger adults. The few concessions towards recognizing alcohol abuse as a public health problem, including restrictions on the sale of alcoholic beverages to minors and a provision against drunk driving (in the Highways Act of 1956), should be appreciated in this context.

Finding the resources for major investments in new infrastructure proved an even greater challenge in the inter-war period, for reasons less political than social and economic. The persistence of a backward rural sector slowed the introduction of pure water supplies and sewer systems, and even in urban areas an ageing housing stock survived with little renewal into the second half of the century. Although in 1940 Paris could boast that 97.6 per cent of its buildings had running water and 94.1 per cent a sewer connection, the situation was very different in the provinces, where almost two-thirds of *communes* lacked adequate supplies of drinking water and outdoor privies were in common use throughout the countryside. The period following the Second World War, however, saw the greatest sustained economic growth in modern French history, attributable in part to government planning and subventions. State-sponsored modernization[107] arguably contributed as much as state-sponsored medical programmes to the sometimes remarkable improvements in public health that France enjoyed after the war (infant mortality, for example, declined from 53 to 8.3 deaths per 1,000 births between 1950 and 1984). It has also, of course, contributed to the construction of a vast health-care system, heavily reliant on advanced technology and increasingly centred in the hospital (which in the process has become a purely medical centre, shedding the last of its old functions as hospice and instrument of public assistance).[108] Like other industrialized countries, France has experienced what might be called the medicalization of public health services and the decline of a vision of social hygiene, in the broadest sense, that emphasized prevention, on the one hand, (sanitary improvements, behaviour modification) and, on the other hand, disinfection, quarantine and other measures designed to contain what were essentially untreatable diseases. The new approach was already apparent after the First World War in a public campaign against cancer, launched in 1918 by a Franco-Anglo-American Anti-Cancer League, which emphasized early detection and aggressive treatment with surgery and radiation therapy.[109] The introduction of antibiotic therapies dramatically transformed the approach to tuberculosis, venereal disease and many of the other major infectious diseases. In retrospect the period from the end of the nineteenth century to the 1940s would appear to have been the classic age of Pasteurian public health, though the emergence of AIDS and of antibiotic-resistant strains of tuberculosis should be enough to remind us that social hygiene is more than a museum piece.

In the last half-century, French exceptionalism in public hygiene has diminished substantially. In the late 1930s, a Belgian minister of public health, who found much to regret in his own country's recalcitrance in matters of public health, pointed to 'the well developed (I would not hesitate to say excessively developed) sense of individual liberty [in France], which until now has [successfully] opposed the premarital certificate and obligatory treatment of venereal diseases, [and] which limits the isolation of patients with contagious diseases, notably tuberculosis.'[110] It would be difficult to imagine a foreign observer making a similar comment in the late 1980s.

Some traces of older patterns do persist. The French response to AIDS is perhaps a case in point, illustrating once again French leadership in theory and research coupled with a lag in public policy and effective action.[111] The team at the Pasteur Institute headed by Luc Montagnier is now generally recognized as the discoverer of the human immunodeficiency virus, and the French have ranked second only to the United States in expenditures for AIDS research. Yet France, which also has the highest number of AIDS cases and the second highest incidence of the disease in Europe, was criticized in the mid 1980s for its relative slowness in adopting a national programme to fight the disease and for not focusing on risk groups. As elsewhere, strong opposition has greeted all suggestions for mandatory national testing; even a proposal in 1988 to test all pregnant women and surgery patients for the HIV virus provoked a storm of controversy and forced the resignation of the government minister who had made it. (The question was a politically loaded one; the right-wing National Front had made AIDS a major issue, and the *département* of the Alpes-Maritimes, a National Front stronghold, proposed its own plan for general screening of the population.) The notorious scandal involving officials who, it was discovered, had allowed HIV-contaminated blood products to be administered to haemophiliacs for nine months in 1985 further undermined confidence in the government. Every country touched by this scourge has witnessed similar contradictory impulses and demands for both privacy and individual liberty, disclosure and compulsion: it raises in their starkest form the most fundamental dilemmas of public health, which are universal. France shares in this experience, to which it adds, perhaps, a sense of *déjà vu;* even the Rockefeller commission, after all, did not persuade the French to make tuberculosis a reportable disease (a legislative proposal making declaration obligatory failed in 1919, despite the support of France's most eminent physician-politician, premier Georges Clemenceau, and it was added to the list only in 1968, well after the development of effective antibiotic therapies).

By the beginning of the new decade, however, France had launched a much more substantial campaign of AIDS education and prevention, coordinated by a semi-autonomous French Agency to Combat AIDS, established in 1989.[112] More remarkable, for its direct infringement of individual freedom, was the measure restricting smoking in public places that went into effect on 1 November, 1992, to be followed in 1993 by a ban on tobacco advertising. Characteristically, perhaps, the restrictions have been widely ignored, and the fines, which run into the hundreds of francs for offending smokers and substantially more for proprietors of establishments that do not enforce the regulations, have rarely been imposed. Still, the new measures made France a leader in anti-smoking legislation – all the more striking in a country where the cigarette, almost a symbol in itself of stubborn Gallic individualism, seemed an integral part of the national culture, and where the government retains its tobacco monopoly and derives considerable revenue (over 27 billion francs in 1992) in taxes from the tobacco trade.[113]

National Health Insurance: the Inter-war Years

A more compelling indication of French distinctiveness can be found in the twentieth-century history of medical assistance. Whereas Britain emulated the German model of social insurance in the years immediately preceding the First World War, France moved only after the war to establish a national programme. The impetus came from the recovery of the territories in Alsace and Lorraine ceded to Germany in 1871, where the programmes instituted by Bismarck remained in force. The French accepted the basic principle that, at least for certain designated groups, coverage would be comprehensive and compulsory; it would be insurance against the risk of illness rather than charity. But the specific forms that social insurance took reflected long-standing French debates.[114]

National health insurance took a decade to bring about, from the establishment of a special commission in 1920 to final passage of a social insurance law in 1930 (modifying a law adopted in 1928 but not yet implemented) covering sickness, disability and old age. The project's long and tortuous trajectory was due in part to opposition from the Left, concentrated in the newly formed Communist Party, but even more to the objections of interest groups, most prominently the medical profession. The original plan resembled its German model in calling for contracts between groups of beneficiaries and groups of physicians, who would provide services in return for a fixed annual payment. The medical profession was divided in its response – the union of medical *syndicats* underwent a schism on this issue – but the majority of private practitioners favoured greater freedom than the bill would have allowed. A declaration generally known as the 'Medical Charter', adopted by the Congress of Medical *Syndicats* of France in 1927, affirmed the profession's commitment to confidentiality and the four cardinal principles of liberal medicine: a doctor–patient relationship freely chosen by both parties, freedom for physicians to diagnose and prescribe according to their own best professional judgement, the direct contract between patient and practitioner (*l'entente directe*), and direct payment of the physician by the patient. The final settlement of 1930 granted major concessions to the physicians, including the four cardinal principles as well as guarantees of professional confidentiality and the profession's right to discipline its own members; physicians, moreover, would be represented in the administration of the system. Insurance would be compulsory only for industrial and commercial employees whose income fell below a certain level (roughly 14 per cent of the population); their payroll deductions, together with contributions from employers and a state fund, would finance the programme. Patients would pay their physician directly for each service; participating practitioners agreed in principle to respect a fee scale but were not actually obligated to do so. The patients would then be reimbursed by their chosen insurer (several options existed, including mutual aid societies) at a rate that was normally 80 per cent of the recognized fee, though the patient's actual co-payment was often much larger than 20 per cent. The whole system, as the Senate had insisted, was independent of the state bureaucracy and was governed by private law. As in 1893, the organized medical profession had succeeded in imposing an arrangement that, although clearly very different from nineteenth-century *laissez-faire,* nonetheless retained many of the key features of the liberal model.

The Modern Social Security System (1945)

Where it had required a decade-long struggle to adopt a social insurance plan, it took a matter of months to transform it into something far more ambitious in the heady climate that followed France's liberation from Nazi occupation. An executive ordinance of the National Resistance Council (October 1945) laid the foundations for a new comprehensive social security system embracing family allowances as well as old age pensions and coverage for sickness and disability.[115] The architects of the plan had studied with considerable interest the Beveridge Report of 1942, which helped inspire the English welfare state, including the National Health Service (1946), but French traditions and priorities dictated a different approach. In keeping with precedent, the system was decentralized, independent of the state bureaucracy, and largely self-governing, administered by independent regional boards representing the contributors (employers and employees), who provided the bulk of the funding for the system. (Although the state's share subsequently increased, it remained the lowest in the European Community.) Social security involved a much larger part of the population than the inter-war social insurance system, but not all of it; public assistance still played a major role, dealing with groups and risks not covered under the 1945 ordinance. During the years that followed, the programme expanded into one of the most comprehensive social security systems in the West. In recognition of the state's expanding role, the government created a national social security office and gave the responsible ministry more authority over the regional offices, without, however, changing the basic structure.

The medical component of the social security programme resembled the 'liberal' health insurance system of the 1930s. The most important change was intended to make it likelier that patients would recover a substantial part of their actual costs. Physicians who participated in the system would be held, with some exceptions, to a fee scale negotiated by their *syndicats* at the departmental level and approved by a tripartite commission including representatives of the social security system, the physicians, and the government. Where no accord was reached, no fee schedule would apply, but patients would receive a much smaller reimbursement – a powerful incentive, where they had a choice, to turn to a practitioner who participated in an agreement. This provision represented a significant departure from the principle of the *entente directe* between doctor and patient, even if other important elements of the liberal model remained; physicians, most of whom went along with the innovation, rationalized it as a 'collective' version of the *entente directe*. The medical profession could not hope to exercise as much influence over an executive legislating by decree as over a parliament of the Third Republic: hence the largely unwelcome innovations of 1945. But it remained a powerful lobby, relatively unified under the Confederation of *Syndicats* (restored after being suppressed under Vichy), and could derail legislation in parliament, the key political arena under the constitution of the Fourth Republic, adopted in October 1946. Its efforts contributed to the defeat of a bill presented by the government in 1956 that would have seriously weakened the *syndicats* by allowing physicians to sign individual contracts with the social security system.[116]

Asserting State Control: the Fifth Republic

The influence of the medical profession declined significantly under the new constitution of 1958, which strengthened the executive at the expense of the legislative branch. The Gaullist state purported to represent the national interest by rising above the squabbling of interest groups, which were said to have weakened both the Third and the Fourth Republics; the political system clearly allowed less room than any previous republican regime for lobbies to influence policy by manipulating the parliamentary process. The government also sought to bring independent programmes such as social security under more direct control; once a sort of referee for the regional agencies, the state emerged as a leading player in the health-care field.[117]

The key reform of the social security system came in a decree of May 1960, which effectively shifted the preponderance of power in fee negotiations from the medical profession to the state. The physicians' *syndicats* would enter into agreements at the *département* level, as before, but the government established a model convention and reserved the right to veto any agreement that deviated too drastically from it. For the first time, moreover, practitioners could join individually on the terms of the national model, where no departmental agreement existed. The use of the national model compromised the freedom of even the collective version of *l'entente directe*: in effect, the government was dictating the economic relationship between providers and recipients of medical care. The incentives (including a package of health care and pension benefits for participating physicians) worked as intended; by the fall of 1964, only about a tenth of practitioners remained outside the system. The minority of die-hard resisters split off from the Confederation of *Syndicats* to form a Federation of Physicians of France, dedicated to defending the liberal model. In order to exert further financial control over the system, a set of ordinances promulgated in 1967, towards the end of de Gaulle's presidency, separated the health, pension and family allowance sectors of social security and required each to balance its budget. The reform also created a quasi-public National Health Insurance Fund, under the ministries of health and finance, to oversee the regional agencies (whose boards were now to be appointed rather than elected); it wound up administering about 70 per cent of the French health care budget. The central issue in the subsequent history of French health insurance, under the presidencies of the Gaullist Pompidou, the moderate conservative Giscard d'Estaing, and the Socialist Mitterrand, has been the state's attempt to contain an increasingly expensive system.[118] The combination of very broad coverage and open-ended fee-for-service (with numerous *dépassements*, or authorized exceptions to the fee schedule, mainly for prestigious specialists) was a recipe for high costs, particularly as the number of medical personnel was rapidly expanding. Health care expenditures increased sharply in absolute terms and rose as a proportion of GDP to near the top of the European scale (from 3 per cent in 1950 to 4.2 per cent in 1960, 5.8 per cent in 1970, 7.6 per cent in 1980, and 8.6 per cent in 1987), still a little behind Sweden and well below the American level, but growing rapidly, generally between 8 and 10 per cent a year.[119]

The framework for agreements with the medical profession underwent successive design changes in 1971 and 1980. The 1971 convention was the first negotiated at the national level, between the government and the Confederation of *Syndicats* (the dissident Federation of French Physicians then grudgingly accepted it); the Confederation, indeed, had sought out the new arrangement, hoping in this way to avert possibly more drastic measures imposed from above. The national plan applied to all physicians, unless they opted out (thereby forfeiting their own benefit package). No part of France would lack a collective agreement, and practitioners would no longer be able to make individual deals with the government. In return for a national fee schedule, the government promised to respect the basic principles of liberal medicine, and the National Health Insurance Fund agreed not to promote health maintenance organizations. By 1980 the overwhelming majority of private practitioners (over 97 per cent) participated in the system.

The financial pressures on the social security system continued to mount, however, exacerbated by the oil crisis of 1974. President Giscard d'Estaing and Raymond Barre, his prime minister for 1976–81, committed to a 'neo-liberal' doctrine of limiting social expenditures to stimulate business and help lift the French economy out of recession, pressed for further restrictions on health care costs. One plan, a proposal to link increases in health care expenditures to growth in the GDP, led to a nationwide doctors' strike and a retreat by the government; Barre was more successful in a sustained effort to undercut the Confederation and further divide the profession by negotiating with the Federation of French Physicians, the smaller of the two major physicians' unions. The agreement concluded in 1980 with the Federation (and accepted the following year by the Confederation) introduced a new model comprising two sectors, between which physicians would choose as individuals. The first would give physicians a benefits package as the *quid pro quo* for adhering to a fee schedule (with no possibility for *dépassements*); physicians in the second sector, which accorded with the government's 'neo-liberal' policies of ending price controls, could charge what they wished but would not receive the benefits. In either case, patients would be reimbursed 70 per cent of the rates set by the fee schedule.

The Socialists came to power in 1981 promising real socialism and an extension of the benefits put in place by the Left coalition of 1945. The first minister of health, the Communist Jack Ralite, presented a 'charter of health', which stressed prevention, health maintenance, more free care and equal care (inequalities in medical consumption had increased rather than decreased under the social security system). A law of March 1982 established several regional health committees emphasizing preventive medicine, in keeping with the Socialists' theme of devolution and decentralization. A law of January 1983 called for 'integrated health centres', essentially HMO's with salaried primary-care physicians, but produced only limited results. In practice, economic pressures forced the Socialists to retreat in health care, as in other domains, to a programme of 'socialist rigour', starting in July 1982. The conservative majority produced by the parliamentary elections of 1986 reversed what remained of the reforms of the early 1980s. Back in power from 1988 until their electoral defeat in the spring of 1993, the Socialists had once again to confront the overriding problem of containing costs.

Despite some major concessions, particularly on fee schedules, the French medical profession has succeeded in maintaining many elements of liberal medical practice, and the French health insurance system remains the furthest removed from socialized medicine of any of the major Western national programmes. One indication, apart from the retention of fee-for-service in the national health insurance system, is the relatively limited number of medical personnel employed full-time by the government, compared with northern Europe (the public medical sector consists chiefly of hospital staff), and the long dominant role of private practitioners in providing patient care. One survey in 1984 indicated that 70.8 per cent of active physicians still practised privately, 59.8 per cent exclusively so.[120] There has been talk at various points in the last decade and a half of containing costs by rationing services, capping total expenditures, or even nationalizing the pharmaceutical industry (though not medicine). In 1992, the government signed an accord with the Confederation of *Syndicats* to impose limits on the growth of expenditures in the 'liberal' sector of medical practice, involving some 108,000 physicians, but the cumbersome machinery proposed to enforce the guidelines quickly proved controversial.[121] An effective mechanism to contain global consumption has yet to be devised.

To be sure, the United States represents an even more striking example of an expanding and unregulated health care system driven by third-party payments. In comparison with its American counterpart, the French profession looks weak, with its divided organizations (to which only a minority of practitioners actually belong); the French state, in contrast, looks quite strong, with a powerful executive and bureaucracy enjoying extensive decree powers facing a relatively weak legislature and a limited judiciary. From an American perspective, the salient features of the French case have been the steady decline in professional power since 1960 and the expansion of government control over health care.[122] In the European context, however, France is remarkable not for state interference but for the degree to which the liberal model of medical practice has survived in the context of a comprehensive social security programme.

French public health in the late twentieth century is far removed from nineteenth-century *laissez-faire*. A series of measures, starting in the nineteenth century itself, have involved the state directly in programmes to reduce morbidity and mortality and have increasingly required French citizens to cooperate – though all this has stopped well short of realizing the vision of an equal right to health for all citizens entertained by the revolutionaries of 1789. The laws of 1822, on the sanitary defence of France's frontiers, and of 1902, on protection against domestic sources of disease, raised the spectre of 'dictatorship' and 'tyranny of hygiene', but their proponents successfully defended them on the grounds that the freedom of some should not put the well-being and life of others in jeopardy. The legislation of 1893, 1930 and 1945 took two further critical steps away from *laissez-faire,* first committing public resources to make medical care more widely available and then making participation in the national health programme compulsory; it no longer sufficed not to harm others.

Just as striking, however, is the pattern of resistance, often at least partly successful, to centralization, state intervention, and compulsion: the many decades of leaving public assistance and hygiene in the hands of local and regional authorities; the extensive role of voluntary associations, such as mutual aid societies; the watering down of public hygiene legislation, particularly the provisions for enforcement, throughout the nineteenth century and into the early twentieth (including the epochal law of 1902); staunch adherence to *le secret professionnel* in ways that seriously compromised the government's efforts to gather critical information on threats to public health; the decentralized structure and private-law status of national health insurance; and the remarkable success of the medical profession in maintaining 'liberal medicine' within the social security programme, despite the fiscal consequences obvious to all.

France is not the extreme case. Among Western societies that have struggled with the politics of public health, it could not match the radical libertarianism of certain Swiss cantons or, for that matter, the long successful efforts of organized medicine and allied political forces to block national health insurance in the United States. The perceived backwardness of French sanitary legislation and institutions (like France's much debated lag in industrialization) was a very relative thing, produced by comparing the French experience with that of a handful of industrialized nations and with the hygienists' own lofty ideals. Nor, it should be stressed, are the themes discussed in this chapter uniquely French. Hygienism was from the beginning a highly cosmopolitan movement, well before the regular international congresses that started in the late nineteenth century. The tensions between statist and liberal tendencies in the Enlightenment form part of the common Western heritage; conflicts between the demands of public health and the interests of property, civil liberties and the medical profession emerged in every society in which social medicine had to co-exist with liberal and democratic political institutions. No polity forged an ideological consensus on these issues. *Laissez-faire* England had its Benthamite centralizers à la Chadwick (who often cited French models), and Germany its liberal critics of Prussian authoritarianism, whose inspiration derived in part from a different French tradition. Partly for this reason, the history of public health is rife with seeming incongruities, and not just in France. The other side of the French paradox is the emergence of successful public health movements and strong legislation in countries with vital libertarian traditions and supposedly weak states, notably Britain and the United States, though with some revealing disappointments, such as the amendment to English vaccination legislation, passed in 1898 under relentless pressure from the anti-vaccination forces, which exempted the children of conscientious objectors, or the failure of national health insurance in the United States.

The paradoxes do not end here. In the United States, the United Kingdom and Germany, libertarian arguments contributed to the abolition or weakening of professional monopoly in medicine in the middle decades of the nineteenth century, and although the American states re-established it at the end of the century, when the prestige of Pasteurianism was at its zenith, the British and Germans did not. France, in contrast, remained the unvarying model of tight control of entry into the medical field. Only the inhabitants of a tiny handful of Swiss Protestant cantons seem to have remained fanatically consistent in their hatred of compulsory public health measures and privileges for doctors.[123] The seeming antinomies can to some extent be resolved. In France, a physician's practice was considered a form of property (on which, for much of the nineteenth century, he had to pay the *patente*, or tax on industry), so that repressing unlicensed practice and defending property owners against the intrusion of the state public health apparatus are in a sense congruent. In Britain, the classic liberal argument that individuals have the right to act without constraint so long as they do not interfere with the rights of others accommodated both toleration for alternative medicine, which at worst might lead the individual to harm himself, and compulsory public health measures, which prevented the individual from harming the community; following the argument made familiar by John Stuart Mill, the state had no right to intervene to avert the first type of injury, but an obligation to prevent the second. Clearly, though, any interpretation that seeks simple correlations between the development of public health institutions, on the one hand, and 'strong' or 'weak' states or authoritarian and liberal ideological traditions on the other, quickly slides on to thin ice.

This said, what has perhaps distinguished the French case has been the abiding strength of both the communitarian and individualist traditions inherited from the Revolution, and of the perennial tensions between them, compounded by the even more profound divisions between those who embraced and those who repudiated the revolutionary heritage as a whole. By setting the terms of the conflict and freighting it with so much emotional baggage, the ideological struggles of the Revolution not only coloured French rhetoric on public health but also made it difficult for the debate to evolve; for many decades, atavistic hostilities hampered the realignments and new alliances (between Catholic paternalists and social democrats, for example) crucial to achieving reform. The one post-revolutionary principle on which the political classes could agree, the glue that held the fragile edifice together, was the sanctity of property, proclaimed in the Declaration of the Rights of Man and reaffirmed in the Napoleonic Code, and both the tenacity of those who defended this right against government intervention and the timidity of those who felt compelled to challenge it in the name of public health owed something to memories of 1789 and 1793–4. That the terrain now seems clearer may owe something to the sense, widely shared in the bicentennial year of 1989, which coincided with the collapse of communism in Central and Eastern Europe, that the French Revolution is finally over.

Other societies fought many of the same battles, but on different terrain and with different results. The extraordinary gulf between a grandiose vision of the public good and the stubborn defence of private interest, between the popular demand for services in a democratic polity and governmental foot-dragging and abdication of responsibility, between the appearance of a strong, rationalized central state and the reality of voluntarism, localism, influence-peddling and muddle – all this has long persisted as a characteristic legacy of French history. *Plus ça change, plus c'est la même chose?* Not quite: the public health system of late twentieth-century France, massively committed to supporting high technology therapeutics, is profoundly different from *l'hygiènisme* of the early nineteenth century; the always blurred boundary between medicine and public health has been lost to view, as in all the countries of the industrialized and post-industrial world. These societies, moreover, face common problems of growing health costs and strained resources and seem to be moving towards convergent solutions. As this volume goes to press, the Treaty on European Union has just taken effect, and President Clinton has presented his plan for a national health programme to the US Congress. These and other developments as the century nears its end may tend to efface what long seemed distinctive and perdurable national traits; the confident ambitions of the Enlightenment public health project may themselves yield to post-modern uncertainties. The historian can only conclude that in the history of modern public health, so far, the French have remained quite recognizably and distinctively French.

Notes

1. Among the older surveys, see, for example, George Rosen, *A History of Public Health* (New York: 1958), which gives about equal attention to France and Germany (though substantially less than to Britain and the United States), and René Sand, *The Advance to Social Medicine* (London: 1952), which accords France approximately the same prominence as England, Germany and the United States. There is no adequate general history of French public health, but its general outlines since the Middle Ages, including the most important legislation, may be found in Raymond Girard's *Contribution à l'étude de l'histoire de l'hygiène en France*, published medical thesis, University of Paris, 1936, no. 680. The relevant legislation for the period since the Revolution of 1789 is conveniently gathered in Ministère de la Santé, *Recueil des textes officiels concernant la protection de la santé publique, 1790–1935*, 9 vols. (Paris: 1938952); for a guide, see F. and M. Bourguin and M. Le Bas, *Tables générales de la législation sanitaire francaise, 1790–1955*, 3 vols. (Paris: 1957). For subsequent legislation, consult the serial *Recueil des textes officiels intéressant la santé publique et la population.*

   The author wishes to acknowledge the assistance of a fellowship from the John Simon Guggenheim Memorial Foundation, which greatly facilitated the preparation of this chapter, and the helpful comments of Ann La Berge and George Weisz on a prospectus of the project.
2. See Colin Jones, *The Charitable Imperative: Hospitals and Nursing in Ancien Régime and Revolutionary France* (London: 1989).
3. On hospitals and assistance, see Camille Bloch, *L'Assistance publique et l'État en France à la veille de la Revolution . . . (1764–1790)* (Paris: 1908); Maurice Rochaix, *Contribution à l'étude des problèmes hospitaliers contemporains: Étude sur l'évolution des questions hospitalières de la fin de l'Ancien Régime à nos jours* (Dijon: 1959), and Françoise Hildesheimer and Christian Gut, *L'Assistance hospitalière en France* (Paris: 1992). On the different types of hospitals: Muriel Jeorger, 'The Structure of the Hospital System in France in the Ancien Régime', tr. Elborg Forster, in Robert Forster and Orest Ranum (eds), *Medicine and Society in France*, Selections from the

Annales: Économies, sociétés, civilisations, 6 (Baltimore: 1980), 104–36. For a detailed account of how the system worked in practice, see the excellent local study by Colin Jones, *Charity and Bienfaisance: The Treatment of the Poor in the Montpellier Region, 1740–1815* (Cambridge: 1982).

4. See the essays in Andrew W. Russell (ed.), *The Town and State Physician in Europe from the Middle Ages to the Enlightenment*, Wolfenbütteler Forschungen 17 (Wolfenbüttel: 1981).
5. The powers of the French boards rarely matched those of their counterparts in northern Italy; see Carlo M. Cipolla, *Public Health and the Medical Profession in the Renaissance* (Cambridge: 1976).
6. Alfred Franklin gives an anecdotal but still useful survey of hygienic regulations and practices in *La Vie privée d'autrefois*, Vol. 7, *l'Hygiène* (Paris: 1890).
7. Denis Diderot *et al., Encyclopédie, ou dictionnaire raisonné des sciences, des arts, et des métiers, par une société de gens de lettres*, 17 vols (Paris: 1751–65), s.v. 'hygiène' and 'police'; on hygiene in the *Encyclopédie*, see William Coleman, 'Health and Hygiene in the *Encyclopédie:* A Medical Doctrine for the Bourgeoisie', *Journal of the History of Medicine and Allied Sciences* 29 (1974): 399–421. *Encyclopédie méthodique: Médecine*, 13 vols, (Paris: 1787–1830), s.v. hygiène. On 'police' and 'medical police', see Ludmilla J. Jordanova, 'Policing Public Health in France, 1780–1815', in T. Ogawa, (ed.), *Public Health* (Tokyo: 1981), 12–32. In two classic articles, George Rosen associated medical police with a German cameralist tradition that put the interest of the state before that of society, but the parallels with France are stronger than he suggests; see his 'Cameralism and the Concept of Medical Police' and 'The Fate of the Concept of Medical Police, 1780–1890', both in Rosen, *From Medical Police to Social Medicine: Essays on the History of Health Care* (New York: 1974).

   The semantic history of names for the field of public health, for which there has never been a single generally accepted label, has yet to be written (though some elements can be found in Rosen, 'What is Social Medicine?', *ibid.*, 60–119), but the implications of the changing vocabulary are worth bearing in mind. France produced no treatise comparable to Johann Peter Frank's *System einer vollständigen medicinischen Polizey*, (6 vols, [Mannheim: 1779–1819]); nor was Frank's work translated into French, although his contribution was widely admired. Nevertheless, the term *la police médicale* came into general and rather indiscriminate use to refer to the large domain where administrative and medical concerns intersected with sanitary regulations but also public health as a discipline, the regulation of medical practice (*la police de la médecine*), and legal medicine. See, for example, Nicolas-Philibert Adelon *et al., Dictionnaire des sciences médicales par une société de médecins et de chirurgiens*, . . . , 60 vols, (Paris: 1812–22), s.v. 'police médicale', article by François-Emmanuel

Fodéré; Fodéré defines the term very broadly as the regulation and oversight of the medical field and treats *la police de santé*, the responsibility of public officials (especially mayors), as a special branch. In the nineteenth century, *la police médicale* (or, with increasing frequency, *la police sanitaire*), continued to be used to designate regulatory measures designed to contain or eliminate sources of disease. *L'hygiène publique*, together with the expressions incorporating the terms for health, *santé* and *salubrité* (both much favoured by the revolutionaries of the 1790s), located the field in the medical rather than the administrative domain and suggested a comprehensive programme to promote health that went well beyond sanitary regulations. A common though not universal or always consistent semantic strategy treated medical police as the practical application of the principles of public hygiene in order to promote public health; see, for example, the use of the term *police médicale* in J.-B. Demangeon, *Des moyens de perfectionner la médecine, et d'asseoir les bases les plus sûres de la salubrité publique*... (Paris: Year XII/1804).

A smaller number of writers favoured *la médecine politique*, which bore the same relation to individual medicine that 'political economy' did to domestic economy, and public to private hygiene. ('State medicine' had no direct equivalent in French.) The term *médecine politique*, in contradistinction to clinical or private medicine, was favoured by Clément-François-Victor-Gabriel Prunelle (1777–1853), librarian and professor of medical history, legal medicine, and medical police at Montpellier, where his liberal opinions cost him the librarianship and then his chair under the Restoration; see his *De la médecine politique en général et de son objet*... (Montpellier: 1814), and *De l'action de la médecine sur la population des états*... (n.p., 1818). A subsequent professor and librarian at Montpellier, Henri-Marcel Kühnholtz, devoted an entire book to straightening out what seemed to him the confused terminology and sub-disciplinary boundaries of the field *(Coup d'oeil sur l'ensemble systématique de la médecine judiciaire, considérée dans ses rapports avec la médecine politique* [Montpellier: 1834]). Kühnholtz objected in particular to what he saw as the common misuse of the term 'legal medicine'; he counted public hygiene, *la médecine judiciaire* (forensic medicine), *la police médicale* (regulation of medical practice), and *la médecine législative/administrative* (advice to the legislative and executive branches of government) among the branches of *la médecine politique*. 'Political medicine' suggested the many connections between medicine and government, and often the role that medical professionals ought to play in guiding the latter; Prunelle was closely linked to the Ideologues, with whom he shared, among other things, an emphasis on the role of the expert in formulating rational public policy and an expansive view of the cognitive claims of medicine and physiology. (Cf. Eusèbe de Salverte, *Des rapports de la médecine avec la politique* [Paris: 1806], a work dedicated to Cabanis and later cited approvingly by Kühnholtz; on the influence of the Ideologues, see the discussion of the early hygiene movement, below.) We should perhaps avoid, however, reading too much significance into this fluid vocabulary; whatever term they used, the great majority of writers on public health favoured active state intervention along lines laid down by medical doctors and shared similarly broad conceptions of hygiene.

The more recent term *médecine sociale*, which came into current use in the mid nineteenth century and typically implied the need for social change as a precondition for improvements in health, and *hygiène sociale*, dating from the late nineteenth century, which connoted a focus on 'social' diseases and disorders (alcoholism, venereal disease, tuberculosis) that seemed to undermine the health of future generations as well as present victims, are discussed later in this chapter.

8. Brief overviews of the growing role of the state in public health can be found in Jean-Pierre Gutton, 'Aux origines d'un ministère de l'assistance et de la santé dans la France de l'Ancien Régime', in Jean-Louis Harouel (ed.), *Histoire du droit social: mélanges en hommage à Jean Imbert* (Paris: 1989), 287–93, and Caroline Hannaway, 'From Private Hygiene to Public Health: A Transformation in Western Medicine in the Eighteenth and Nineteenth Centuries', in Ogawa, *op. cit.* (note 7), 108–27. See also Shelby T. McCloy, *Government Assistance in Eighteenth-Century France* (Durham, N.C.: 1946), chs 6–10, and Bloch, *op. cit.* (note 3), Book II. A still useful regional study is Paul Delaunay, *Études sur l'hygiène, l'assistance et les secours publics dans le Maine sous l'Ancien Régime* (Le Mans: 1923).
9. On mercantilist ideas and their transformation in the Enlightenment, see George Rosen, 'Mercantilism and Health Policy in Eighteenth-Century French Thought', in Rosen, *op. cit.* (note 7), 201–19.
10. For an overview, see Jean-Pierre Goubert, 'Épidémies, médecine et état en France à la fin de l'Ancien Régime', in *Maladie et société (XIIe–XVIIIe siècles): Actes du Colloque de Bielefeld* (Paris: 1989), 393–401. Goubert analyses in detail the workings of this system in one province in his *Malades et médecins en Bretagne, 1770–1790* (Paris: 1974).
11. Matthew Ramsey, 'Traditional Medicine and Medical Enlightenment: The Regulation of Secret Remedies in the Ancien Régime', *Historical Reflections/Réflexions historiques*, 9, nos 1–2 (1982), 215–32.
12. Caroline C. Hannaway, 'Medicine, Public Welfare, and the State in Eighteenth-Century France: The Société Royale de Médecine of Paris (1776–1793)', (Ph.D. Dissertation, The Johns Hopkins University, 1974), remains the fullest study of the Society. For an overview, see *idem*, 'The Société Royale de Médecine and Epidemics in the Ancien Régime', *Bulletin of the History of Medicine*, 46 (1972), 257–73.

13. See Jean Meyer, 'L'Enquête de l'Académie de Médecine sur les épidémies, 1774–1794', in *Études rurales*, 34 (1969), 7–69, and Jean-Paul Desaive *et al., Médecins, climat et épidémies à la fin du XVIII*[e] *siècle* (Paris and The Hague: 1972). For an overview of environmental medicine in Europe and its implications for public health, see James C. Riley, *The Eighteenth-Century Campaign to Avoid Disease* (New York: 1987).
14. It played an active role, for example, in the campaign that led to the closing of the capital's most important burial ground, the desperately overcrowded Cemetery of the Holy Innocents, in the centre of the city, and the removal of the remains of many thousands of Parisians to catacombs in what were then the suburbs. See Owen and Caroline Hannaway, 'La Fermeture du cimetière des Innocents', *Dix-huitième siècle,* 9 (1977), 181–91.
15. Harvey Mitchell explores some of the conflicting views in 'Politics in the Service of Knowledge: The Debate Over the Administration of Medicine and Welfare in Late Eighteenth-Century France', *Social History,* 6 (1981), 185–207. On changing conceptions of welfare, see Thomas McStay Adams, *Bureaucrats and Beggars: French Social Policy in the Age of the Enlightenment* (New York: 1990).
16. On perceptions of hygiene and self-help, see Coleman, *op. cit.* (note 7).
17. George Rosen provides a brief overview in 'Hospitals, Medical Care, and Social Policy in the French Revolution', in Rosen, *op. cit.* (note 7), 220–45. On medicine in the Revolution, see also Jean-Charles Sournia, *La Médecine révolutionnaire* (Paris: 1989).
18. Dora B. Weiner, 'Le Droit de l'homme à la santé: une belle idée devant l'Assemblée Constituante, 1790–91', *Clio Medica* , 5 (1970), 209–23
19. On the debates, see Michel Foucault, *The Birth of the Clinic: An Archaeology of Medical Perception,* tr. A. M. Sheridan Smith (New York: 1973), chs 2–3.
20. On the work of the health committee, see Henry Ingrand, *Le Comité de Salubrité de l'Assemblée Nationale Constituante (1790–1791): un essai de réforme de l'enseignement médical, des services d'hygiène et de protection de la santé publique* . . . (Paris: 1934).
21. On public assistance under the Revolution, see Alan Forrest, *The French Revolution and the Poor* (New York: 1981), and Jean Imbert (ed.), *La Protection sociale sous la Révolution française* (Paris: 1990).
22. Dora B. Weiner, 'The French Revolution, Napoleon, and the Nursing Profession', *Bulletin of the History of Medicine* , 46 (1972), 274–305.
23. See Jean Imbert, *Le Droit hospitalier de la Révolution et de l'Empire* (Paris: 1954).
24. On the Faculty's ambitions as a medical academy, see George Weisz, 'Les Professeurs parisiens et l'Académie de Médecine', in Christophe Charle and Régine Ferré (eds), *Le Personnel de l'enseignement*

supérieur en France aux XIXe et XXe siècles (Paris: 1985), 47–65. On the medical societies, see Erwin H. Ackerknecht, *Médicine at the Paris Hospital, 1794–1848* (Baltimore: 1967), ch. 9. On the Société de Médecine de Paris, see *Société de Médecine de Paris, 1796–1896, centenaire: 22 mars 1896* (Paris: 1896), 'Histoire de la Société . . . par le docteur P. Duroziez', 87–106. Cf., on the Academy of Medicine of Paris, R. Pichevin, 'La première Académie de Médecine de Paris (1804–1819)', *Bulletin de la Société Française d'Histoire de la Médecine,* 12 (1913), 196–231.

25. See, for example, Simon Schama, *Citizens: A Chronicle of the French Revolution* (New York: 1989).
26. See, for example, Cissie C. Fairchilds, *Poverty and Charity in Aix-en-Provence, 1640–1789* (Baltimore: 1976).
27. We have no comprehensive account of French public health in the nineteenth century. Elements of a survey can be found in Jacques Léonard, *La Médecine entre les savoirs et les pouvoirs: Histoire intellectuelle et politique de la médecine française au XIXe siècle* (Paris: 1981), and Alain Bideau *et al.*, 'La Mortalité', in J. and M. Dupâquier (eds), *Histoire de la population française,* 4 vols, (Paris: 1988), Vol. 3, ch. 6. For a useful brief overview, see Olivier Faure, 'Les Politiques sociales de la santé au XIXe siècle', *Cahiers de la recherche en travail social,* no. 16 (1989), 29–38. An excellent monographic study of public health at the local level, showing how laws and institutions worked in practice and the social context in which they operated, can be found in Evelyn Bernette Ackerman, *Health Care in the Parisian Countryside, 1800–1914* (New Brunswick: 1990), which deals with the department of Seine-et-Oise. See also Chantal Beauchamp, *Délivrez-nous du mal: Épidémies, endémies, médecine et hygiène au XIXe siècle dans l'Indre, l'Indre-et-Loire et le Loir-et-Cher* (n.p., 1990), and Jacques Léonard, 'La Santé publique en Bretagne en 1889', *Annales de Bretagne* 91 (1984), 287–307.
28. See Ann F. La Berge, 'Edwin Chadwick and the French Connection', *Bulletin of the History of Medicine,* 62 (1988): 23–41.
29. For this interpretation, see Allan Mitchell, *The Divided Path: The German Influence on Social Reform in France after 1870* (Chapel Hill: 1991).
30. Erwin H. Ackerknecht made the case for the significance of the French hygienists in a seminal article, 'Hygiene in France, 1815–1848', *Bulletin of the History of Medicine,* 22 (1948), 117–55; see also *idem, op. cit.* (note 24), ch. 13. The most important contribution to the history of the early French public health movement, however, is the work of Ann F. La Berge, beginning with her 1974 dissertation, 'Public Health in France and the French Public Health Movement, 1815–1848' (University of Tennessee), followed by a series of pioneering articles and ultimately a book: *Mission and Method: The Early Nineteenth-Century French Public*

Health Movement (Cambridge: 1992). (I am grateful to La Berge for sharing excerpts from the unpublished manuscript at an earlier stage of the preparation of this chapter.) See also *idem,* 'The French Public Health Movement, 1815–1848', *Proceedings of the Western Society for French History, 1975*, 337–53, and 'The Early Nineteenth-Century French Public Health Movement: The Disciplinary Development and Institutionalization of *hygiène publique*', *Bulletin of the History of Médicine,* 58 (1984), 363–79. The useful overview by Bernard Lécuyer, 'L'Hygiène en France avant Pasteur, 1750–1850', in Claire-Salomon Bayet and Bernard Lécuyer (eds), *Pasteur et la Révolution pastorienne* (Paris: 1986), 67–139, relies extensively (as does the present account) on La Berge's work.

31. Fodéré, *Traité de médecine légale et d'hygiène publique, ou de police de santé adaptée aux lois de l'Empire Français,* 6 vols, (Paris: 1813); an earlier edition appeared under a different title in 1799. *Idem, Leçons sur les épidémies et l'hygiène publique,* 4 vols, (Paris: 1822–4).
32. See Bernard Lécuyer, 'Médecins et observateurs sociaux: Les *Annales d'hygiène publique et de médecine légale* (1820–1850)', in *Pour une histoire de la statistique* (Paris: 1977), 445–75.
33. On the medical profession and public health programmes, see Jacques Léonard, 'Les Relations entre le corps medical et les instances administratives locales en France de 1803 à 1892', *Histoire des sciences médicales,* 22 (1988), 289–99.
34. See Robert G. Dunbar, 'The Introduction of the Practice of Vaccination Into Napoleonic France', *Bulletin of the History of Medicine,* 10 (1941), 635–50.
35. See Matthew Ramsey, 'Property Rights and the Right to Health: The Regulation of Secret Remedies in France, 1789–1815', in W. F. Bynum and Roy Porter (eds), *Medical Fringe & Medical Orthodoxy, 1750–1850* (London: 1987), 79–105.
36. The capital was, of course, a special case: post-revolutionary Paris, deprived of a mayor and subject to the oversight of a prefect of police and the prefect of the *département* of the Seine, both answerable to the Minister of the Interior, was in a sense both the chief victim and the prime beneficiary of centralization. On the history of the Council, see Dora B. Weiner, 'Public Health under Napoleon: The Conseil de Salubrité de Paris, 1802–1815', *Clio Medica,* 9 (1974), 271–84, and Ann F. La Berge, 'The Paris Health Council, 1802–48', *Bulletin of the History of Medicine,* 49 (1975), 339–52.
37. See Françoise Hildesheimer, 'Marseille, capitale sanitaire de la France', *Actes du 101e Congrès National des Sociétés Savantes, Montpellier, 1985, histoire moderne et contemporaine,* Vol. 1 (Paris: 1985), 135–49.
38. See George Weisz, 'Constructing the Medical Elite in France: The Creation of the Royal Academy of Medicine, 1814–20', *Medical History,* 30 (1986), 419–43.

39. On responses to yellow fever and Restoration medical institutions, see George D. Sussman, 'From Yellow Fever to Cholera: A Study of French Government Policy: Medical Professionalism and Popular Movements in the Epidemic Crises of the Restoration and the July Monarchy', (Ph.D. Dissertation, Yale University, 1971), chs 1–3.
40. For the text, see *Recueil des textes officiels* 1 (1938), 243–8; see also 'Ordonnance du 7 août 1822 qui, en exécution de la loi du 3 mars 1822, détermine les mesures relatives au régime et à la police sanitaire', *ibid.*, 248–71.
41. Say, *Traité d'économie politique* (1803); Sismondi, *Nouveaux principes d'économie politique* (1819).
42. See the detailed analysis, focusing on Villermé, in William Coleman, *Death is a Social Disease: Public Health and Political Economy in Early Industrial France* (Madison: 1982).
43. The starting point is Erwin H. Ackerknecht, 'Anticontagionism between 1821 and 1867', *Bulletin of the History of Medicine,* 22 (1948), 562–93. For an assessment of the debates and an attempt to revive the analysis of 'epidemiology's social constitution', see Roger Cooter, 'Anticontagionism and History's Medical Record', in *The Problem of Medical Knowledge,* P. Wright and A. Treacher (eds), (Edinburgh: 1982), 87–108, (quotation, 93).
44. On the pervasive belief in the pathogenic properties of stenches and noxious gases, see Alain Corbin, *The Foul and the Fragrant: Odor and the French Social Imagination* (Cambridge, Mass.: 1986).
45. On the functions of the early nineteenth-century hospital, see the useful local studies by Evelyn Ackerman, 'The Hospital of Mantes-la-Jolie in the First Half of the Nineteenth Century', *Proceedings of the Consortium on Revolutionary Europe,* 1978, 200–7, and Olivier Faure, *Genèse de l'hôpital moderne: les hospices civils de Lyon de 1802 à 1845* (Lyons: 1982).
46. On the workings of this system, see Evelyn Ackerman, 'Medical Care in the Countryside Near Paris, 1800–1914', *Annals of the New York Academy of Sciences,* 412 (1983), 1–18.
47. Dora B. Weiner, 'The Role of the Doctor in Welfare Work: The Philanthropic Society of Paris, 1780–1815', *Historical Reflections/Réflexions historiques,* 9 (1982), 279–304.
48. See George D. Sussman, 'Enlightened Health Reform, Professional Medicine, and Traditional Society: The Cantonal Physicians of the Bas-Rhin, 1810–1870', *Bulletin of the History of Medicine,* 51 (1977), 565–84.
49. See Matthew Ramsey, *Professional and Popular Medicine in France, 1770–1830: The Social World of Medical Practice* (Cambridge, 1988), ch. 2.
50. See Ramsey, *op. cit.* (note 35).
51. See Jill Harsin, *Policing Prostitution in Nineteenth-Century Paris* (Princeton: 1985), and, on France as a whole in the later part of the

century, Alain Corbin, *Women for Hire: Prostitution and Sexuality in France after 1850,* tr. Alan Sheridan (Cambridge, Mass.: 1990).

52. On the early history of the vaccination campaign, see Yves-Marie Bercé, *Le Chaudron et la lancette: croyances populaires et médecine préventive, 1798–1830* (Paris: 1984); for a longer perspective, see Pierre Darmon, *La Longue Traque de la variole: les pionniers de la médecine préventive* (Paris: 1986).
53. See Sussman, *op. cit.* (note 39), ch. 3.
54. The record of prosecutions and their results can be traced in the annual reports of the Ministry of Justice, *Compte général de l'administration de la justice criminelle en France.* The numbers were in some cases derisory – only one case, for example, in 1830, the year in which the Bourbon monarchy, which had promulgated the legislation of 1822, collapsed.
55. Parent-Duchâtelet, *De la prostitution dans la ville de Paris,* 2 vols, (Paris: 1836), and *Hygiène publique,* 2 vols, (Paris: 1836); Villermé, *Tableau de l'état physique et moral des ouvriers employés dans les manufactures de coton, de laine, et de soie,* 2 vols, (Paris: 1840).
56. On the cholera in Paris, see François Delaporte, *Disease and Civilization: The Cholera in Paris, 1832,* tr. Arthur Goldhammer (Cambridge, Mass.: 1986), and Catherine Jean Kudlick, 'Disease, Public Health, and Urban Social Relations: Perceptions of Cholera and the Paris Environment, 1830–1850', (Ph.D. Dissertation, University of California, Berkeley, 1988). For a national perspective, see Patrice Bourdelais and Jean-Yves Raulot, *Une peur bleue: Histoire du choléra en France, 1832–1854* (Paris: 1987).
57. See Sussman, *op. cit.* (note 39), ch. 5.
58. For an instructive account of how the system functioned in practice at the local level, see Guy Thuillier, 'Hygiène et salubrité en Nivernais au dix-neuvième siècle', *Revue d'histoire économique et sociale,* 45 (1967), 306–25.
59. This is the theme of Vincent-Pierre Comiti, 'Les modalités du contrôle des structures et des actions de santé en France de 1850 à 1920', *Histoire des sciences médicales,* 22 (1988), 277–81.
60. See Katherine A. Lynch, *Family, Class, and Ideology in Early Industrial France: Social Policy and the Working-Class Family, 1828–1848* (Madison: 1988), and Peter Stearns, *Paths to Authority: The Middle Class and the Industrial Labor Force in France, 1820–48* (Urbana, Ill.: 1978).
61. See Ann F. La Berge, 'A Restoration Prefect and Public Health: Alban de Villeneuve-Bargemont at Nantes and Lille, 1824–1830', *Proceedings of the Western Society for French History, 1977,* 128–37.
62. Buret, *De la Misère des classes laborieuses en Angleterre et en France...,* 2 vols, (Paris: 1840).
63. See Dora B.Weiner, *Raspail: Scientist and Reformer* (New York: 1968).

64. See William Coleman, *Yellow Fever in the North: The Methods of Early Epidemiology* (Madison: 1987).
65. Bénédict-Augustin Morel, *Traité des dégénérescences physiques, intellectuelles, et morales de l'espèce humaine* (Paris). On Morel and degeneration, see Ian Dowbiggin, 'Degeneration and Hereditarianism in French Mental Medicine, 1840–1900', in William P. Bynum, Roy Porter and Michael Shepherd (eds), *The Anatomy of Madness: Essays in the History of Psychiatry*, 2 vols, (London: 1985), 1, 188–232, and, for the European context, Daniel Pick, *Faces of Degeneration: A European Disorder, c.1848–c.1918* (Cambridge: 1989).
66. On this programme and subsequent medical assistance measures, see Olivier Faure, 'La Médecine gratuite au XIXe siècle: de la charité à l'assistance', *Histoire, économie, société* 3 (1984), 593–608.
67. See George Weisz, 'The Politics of Medical Professionalization in France, 1845–48', *Journal of Social History*, 12 (1978–79), 3–30.
68. Jeanne Gaillard, 'Une expérience de médecine gratuite au XIXe siècle: l'arrêté d'Haussmann du 20 avril 1853', *Actes du 103e Congrès National des Sociétés Savantes, Nancy, 1978: Colloque sur l'histoire de la sécurité sociale* (Paris: 1978), 61–73.
69. See Lee Shai Weissbach, *Child Labor Reform in Nineteenth-Century France: Assuring the Future Harvest* (Baton Rouge: 1989), and, for a useful discussion of the debates, Philippe Sueur, 'La Loi du 22 mars 1841: un débat parlementaire: l'enfance protégée ou la liberté offensée', in Harouel, *op. cit.* (note 8), 493–508.
70. On this and subsequent legislation on unhealthful housing, see Anne-Louise Shapiro, *Housing the Poor of Paris, 1850–1902* (Madison: 1985).
71. See David Pinkney, *Napoleon III and the Rebuilding of Paris* (Princeton: 1958), chs 5–6, and Donald Reid, *Paris Sewers and Sewermen: Realities and Representations* (Cambridge, Mass.: 1991), which surveys the entire history of the Paris sewer system and the men who maintained it from its Old Régime beginnings to the present.
72. Jean-Pierre Goubert, *La Conquête de l'eau: l'avènement de la santé à l'age industriel* (Paris: 1986). This work has appeared in English as *The Conquest of Water: The Advent of Health in the Industrial Age*, tr. Andrew Wilson (Princeton: 1989).
73. See Julia Csergo, *Liberté, égalité, propreté: la morale de l'hygiène au XIXe siècle* (Paris: 1988).
74. For an excellent treatment of French welfare and public health policies in comparative context, see Mitchell, *op. cit.* (note 29). A useful analysis of the key reforms of the end of the century and the constraints that limited French emulation of the German model can be found in Martha Lee Hildreth, *Doctors, Bureaucrats, and Public Health in France, 1888–1902* (New York: 1987). The discussion that follows owes much to both Mitchell and Hildreth. A more optimistic

view of French social welfare measures in the nineteenth century (particularly the last decades) may be found in Douglas E. Ashford, 'In Search of the État Providence', in James F. Hollifield and George Ross (eds), *Searching for the New France* (New York and London: 1991), ch. 6. In an effort rehabilitate the French record *vis-à-vis* the English and the German, Ashford notes the importance in France of a republican tradition that remained distrustful of voluntarism, philanthropy and Christian charity and sought, in the late nineteenth century, to create a welfare system consistent with French democracy. Social insurance systems as they developed in Germany and Britain were, in the first case anti-democratic, designed to undercut the Social Democratic Party, and, in the second case, élitist and 'quite consistent with punitive social assistance as it had developed throughout Victorian times'.

75. On the history of nursing, see Yvonne Knibiehler *et al., Cornettes et blouses blanches: les infirmières dans la société française (1880–1980)* (Paris: 1984).
76. On the puericulture movement and related phenomena, see Jane Ellen Crisler, '"Saving the Seed": The Scientific Preservation of Children in France during the Third Republic', (Ph.D. Dissertation, University of Wisconsin, Madison 1984).
77. See, for example, Alain Riols, 'Enseignement populaire et hygiénisme au début du XXe siècle', *Le Corps humain: nature, culture, surnaturel, Actes du 110e Congrès National des Sociétés Savantes, Montpellier, 1985, Commission d'Anthropologie et d'Ethnologie Françaises* (Paris: 1985), 209–19, on the work of the popular university of Montpellier, one of many such institutions established in France at the end of the nineteenth century.
78. Richet, *La Sélection humaine* (Paris: 1919). On the French eugenists, see William Schneider, 'Toward the Improvement of the Human Race: The History of Eugenics in France', *Journal of Modern History,* 54 (1982), 268–91; *idem,* 'The Eugenics Movement in France, 1890–1940', in Mark B. Adams, *The Wellborn Science: Eugenics in Germany, France, Brazil, and Russia* (New York: 1990); and *idem, Quality and Quantity: The Quest for Biological Regeneration in Twentieth-Century France* (Cambridge: 1990).
79. On the links between hygiene and social science in the first half of the twentieth century, see the interesting study by Lion Murard and Patrick Zylberman, 'La Raison de l'expert, ou l'hygiène comme science sociale appliquée', *Archives européennes de sociologie,* 26 (1985), 58–89; they focus on Durkheimian sociology and the case of Robert-Henri Hazemann (1897–1976), whose long career in public health took him from the hygiene bureau of Vitry-sur-Seine to the hygiene division of the League of Nations.
80. See Martha L. Hildreth, 'The French National Public Health Bureaucracy and the Bacteriological Revolution', *Proceedings of the*

Nineteenth Annual Meeting of the Western Society for French History, 1983 (1984), 316–27.

81. See Jack D. Ellis, *The Physician-Legislators of France: Medicine and Politics in the Early Third Republic, 1870–1914* (Cambridge: 1990).
82. See Martha L. Hildreth, 'Medical Rivalries and Medical Politics in France: The Physicians' Union Movement and the Medical Assistance Law of 1893', *Journal of the History of Medicine,* 42 (1987), 5–29.
83. The expression dates from the 1860s, when those who employed it (such as the liberal republican Émile Ollivier) characteristically contrasted French individualism and dependence on a paternalist state with the intermediate-level organizations and mutualism that they thought prevailed in Britain. See Alain Cottereau, 'Providence ou prévoyance? Les prises en charge du malheur et la santé des ouvriers au cours des XIXe siècles britannique et français', *Prévenir,* no. 19 (1989), 21–77.
84. See Judith F. Stone, *The Search for Social Peace: Reform Legislation in France, 1890–1914* (Albany: 1985).
85. On Pasteur, microbiology, and public health, see Bruno Latour, *The Pasteurization of French Society,* tr. Alan Sheridan and John Law (Cambridge, Mass.: 1988), and the articles by Latour ('Le Théâtre de la preuve'), Claire Salomon-Bayet ('Penser la révolution pasteurienne'), and Robert Carvais ('La Maladie, la loi, et les moeurs'), in Salomon-Bayet and Lécuyer, *Revolution pastorienne.*
86. See Hildreth, *op. cit.* (note 82).
87. For a historical overview of mutual aid societies and their relation to public social welfare programmes, see Bertrand Gibaud, *De la mutualité à la sécurité sociale: conflits et convergences* (Paris: 1986).
88. On the place of these early measures in the larger history of French social insurance, see Yves Saint-Jours, 'France', in Peter A. Köhler and Hans F. Zacher (eds), *The Evolution of Social Insurance, 1881–1981: Studies of Germany, France, Great Britain, Austria, and Switzerland* (London and New York: 1982), 93–149.
89. See Martha L. Hildreth, 'The Foundations of the Modern Medical System of France: Physicians, Public Health Advocates, and the Medical Legislation of 1892 and 1893', *Proceedings of the Western Society for French History,* (1980), 311–27.
90. On the history of regulation of wet-nursing, see George D. Sussman, *Selling Mothers' Milk: The Wet-Nursing Business in France, 1715–1914* (Urbana, Ill.: 1982).
91. On the French temperance movement and anti-alcoholism legislation, see Patricia Prestwich, *Drink and the Politics of Social Reform: Anti-alcoholism in France since 1870* (Palo Alto: 1988); *idem,* 'Temperance in France: The Curious Case of Absinthe', *Historical Reflections/Réflexions historiques,* 6 (1979), 301–19; and Allan Mitchell, 'The Unsung Villain: Alcoholism and the Emergence of Public Welfare in France, 1870–1914', *Contemporary Drug Problems,* 13 (1986),

447–71. See also Didier Nourrisson, *Le Buveur du XIXe siècle* (Paris: 1990), on the place of alcohol in the economy, society, and culture of nineteenth-century France as well as the campaign for reform.

92. On the history of water and water supplies in France, see Goubert, *op. cit.* (note 72), and 'Équipement hydraulique et pratiques sanitaires dans la France du XIXe siècle', *Études rurales,* (1984), 123–42. For an anecdotal historical overview of latrines, sewerage, and related subjects (including the role of the public hygiene movement in promoting modern methods for the disposal of human waste), see Roger-Henri Guerrand, *Les Lieux: Histoire des commodités* (Paris: 1986).
93. See Allan Mitchell, 'Obsessive Questions and Faint Answers: The French Response to Tuberculosis in the Belle Époque', *Bulletin of the History of Medicine,* 62 (1988), 215–35. David S. Barnes challenges one aspect of Mitchell's interpretation in 'The Rise or Fall of Tuberculosis in Belle-Époque France: A Reply to Allan Mitchell', *Social History of Medicine,* 5 (1992), 279–90; see also Mitchell's reply, 'Tuberculosis Statistics and the McKeown Thesis: A Rebuttal to David Barnes', *ibid.,* 291–6. Barnes suggests that higher mortality rates in France, compared with England and Germany, should be attributed to a lower standard of living rather than to less successful intervention; but he does not dispute Mitchell's basic characterization of the French anti-tuberculosis campaign.
94. A full account of the 1902 law and its background, together with the key texts, can be found in Henri Monod, *La Santé publique (législation sanitaire de la France)* (Paris: 1904); other useful contemporary publications include Ernest Mosny (physician), *La Protection de la santé publique: Loi, commentaires de la loi, règlements d'administration* (Paris: 1904), and Albert Guerlin de Guer (lawyer), *La Protection de la santé publique: les pouvoirs des maires et la loi du 15 février 1902* (Caen: 1903). See also Vincent-Pierre Comiti, 'Histoire de la loi de la santé publique de 1902', *Revue française des affaires sociales,* 37 (1983), 81–8.
95. See François Burdeau, 'Propriété privée et santé publique: étude sur la loi du 15 février 1902', in Harouel, *op. cit.* (note 8), 125–33. After surveying the impediments to the public health programme in the period before 1902, Burdeau notes the obstacles that remained after adoption of the new legislation but also the evolution of jurisprudence in a more favourable direction.
96. See E. P. Hennock, *British Social Reform and German Precedents: The Case of Social Insurance, 1880–1914* (Oxford: 1987).
97. See Richard Evans, *Death in Hamburg: Society and Politics in the Cholera Years, 1832–1910* (Oxford: 1987).
98. Hoffmann, 'Some Paradoxes of the French Political Community', in Hoffmann *et al.* (eds), *In Search of France: The Economy, Society, and Political System in the Twentieth Century* (New York: 1963), 1–117.
99. See Stanley Hoffmann, 'The Vichy Circle of French Conservatives',

in his *Decline or Renewal? France Since the 1930s* (New York: 1974), ch. 2, and Robert O. Paxton, *Vichy France: Old Guard and New Order, 1940–1944* (New York: 1972).

100. Léon Bernard, *La Défense de la santé publique pendant la guerre* (Paris and New Haven: [1929]).

101. See Alexandre Bruno, *Contre la tuberculose: la mission américaine en France et l'effort français* (1925), and, for a broader historical perspective, Lion Murard and Patrick Zylberman, 'La Santé publique en France sous l'oeil de l'Amérique', *Revue historique,* 276 (1986), 367–97

102. On the development of the French anti-tuberculosis campaign, see France Lert, 'Émergence et devenir du système de prise en charge de la tuberculose en France entre 1900 et 1940', *Social Science and Medicine,* 16 (1982), 2073–82, and D. Dessertine and Olivier Faure, *Combattre la tuberculose, 1900–1940* (Lyons: 1988), which focuses on the Lyons region but also provides a useful overview of national developments.

103. On the French social work profession, see Yvonne Knibiehler, *Nous les assistantes sociales* (Paris: 1980).

104. Allan M. Brandt, *'No Magic Bullet': A Social History of Venereal Disease in the United States since 1880* (New York: 1985), ch. 3.

105. See, for example, Georges Duhamel, 'Les Excès de l'étatisme et les responsabilités de la médecine', *Revue des deux mondes,* 21 (1934), 277–99.

106. Distrust of the public hygiene programme and public health professionals was of long standing on the Left and among workers. See, for example, Madeleine Rebérioux, 'Mouvement syndical et santé: France, 1880–1914', *Prévenir,* no. 18 (1989), *Mouvement ouvrier et santé: une comparaison internationale,* Vol. 1, 15–30, and, for a useful local study, Yannick Marec, 'Monde ouvrier, santé et protection sociale à Rouen du milieu du XIXe siècle à 1914', *ibid.,* 45–55.

107. On the transformed economic role of the state, see Richard F. Kuisel, *Capitalism and the State in Modern France: Renovation and Économic Management in the Twentieth Century* (Cambridge: 1981).

108. On this last development, see Danièle Voldman, 'Guérir du cancer et mourir de vieillesse: Histoire de l'hospice Paul-Brousse de 1905 à 1975', *Asclepio,* 35 (1983), 317–26. On the contemporary French hospital system, see also Christian Maillard, *Histoire de l'hôpital de 1940 à nos jours: comment la santé est devenue une affaire d'État* (Paris: 1986).

109. Patrice Pinell, *Naissance d'un fléau: Histoire de la lutte contre le cancer en France (1890–1940)* (Paris: 1992). The practical results, it must be said were limited.

110. Émile Vandervelde, preface to Henri Sellier and R.-H. Hazemann, *La Santé Publique et la collectivité: Hygiène et service social . . .* (1937), 3–4. Hazemann was Sellier's deputy for technical affairs; see above, note 79.

111. See the series of short articles by Peter Coles in *Nature*, 1987–8.
112. See the official publication, *La Luttre contre le sida en France* (Paris: 1992).
113. See Judson Gooding, 'An Ambivalent War Against Smoking', *Atlantic*, (1992), 50–5. Among the press reports on the initial reaction to the Evin law of 1992, see Alan Riding, 'Paris Journal', *New York Times*, 9 November, 1992.
114. On the history of French social insurance, see Saint-Jours, 'French Social Insurance', in Henri Hatzfeld, *Du Paupérisme à la sécurité sociale* (Paris: 1971).
115. On the French social security system, see Henry C. Galant, *Histoire politique de la sécurité sociale française, 1945–1952* (Paris: 1955); Douglas Ashford, *Policy and Politics in France: Living With Uncertainty* (Philadelphia: 1982), ch. 6: 'Social Security: Success by Default', and *idem*, 'In Search of the État Providence'; and André Getting, *La Sécurité sociale*, 7th edn, (Paris: 1966).
116. On the medical profession and social security, see Henry C. Galant, *The French Doctor and the State*, Skidmore College Bulletin, Vol. 52, no. 1 (1966), and Henri Hatzfeld, *Le Grand Tournant de la médecine libérale* (Paris, 1963).
117. On the changing role of the state in the national health plan, see Galant, *op. cit.* (note 116), and François Steudler, 'The State and Health in France', *Social Science and Medicine*, 22 (1986), 211–21.
118. On the state, the medical profession, and problems of cost containment, see Victor G. Rodwin, 'The Marriage of National Health Insurance and *La Médecine Libérale* in France: A Costly Union', *Milbank Memorial Fund Quarterly, Health and Society*, 59 (1981), 16–43, and Paul J. Godt, 'Doctors and Deficits: Regulating the Medical Profession in France', *Public Administration*, 63 (1985), 151–69.
119. Estimates vary somewhat. See S. Sandier, *Comparison of Health Expenditures in France and the United States, 1950–78*, US Department of Health and Human Services, Public Health Service, National Center for Health Statistics, Vital and Health Statistics, ser. 3, *Analytical Studies*. no. 21 (Hyattsville, Md.: 1983); M. Duriez, 'La Croissance des dépenses médicales depuis 1970', *Solidarité, santé: études statistiques*, no. 6, 1985, 19–38; Caisse Régionale d'Assurance Maladie d'Île-de-France, *Indicateur statistique*, 1990, p. 196 (statistics from Caisse Nationale d'Assurance Maladie des Travailleurs Salariés); and Centre de Recherche, d'Étude et de Documentation en Écconomie de la Santé, *Socio-économie de la santé: une année de recherche*, 1989/1.
120. Michel Arliaud, *Les Médecins* (Paris: 1987), 68 and *passim*. Although overcrowding has driven some practitioners to seek the security of salaried employment, opportunities have been limited, particularly outside the hospital setting. Bui Dang Ha Doan, *Les Médecins en France: perspectives de démographie professionnelle et d'organisation*

sanitaire (Paris: 1984), reporting on a survey of 1979, notes that both private practice and non-hospital salaried practice were less common among younger physicians; Jean Terquem, *Les Médecins dans la société française*, (Paris: 1992), reports a six per cent decline in salaried practitioners between 1987 and 1989. On the liberal model, see also Jacqueline Pincemin and Alain Laugier, 'Les Médecins', *Revue française de science politique*, 9 (1959), 881–900.

121. Jean-Michel Normand, 'De nouvelles règles du jeu pour la médecine libérale', *Le Monde*, 2 June, 1992.

122. For a suggestive development of this argument, see David Wilsford, 'The Cohesion and Fragmentation of Organized Medicine in France and the United States', *Journal of Health Politics*, 12 (1987), 481–503, and 'Physicians and the State in France', in Giorgio Freddi and James W. Bjorkman (eds), *The Comparative Politics of Health Governance* (London: 1988), 130–56. Wilsford explores the more general question of the powers of the French state in 'Tactical Advantages versus Administrative Heterogeneity: The Strengths and Limits of the French State', *Comparative Political Studies*, 21 (1988), 126–68, and develops an extended comparative analysis of the political economy of health care in France and the United States in *Doctors and the State: The Politics of Health Care in France and the United States* (Durham, N.C.: 1991) .

123. For an extended comparative analysis of this question, see Matthew Ramsey, 'The Politics of Professional Monopoly in Nineteenth-Century Medicine: The French Models and Its Rivals', in Gerald L. Geison (ed.), *Professions and the French State, 1700–1900* (Philadelphia: 1984), 225–305.

2

Public Health in Germany

Paul Weindling

Although public health in Germany has been associated with aspirations for national unity, the notion of any monolithic German welfare state is highly misleading. While the concept of the 'Bismarckian welfare state' has long been regarded as a seminal turning point in the evolution of the modern welfare state, the historical reality has been of a great array of systems with considerable local and regional diversity. Public health training, administration and career structures have often lagged behind other countries. Even at times of great political centralization, public health systems have remained regionalized and administratively fragmented. Despite the movement for a national ministry of health with a physician as minister – demanded by the liberal doctor Rudolf Virchow in the wake of the revolutions of 1848 – this combination of centralization and professional power has only been attained for brief periods. In the unified nation-state from the 1870s, health remained a responsibility of the constituent federal states. Although from the 1890s eugenically minded doctors supported comprehensive schemes for all doctors becoming state officials, in reality full-time public health appointments remained rarities. The Weimar welfare state was never a monolithic unity, instead resting on complex voluntary, municipal and state schemes. The Nazi period saw increasing centralization, yet also rivalries between competing state and part authorities as well as continuing regional variations. Even in the highly centralized GDR various aspects of hospital provision, health insurance and health care were immune from state intervention. Moreover, since at least the fourteenth century and with the Reformation as a stimulus, there has been a tradition of municipal initiatives in public health.

There are strong arguments for tracing the evolution of public health within the administrative confines of modern Germany. As in many other areas of German history, public health is revealing of the rise of Prussian hegemony over the rest of Germany. Comparison of the archives of the Prussian medical administration with those of other German states gives the impression that in addition to the greater scale of the Prussian administration, here was more elaborate administrative machinery with highly developed routines. Prussia consequently offers a well-documented – albeit highly complex – state, with numerous instances when the Prussian administration was influential over developments elsewhere in Germany.[1] Yet this should not obscure the varying pace of innovation in other German states. Saxony provides a good example of an innovative administration since the early eighteenth century in a state combining early industrialization with high population density.[2] Smaller states are particularly appropriate for in-depth studies, although these have been rarely undertaken. A notable exception are studies of Sachsen-Anhalt.[3] The various German states reveal wide differences, for example concerning permissive and coercive legislation for sexually transmitted diseases, or in terms of administrative personnel and practices. It has been shown that such differences persisted during the centralization of the Nazi period, when conflicts between various state and party agencies resulted in new forms of pluralism. However, long-term historical studies of the various state public health administrations as well as prosopographical studies of medical officers are lacking. This means that it is difficult to assess the career patterns and social and educational background of medical officers of health, as well as the underlying historical causality for processes of reform and innovation in public health. Studies have tended to concentrate selectively on innovative individuals rather than to identify standard routines and normal types of MOHs. Although there are some studies of central administrators and of policy formulation, peripheral practices have not been analysed. Moreover, the dearth of studies on factors affecting changes in morbidity and mortality means that correlation of administrative and sanitary improvements with health outcomes has so far eluded historians.

The diversity of German public health is even more apparent in the various towns and cities, which since the Middle Ages have been innovative in public health. Here it is necessary to take account of wide variations between urban districts of complex metropolitan centres like Berlin, Dresden and Munich and the industrial region of the Ruhr as they interacted with diverse state and municipal authorities. Further problems of the various tiers of districts and central urban administration emerge. Although the Hansa cities of Bremen, Hamburg and Lübeck provided unique instances of co-terminous state and municipal administrations, public health structures were remarkably diverse. The problem of local variation was further compounded by variations in the organization and scope of sickness insurance provisions. Thus while Berlin remained administratively fragmented prior to 1918, in the newly unified greater Berlin of the Weimar period there were tensions between the central municipal health administration and the districts which often combined greater political radicalism with a drive to introduce health centres and other innovative forms of primary health care.[4] Moreover, the local sickness insurance fund *(Berliner Ortskankenkasse)* undertook certain public health activities – for example supporting maternal and infant welfare provision, and measures against tuberculosis.

Developments within the Habsburg Empire, and the successor state of Austria, are only occasionally mentioned in this chapter, while comments on Nazi public health apply to Austria after its incorporation into Germany in 1938. This omission is unfortunate given that the Habsburg Empire was a natural casualty of the emergence of modern nation states. Habsburg public health measures – with a strong emphasis on quarantine and medical policing – exercised widespread influence during the Enlightenment. Despite the rising clinical prestige of the Vienna medical school, the public health systems of the Austro-Hungarian Empire have received scarcely any historical study. Although lagging in terms of input into the Prussian-dominated bacteriological revolution, there continued to be considerable interchange between major medical centres like Vienna and Prague with rest of Germany. Examples of Austrian public health experts working in Germany have included Max Gruber and Ignaz Kaup who were both in Munich, and Ludwig Teleky in Düsseldorf during the Weimar period.[5] That these must be ranked – with the Vienna anatomist and public health reformer Julius Tandler – as among the most innovative contributors to social medicine in the first three decades of the twentieth century, suggests that Austria should be seen as a major centre of innovation.[6]

From Territorial Fragmentation to Unification

In the early modern period state-sanctioned colleges of physicians with a supervisory control over public health were established in the multitude of small German states. For example, in 1685 Brandenburg-Prussia established state supervision of medical matters, and in 1724 a *Collegium medicum chirurgicum* was established. These supervised elaborate hierarchies of various grades of practitioners including barber surgeons and midwives. How much these theoretical hierarchies corresponded to the actuality of medical practice has only begun to be investigated. In 1776 Frederick of Prussia provided certain guidelines for state medical officials (or *physicus*), but their exact responsibilities continued to be unclear.[7]

The Enlightenment fostered an interest in the theoretical underpinnings of medicine as an integral part of state activity and of civil society. Concepts of supervision and rational administration gave rise to the concept of a state police, which was then applied to medicine. The term 'medical police' was apparently first employed in 1764 by Wolfgang Thomas Rau. The system of medical police was fully elaborated by Johann Peter Frank between 1779 and 1817 in the context of Habsburg Northern Italy, and for the Palatinate in 1800 by Franz Anton Mai. Both authors saw the need for the state to support pro-natalist population policies, and so state supervision of midwifery was a priority.[8]

Since 1808 the Prussian Ministry of the Interior had a medical department. In 1817 the Prussian state established a Ministry for Educational, Religious and Medical Affairs. While medicine developed more formal bureaucratic and administrative structures the linked responsibilities of this ministry shows the artificiality of any modern concept of a discrete medical sphere.[9] Medical administration remained in the hands of legally trained civil servants. However, university professors and other professional leaders had an input on policy through the advisory council *(wissenschaftliche Deputation für das Medicinalwesen)* established in 1808. From 1852 its deliberations were published in *Vierteljahrsschrift für gerichtliche und öffentliche Medicin.* By the late nineteenth century this academic body was of considerable prestige as a policy-making think-tank, and membership was extended to include professional leaders. A broader forum was called for in the changed political circumstances of the 1920s involving non-physicians.

State examinations led to accreditation as a *Kreisarzt* or *physicus.* These were not full-time posts, but provided physicians with extra responsibilities (and income). Much of these responsibilities were for forensic medicine. Only towards the end of the century was the division between forensic medicine and public health – conveniently linked under the rubric of medical police – becoming clearer with the advent of bacteriology. It should be noted that the administration of psychiatry in Prussia was carried out at a provincial level.[10]

State medicine was primarily oriented to infectious diseases. The law of 1835 arose from the cholera epidemics of 1831–2 giving the state extensive powers regarding sickness registration, isolation and disinfection. However, the medical reform movement dating from the 1840s represented a process of the wresting of power away from legally trained civil servants – and thereby dismantling the administrative and ideological structures of medical police. There was much admiration of English and Scottish reformers with emphasis on disease as a result of socio-economic conditions. The radical demand for a ministry of health headed by a doctor was only partially realized. Whereas commentators like Ackerknecht emphasized the democratic content of the medical reformers' programme, more recently the issue of professional power and rejection of accountability has been emphasized.[11] It was only in 1911 that a doctor took over as chief official of the Prussian medical department when it moved to the Ministry of the Interior (where it remained until 1919).[12]

The system of poor law doctors, introduced in the nineteenth century, was greatly extended with doctors assigned to districts from the 1850s until it encountered increasing hostility during the 1890s. This class of practitioner requires further investigation. Initially intended as a progressive measure, deprivation of civil rights under the poor law meant that the system became discredited.[13]

In 1855 Max Pettenkofer, a Munich chemist, replaced lectures on 'medical police' by lectures on the science of hygiene. This marked a transfer of authority from the state to the professional academic sphere. Pettenkofer was appointed to the first German chair in 'hygiene' in 1865, and by 1879 was in command of an institute.[14] New university chairs and hygiene institutes were established. Pettenkofer approached health from the perspectives of political economy. He encouraged municipal improvements, civic welfare associations and education for the purpose of improving health. He initiated a period when experts with technical qualifications in subjects like chemistry and engineering took a lead in public health improvements. Physicians also had to keep up with improvements in plumbing, drainage, ventilation, heating, lighting, disinfection techniques, washing, laundering, cooking and housing design.

In 1873 a National Society for Public Health was founded, as an offshoot of the German Association of Scientists and Doctors. Local public health associations were founded in industrializing areas like the Ruhr. The liberal faith in economic improvement was reflected in the strong interest in water supply and sewers – with intense admiration of British public health reformers.

The Reich Health Office founded in 1873 and functioning from 1876 had only a very limited monitoring and coordinating role. The office collected statistics, and subsequently established a laboratory. From 1881 the bacteriologist Koch was employed by this office. Although initially with Bismarck's physician, Heinrich Struck, as Director, he was suceeded by two legally trained general administrators. (A medically qualified Director was again appointed only in 1925.)[15] The instituting of an advisory health council (*Reichsgesundheitsrat*) of 77 medical experts in 1900 was a sign of increasing professional assertiveness.[16]

Bacteriology facilitated the transition to a more interventive approach in public health. Military and colonial interests were supportive of bacteriology, and military medical officers like Emil Behring were seconded to the new hygiene institutes. Moreover, bacteriology appealed to state administrators like Althoff as a means of improving public health without involving intervention in economic or living conditions, while facilitating administrative centralization. A good example is the case of Bernhard Nocht, a nationalistic Koch pupil, being delegated to Hamburg where he subsequently established the Hamburg Institute for Maritime and Tropical Diseases.[17]

The Prussian Medical Officers Law of 1899 provided for full-time MOHs (*Kreisarzt*) in state employment. It took many years for the transition from part-time appointments to full-time to become effective, and here Germany should be seen as lagging behind the professionalization of MOHs in Britain. In the pioneering outlying municipalities around Berlin, full-time municipal medical departments were established at Charlottenburg under Gottstein, Schöneberg under Rabnow and Neukölln under Raphael Silberstein.[18] The result was a dual system with overlapping administrative responsibilities. Taking a cue from the *Assistance Publique* in Paris, municipal hospitals made rapid developments from the 1880s.

The theoretical counterpart to these innovations were new theories of social hygiene and social medicine. Although the most notable theoreticians were Alfred Grotjahn and Alfons Fischer in Baden, there were virtually as many different theories as theoreticians.[19] A trend was the move away from economically based theories of the aetiology of illness to biologically determined theories. Eugenics and population policy became integral aspects of social medicine. These theories can also be seen in terms of extending the powers and boosting the status of public health officials. The medicalized totalitarianism of the eugenic theorist, Wilhelm Schallmayer, that all doctors be state officials and all citizens carry a health passport requiring annual medical examinations moved a stage nearer realization. Socialists like Karl Kautsky also supported demands for the socialization of the medical profession.

While theories of the social causation of disease promoted expansion of services, the administrative framework for state public health in Imperial Germany was narrow. This was a result of the liberal constitution, formalizing the reaction against the intrusive policing legacy in public administration. Apart from the poor law, family welfare was designated a matter for private philanthropic agencies rather than the state. This meant that Prussian initiatives for infant and child health as well as against chronic diseases were severely hampered from the 1890s by rigid controls from the Finance Ministry. This situation was overcome by the establishing of semi-official intermediary agenicies: nominally voluntary but dominated by medical officials, aristocrats, and senior civil servants like the mastermind of the higher education system, Friedrich Althoff. Voluntary but semi-official organizations for infant welfare, as well as for combating so-called racial poisons like alcoholism, tuberculosis and sexually transmitted diseases.[20] These organizations sponsored the introduction of dispensaries – known as *Fürsorgestellen* – for tuberculosis, infant welfare, alcoholism and sexually transmitted diseases (from 1914).

The First World War saw increasing centralization of these agencies. Prussian ministerial officials endeavoured to develop a wide-ranging programme of legislative reforms for health and population policies through an inter-ministerial council, which had the backing of military medical authorities. The programme included state health offices (*Kreisfürsorgestellen*) and the combining of services into integrated health centres. These developments can be seen as laying the foundations for the Weimar welfare state. Ironically, unification in the welfare sphere was achieved only when the imperial order was in its death throes.

The Welfare State from Weimar to National Socialism

The post-war turmoils saw the failure of efforts to institute a national ministry of health. However, the Weimar constitution made welfare work a formal state responsibility, and this provided the economically impoverished middle classes with new professional identities. Professional disputes ensued between medical officers, educationalists and social workers seeking control over family welfare provision. Eugenics offered a rationale for attaining medical control over a vast range of welfare services. Women's groups and nature therapists also objected to the profesional imperialism of the public health lobby, abortion being a major issue of controversy.[21]

Radical reformers sought to use the administrative machinery of public health to develop comprehensive systems of primary health care, linked to birth control, welfare services and education.[22] On the one hand such initiatives can be seen as pioneering in the field of social medicine with many innovations like child guidance and birth control clinics.[23] While Rockefeller observers condemned German public health work as too oriented to the provision of hospitals and large-scale institutions, municipal initiatives can be seen as an area of rapid expansion and innovation during the 1920s. The municipal outsiders became insiders within the central state: for example, the municipal health official, Gottstein, was until 1925 Prussian ministerial director. The curricula of the new state academies for training medical officers at Breslau (Wroclaw), Charlottenburg-Berlin, and Düsseldorf provide a convenient source for the professional agenda of Weimar public health.

The Weimar welfare state was a highly complex entity with a plurality of authorities. For example, there was an overlap between the jurisdictions of municipal and state medical officers. Voluntary agencies were grouped into larger associations, which worked closely with the state. There were groupings for Catholic, Protestant, Jewish and socialist welfare work.[24] A notable example is provided by the Protestant eugenicist Hans Harmsen (a post-war professor of public health in Hamburg). Thus American imports like Mothers Days and Health Weeks were given a distinctive nationalistic twist.[25] Indeed, the work of left-wing MOHs should be set against an increasingly conservative profile among the profession as a whole. Eugenics in all its varieties cemented professional links between left and right among public health professionals. In this sense Weimar social hygiene laid foundations for the nazification of public health.

Weimar public health has left an ambivalent legacy. It was theoretically innovative in fusing social sciences and medicine, also in development of health centres and service provision. Yet it had authoritarian implications, seen with its central eugenic component, and in coercive and unaccountable professional structures. It was thus possible for databanks for community care to be used by Nazis for segregation of the chronically poor and mentally ill.

The continuity of Nazi public health raises interesting problems. On the one hand many innovative medical officers were dismissed for political reasons, resulting in loss of livelihood, enforced emigration, persecution and death. Race became a major factor in public health.

Nazi public health was underpinned by a law of July 1934 uniting municipal and state health services. The Nazis dissolved Prussian autonomy with the fusion of the Reich and Prussian Interior Ministries, and there was fusion between the Reich and the various federal states. Apart from political hostility towards municipal medical officials as left wing, the law was racially motivated. The new health offices (*Gesundheitsämter*) were to administer the Nazi sterilization law of July 1933, and marriage health laws of October 1935. Medical officers were given an increasingly important role in implementing the racial and population policies.[26] Despite the drive towards centralization, there persisted a plurality of state ministerial, party and professional authorities, compounded by bitter personal rivalries.[27]

Nazism allowed a resurgence of the medical police tradition although on a modern biological, administrative and professional basis. It thus represented an antithesis to the radical populist measures of the 1848 reformers, although not to the emphasis on professional power. Calculation and efficiency dictated the need to root out burdensome and worthless lives. These lethal forms of health economics were linked to racial ideology leading to extermination and military conquest. The case of Thuringia with a model public health administration in a state which had the first Nazi government shows a fusion of racial-ideological with scientific-eugenic procedures.[28] Medical officers facilitated the Holocaust isolating Jews into ghettoes by stigmatizing them as epidemiological risks, and authorizing draconian measures of the extermination of the sick, infirm and 'racially degenerate' in occupied territories. The SS developed its sanitary service, deployed in concentration camps. Here Zyklon a disinfectant for eradicating lice as a typhus control measure, was used to murder millions in the gas chambers.

From Cold War to Unification

The Soviet Military Administration had a health department staffed by Russian medical experts, and in 1946 a central administrative authority was established. At the time it was claimed that the latter was the first fully centralized health authority responsible for the totality of the health system in Germany. The proclamation of the GDR in October 1949 resulted in the establishment of a department of health in the Ministry of Labour and Social Welfare. This came close to fulfilling the demand for a unified ministry of health, social insurance and population policy. However, a separate Ministry of Health was soon formed.

The GDR continued the traditions of social hygiene with

medicine organized on a socialized basis. Primary care was based in polyclinics located either at the workplace or in residential areas. The continuing of the insurance system, private medical practice and church-owned hospitals and welfare institutions should be noted as factors offsetting any monolithic system of socialized medicine. In theory the systems of care were well thought out. In practice the system was underfunded, problematic regarding the provision of health care at the work-place as potentially undermining confidentiality and personal privacy, and could not counteract massive environmental pollution. Apart from certain residual exceptions, unification in 1989 has meant the virtual extinction of socialized forms of health care provision, with only residual continuity of polyclinics where no alternative form of care is practicable.

By way of contrast the Western allies had no separate health department, and health was a much lower priority. Initially concern was limited to the control of epidemic diseases. In 1946 the Americans instigated a Health Committee with the brief to ensure even promotion of medicines.[29] On the whole the Allies left health matters to the Germans, somewhat unwisely given the central importance of health policies under Nazism. It meant that anomalies remained regarding the sterilization laws and there was a lack of will to de-nazify medical, administrative and professional structures. The Nazi law for the unification of health services remained in force in the Federal Republic. This was confirmed by a decision of the supreme court in February 1957.

Considerable variation has continued to characterize public health. The varying responses to AIDS well shows a division among medical officers between chilling calls emanating from Bavaria for tatooing of those with HIV and AIDS, to progressive calls for education and a changing lifestyle. From the political patchwork of the early modern period to the economically strong and unified state of the later twentieth century public health administration in Germany has been strongly shaped by the fragmentation of political structures. Initially this was because of a lack of political unity, and latterly this was because of the preservation of federal structures. While public health has been associated with regional and civic autonomy, there has been a dilemma: professional efficiency and the application of modern scientifically based approaches has undermined democratic accountability and popular participation in the development of community health services.

Notes

1. For the Prussian medical administration see M. Pistor, *Geschichte der Preussischen Medizinalverwaltung* (Berlin: 1909). *Fünfundzwanzig Jahre preussischer Medizinalver waltung seit Erlass des Kreisarztgesetzes 1901–1926* (Berlin: 1927).
2. Sächsische Landesgesundheitsamt, *Einrichtungen auf dem Gebiete der Volksgesundheits-und Volkswohlpflege im Freistaat Sachsen* (Dresden: 1922).
3. W. Kaiser and A. Völker, 'Die Entwicklung von Medizinalorganisation und Apothekenwesen am territorialen Beispiel von Anhalt', *Wiss. Beiträge Univ. Halle*, no. 54 (1987), 1–227. For a bibliography of the the numerous local studies by Kaiser and Völker see A. Völker (ed.), *Dixhuitième; zur Geschichte von Medizin und Naturwissenschaften im 18. Jahrhundert* (Halle: 1988), 214–45.
4. A bibliography of the numerous publications by Manfred Stürzbecher on public health in Berlin is much needed.
5. M. Hubenstorf, 'Die Genese der Sozialen Medizin als universitares Lehrfach in Osterreich bis 1914. Ein Beitrag zum Problem der Disziplinbildung und wissenschaftlichen Innovation' (MD thesis, Free University Berlin, 1992). This thesis augments and corrects distortions in E. Lesky (ed.), *Sozialmedizin. Entwicklung und Selbsterverstandnis* (Darmstadt: 1977).
6. Karl Sablik, *Julius Tandler. Mediziner und Sozialreformer* (Vienna: 1983).
7. Alfons Fischer, *Geschichte des deutschen Gesundheitswesens* (Berlin: 1933), Vols 1 and 2 and A. Labisch, *Homo Hygienicus. Gesundheit und Medizin in der Neuzeit* (Frankfurt am Main: 1992) for overviews of developments.
8. G. Rosen, *A History of Public Health* (New York: 1958), 160–7. U. Frevert, *Krankheit als politisches Problem 1770–1880. Soziale Unterschichten in Preussen zwischen medizinischer Polizei und staatlicher Sozialversicherung* (Göttingen: 1984).
9. For the complex administrative history of this department see Labisch and Tennstedt, *GVG*, 10–12.
10. D. Blasius, *Der verwaltete Wahnsinn* (Frankfurt am Main: 1980).
11. E. Ackerknecht, *Rudolf Virchow. Doctor. Statesman and Anthropologist* (Madison: 1953). P. Weindling, 'Was Social Medicine Revolutionary? Virchow on Famine and Typhus in 1848', *Bulletin of the Society for the Social History of Medicine*, no. 34 (1984), 13–18.
12. For prior legally trained ministerial directors of the Prussian medical department see P. J. Weindling, 'Bourgeois Values, Doctors and the State: the Professionalization of Medicine in Germany 1848–1933', D. Blackbourne and R. J. Evans (eds), *The German Bourgeoisie* (London: 1991), 198–223 (207).
13. Fischer, *Gesundheitswesens*, Vol. 2, 413–21.

14. There is no adequate biography of Pettenkofer. For a sketch see H. Breyer, *Max von Pettenkofer* (Leipzig: 1980).
15. There is no adequate study of the Imperial Health Office, *Das Reichsgesundheitsamt 1876–1926* (Berlin: 1926). For a memoir see G. Kärber, *Aus der Zeit des Reichsgesundheitsamts* (np, nd). Also M. Stürzbecher, '100 Jahre Forschung für die Gesundheit. Vom Kaiserlichen Gesundheitsamt zum Bundesgesundheitsamt', *Die Berliner Ärztekammer*, Vol. 13 (1976), 147–54.
16. Kurt Glaser, *Vom Reichsgesundneitsrat zum Bundesgesundheitsrat* (Stuttgart: 1960).
17. Nocht's significance has been overlooked by R. J. Evans, *Death in Hamburg* (Oxford: 1987).
18. See for example M. Stürzbecher, 'Aus der Geschichte des Charlottenburger Gesundheitswesens', *Bär von Berlin* (1980), 43–113.
19. For an overview see E. Lesky (ed.), *Sozialmedizin. Entwicklung und Selbstverständnis* (Darmstadt: 1977). K-D. Thomann, *Alfons Fischer (1873–1936) und die Badische Gesellschaft für Soziale Hygiene* (Cologne: 1980). There is a large and complex literature on Grotjahn. A recent synthesis is C. Kaspari, *Alfred Grotjahn (1869–1931) Leben und Werk* (Bonn: 1989).
20. P. J. Weindling, 'Hygienepolitik als sozialintegrative Strategie im späten Deutschen Kaiserreich', A. Labisch and R. Spree (eds), *Medizinische Deutungsmacht im sozialen Wandel* (Bonn: 1989), 37–56.
21. A. Grossman, 'The New Woman, the New Family and the Rationalization of Sexuality. The Sex Reform Movement in Germany 1928–1933' (Ph.D. Rutgers University 1984).
22. E. Hansen, *et al., Seiteinem Jahrhundert...: Verschütterte Alternativen in der Gesundheitspolitik* (Cologne: 1981). D. S. Nadav, *Julius Moses und die Politik der Sozialhygiene in Deutschland* (Gerlingen: 1985).
23. Feminism has led to study of the former but not the latter. Kristine von Soden, *Die Sexualberatungsstellen der Weimarer Republik 1919–1933* (Berlin: 1988).
24. E. Dietrich, 'Die Organisation der Gesundheitsfürsorge, insbesonders die Aufgaben von Reich, Ländern, Landesteilen und Gemeinden auf dem Gebiete der Gesundheitsfürsorge und die damit betrauten Stellen', A. Gottstein, A. Schlossmann and L. Teleky (eds), *Handbuch der sozialen Hygiene*, Vol. 1 (1925), 401–38.
25. Karin Hausen, 'Mütter zwischen Geschäftsinteressen und kultischer Verehrung. Der 'Deutsche Muttertag' in der Weimarer Republik', G. Huck (ed.), *Sozialgeschichte der Freizeit* (Wuppertal: 1980), 249–80.
26. Labisch and Tennstedt, *GVG.*
27. Foreign Office and Ministry of Economic Warfare, *The Nazi System of Medicine and Public Health Organization* (London: 1944).
28. P. J. Weindling, ' 'Mustergau' Thüringen. Rassenhygiene zwischen Ideologie und Machtpolitik', N. Frei (ed.), *Medizin und Gesundheitspolitik der NS-Zeit* (Munich: 1991), 81–97.

29. S. Kirchberger, 'Public Health Policy 1945–1949', D. W. Light and A. Schuller (eds), *Political Values and Health Care: the German Experience* (Cambridge, Mass.: 1986), 185–238.

3

State Medicine in Great Britain

Christopher Hamlin

As first industrial nation, Britain, it is often suggested, was first to experience the catastrophe of communicable disease in the industrial city, and thus first to respond to it. The responders – Edwin Chadwick, Florence Nightingale, William Farr, John Snow and John Simon – are among the best known figures in the history of public health. Their story is a familiar one, of institutional and state growth, of the development (or recognition) of public responsibility. Beginning in the 1840s, the first generation of sanitarians took on the big problems, the 'filth diseases' that could be conquered by sound sewers and good water. Aided by increasingly comprehensive health statistics and maturing aetiological science, their successors moved on to tackle causes of disease (or sources of ill-health) that were more obscure, or more personal, or requiring greater social readjustments, commitments, or investments. Yet always the move was toward a society in which the circumstances of life facilitated individual well-being.[1]

What drove these changes? In a broad sense, justice and rationality: they were seen to come because they were right and good. Historians have disagreed about the extent to which the coming of state medicine represented the permeation of government service by followers of the utilitarian philosopher Jeremy Bentham, and the extent to which it simply reflected the efforts of a growing cadre of civil servants to uncover and cope with the problems of the day, but their inquiry focused on the rate of progress and the identity of its achievers; the character of the achievement itself seemed unproblematic.[2] Inasmuch as public health arrangements (or aspirations) in much of the world – technologically, scientifically, institutionally and ideologically – seem similar to what was achieved in nineteenth-century Britain, it has been easy to see the British experience as paradigmatic. But to do so misses both what was unique to Britain and what is unique elsewhere. Moreover, in the past decade the fragility of the achievement has become evident. That elements of it could be so easily dismantled, that its rationale no longer seemed unarguably rational, has forced us to attend more closely to the contingency of its construction in the first place. Many recent writers have complemented the older historiography with an exploration of the ways in which public health at various periods reflected contemporary social relations – perceptions of obligation or of danger, and of the distinguishing of one class (the object of public health reforms) by another, that was to undertake those reforms.

Such study of social relations is so central to the history of public health because most of the situations deemed problematic could be justly attributed to a complex network of causes. What one typically sees, however, is the isolation of a single node in that network as *the* problem and correspondingly *the* locus of prevention, the other nodes remaining unproblematic.[3] Such a node may be a part of the physical environment (a source of water or a site of filth), or the habits of people (their consumption of alcohol, mode of housekeeping) or it may be the people themselves (as carriers of contagia or later, of undesirable hereditary characteristics). Designations of problems and solutions varied regionally – public health grew up differently in England, Scotland, and Ireland.[4] It sometimes varied town-to-town, reflecting local physical, social, cultural, or economic factors. But it also varied in time, and I shall organize this discussion in terms of three more-or-less distinct configurations of social relations: one characteristic of the deferent society of the eighteenth century, a second characteristic of the liberal industrial society of the mid nineteenth, and a third characteristic of the incipient (if never fully realized) social democracy of the late nineteenth and early twentieth.[5] I shall give a good deal of attention to the first of these as it has been too little recognized, and perhaps too little attention to the last as twentieth century state medicine merges (and in very complicated ways) into the well-known history of the welfare state. In each case it will be important to explore what 'public health' was (the term itself can mislead insofar as it summarizes modern views of problems, solutions, responsibilities), what was included, what excluded; what made a public health movement politically viable; what people were its insiders, and who remained outside.[6]

The story of public health in Britain often begins with the

famous 1842 *Report on the Sanitary Condition of the Labouring Population* by Edwin Chadwick, barrister, bureaucrat, and follower of Jeremy Bentham. Yet Chadwick was an astute synthesizer, drawing on idioms that had grown up over the previous century, and even co-opting existing institutions and modes of social action. Had he been as revolutionary as he is sometimes presented he surely would have been less successful.[7]

A key pre-requisite for the public action that Chadwick engendered was simply the notion that the people's health was a matter of public concern. The origins of this notion are obscure. During the sixteenth and seventeenth centuries the Privy Council – less so Parliament – adopted continental responses to outbreaks of plague, ordering confinement of the stricken, destruction of vermin, disinfection of household goods. By and large these steps were reactive rather than genuinely preventive, concerned with controlling the spread of plague rather than maintaining health. Only occasionally, as in the advice to Charles I of the Huguenot physician Theodore Turquet de Mayerne (1630), did discussions include steps – such as relief of overcrowdedness and destitution – to make the nation less vulnerable to plague.[8]

Whatever their success, these efforts were neither permanent nor pervasive and do not mark the birth of the state medicine of the nineteenth century. Britain, like other European nations, remained prodigal of people throughout the eighteenth century: despite the enlightenment of John Pringle and James Lind, the fact that soldiers and sailors posted to the tropics – or even to the Low Countries – died at a prodigious rate, was relatively unproblematic; it would have been utterly unacceptable a century later.[9] Moreover, any extension in Britain of a top-down approach, akin to the schemes of medical police that were arising in absolutist continental states, would have been frustrated by the weakness of the state. In England (to say nothing of the other parts of Britain) central control (especially over the kinds of environmental matters that affected health) was virtually non-existent: to a large degree counties, boroughs, and parishes were responsible for their own affairs, each conducting these with its own traditions, institutions, and ineptitude.

Yet a marked concern for the health of the people – a public health movement of sorts – is evident in the second half of the eighteenth century. Though its focus was usually local, it was not tied to innovations or reform movements in local government, or for that matter to changes in social conditions (or fuller knowledge of those conditions), or to the appearance of new patterns of disease, or to the adoption of new aetiological or pathological conceptions. This public health movement arose not out of any narrowly medical concern, but as a focus of a broader concern with social welfare and class relations. Its appearance reflects a broad change in sensibility: the rise of confidence and humanitarianism of the Enlightenment. Thomas Haskell has argued that the new capitalism brought with it crucial preconditions for this humanitarianism: a more extended social network, a notion of contractual obligation, concern for long-term consequences and for disciplined behaviour.[10] Underlying these visions of a new kind of citizen was great confidence that people could change (or be changed) for the better, a confidence traceable in part to the influence of Locke, but manifested widely in eighteenth-century Britain, as much in the rationalism of Unitarians as in the emotional reawakenings of Methodists or the quiet lights in the hearts of Quakers.

Many medical men involved themselves in the new humanitarianism. They wrote pamphlets and books about the needs of the poor, started hospitals or dispensaries and recruited subscribers, initiated or became active in charitable societies. Networks of dissenters and political radicals, excluded both from conventional symbols of professional status (e.g. fellowship in the College of Physicians) and from leadership of Anglican-dominated charities or institutions (e.g. parish institutions) were most visible in such efforts, but concern was widespread.[11] Aside from fever, the focus of much of their effort was smallpox, though the inoculation campaigns they urged remained controversial.[12] Many of these men shared a common theoretical perspective: in the middle of the century they were associated with Sir John Pringle, a Leiden-educated military physician and long-time Royal Society president who attributed fever to a process of internal putrefaction.[13] Slightly later many of them were students (or students of students) of William Cullen, the Edinburgh professor of medicine (many of the next generation of public health-oriented doctors would be students of William Pulteney Alison, in many respects Cullen's successor). For both Pringle and the Cullenians, environment, broadly understood, was central in explaining disease.

Especially important in fostering concern with social causes of disease would be the concepts of environmentally-induced debility of Cullen, Alison and many others. In explaining the pervasiveness of fever among the poor, both Cullen and Alison emphasized a debility induced by the totality of environmental conditions – poor diet, inadequate clothing and shelter, overwork, putrid fumes and insufficient oxygen combined to undermine health constantly and occasionally to throw the constitution into fever.[14] The pharmacopeia might enable one to manage such fevers, isolation of the ill might help prevent their spread, but ultimately they were nothing other than the lawful physiological manifestation of poverty. Wrote John Mason Good, in an essay awarded a prize by the dissenter-dominated and reform-minded London Medical Society: wherever multitudes of people congregated 'and especially where poverty much prevails, the allowance of food is slender, and often improper, and where little attention is paid to cleanliness, pure air, and activity ... a particular class [of diseases] ... must be more or less prevalent, and more or less active, in proportion to the extent or energy of those causes themselves.'[15] Ultimately the cause of such afflictions was price inflation, Good maintained: 'even if the strictest economy be made use of', wages might 'scarcely suffice to procure the bare necessaries of life which are continually called for.' Hence the problem was not strictly medical: 'in the cure of such complaints in such situations, little can be expected from the skill of the surgeon, if he have not influence enough with the chief parishioners to unite their efforts with his to produce a complete reformation.'[16] Although most of this anti-fever concern focused on private charity or the quasi-public charity of the parish, occasionally authors such as Haygarth of Chester would find comprehensive national policy to be the only feasible solution.[17] Dispensary practice itself reinforced such outlooks; men like Alison, R. Baron Howard, and James Phillips Kay found the experience of intervening in the lives and homes of the poor forced their attention to broad matters of social welfare and political economy.[18]

However much its immediate target might be the social and physical environment, increasingly the ultimate focus of such activity was the individual person, considered as a quasi-independent agent. As notions of political and economic liberalism took hold, the issue of the competence of persons – their capability of participating responsibly in markets, and in all other forums of social, moral, and political affairs – became acute. A debilitating environment of illness and poverty undermined that competence, contributed to an irresponsibility that generated social instability. Much of this public medicine, the focus of the concerns of the Cullenians and Good, was with making the individual competent to escape that environment. Such concern for reforming people would be central to the next formation of public health, the great public health movement of the mid nineteenth century, and is as much apparent in efforts to alter physical structures (housing reform, sewers) as in plans for institutions for moral instruction. The prototype of these reform campaigns, however, was the prison reform movement that began in the 1770s.[19]

Prison reform was partly a medical movement – reformers campaigned for architectural, administrative, and dietary improvements to prevent gaol fever – but such efforts were bound up in a changing understanding of what prisons were for. Prisons were no longer to be holding pens for those awaiting trial, or execution, or payment of debt, but sites for the engineering of the new model person. If, through incarceration, a prisoner were to develop remorse for crimes, a conscience, prudence and mental discipline (as well as physical health), all aspects of the prison environment – air, food, odour, noise, sights, contact with others – had to be controlled. Because the physical, mental and moral states of the person were conceived to be integrated and mutually influential, the process of reforming the individual could be understood physiologically. A key metaphor for the interactions that occurred within the prison was that of contagion; the totality of the prison environment, a product both of physical conditions and of the manifold influences of other inhabitants, affected any new person who came into it, its effect transmitted through air, the inescapable medium of contact. This contagion was as much a moral as a physical process; the moral contagion of the master criminal would spread to the innocent youth no less readily (or literally) than would the feverish effluvia from his debauched body.[20]

Enthusiasm for prison reform had largely collapsed by the second quarter of the nineteenth century but, transferred to the urban slum, the same conception of the law-like effect of the total environment – physical and social – on those exposed to it, is evident among first-generation sanitary reformers in the 1830s. Both slum and prison were confined communities; in either the incidence of disease both signalled the social malignancy that was its cause and exacerbated that malignancy as well. Prison reform was also prototypical for public health in reflecting the cooperation of an unusual coalition of reformers, ranging from secular utilitarians with their schemes for engineering human souls (e.g., Chadwick's mentor, Bentham) to evangelical Christians hoping to effect a redemption from bestial passion to the graced state of prudence and heightened sentiment.[21] Such coalitions would be crucial in the public health movement in the nineteenth century. Perhaps most important, prison reform, like Victorian public health, was not mainly reactive (to the existence of disease) but on the contrary was a visionary movement toward production of a new kind of person and a new kind of society.

Contemporary, but quite distinct from the humanitarian medicine of the dispensary and the social engineering of the prison was a growing concern for the fabric of towns. In the Midlands and the north parishes bloomed into industrial towns with only parochial (or even older baronial) instruments to govern themselves. In older towns too there was interest in improvement and reform, electoral, institutional, structural. Immune to the pressure of public will, the old municipal corporations had been more interested in harvesting fees to subsidize banquets than in governing towns. (Besides, they claimed, they lacked legal power to provide the water or paved and lit streets people wanted.) Citizens often opted to circumvent existing local government: they established improvement or police or paving or lighting commissions, or water companies. The means to improvement was a private act of parliament. With enough money and energy (and provided opposition was not too determined) a committee of citizens could gain passage of an act establishing such a commission as a new local governmental institution, defining its composition, stating its obligations and the limits of its powers, permitting it to raise a rate to finance its operations. Some of these commissions quickly succumbed to sloth, for others (Plymouth) brief bursts of activity interrupted long still periods, still others (Leamington, Leeds, Manchester, Birmingham) acquired through amending acts more and more responsibilities and became the principal agencies of local government. Many of these commissions did undertake some sewer-building, and they did administer sweeping and scavenging operations, usually with the hope of profit, occasionally with profit.[22]

While conventions about the virtues of ventilation, drainage, cleanliness and decency sometimes figured in the rhetoric of improvement commissions, improvement was not conceived as state medicine. Crime, public safety, commerce, amenities, seemed more immediate than health.[23] But the commissions did learn much about running a modern city. The clerks and surveyors they employed, to say nothing of the elected members of the commissions themselves worked out by trial-and-error legal, financial and technical aspects of the great sanitary undertakings that would be so important in the coming century; moreover, these improvement commissions, not the short-lived boards of health established during epidemics, would be the models of Chadwick's local boards of health.

As Peter Hennock argued long ago, one should not make too

much of an eighteenth century public health movement.[24] Those medical men concerned with public health and social welfare were few and their efforts occasional and isolated. The activities of improvement commissions were episodic, asystematic, uncoordinated, and often poorly executed. Yet the patterns – professional, technical, financial, legal, administrative, ideological, theoretical – that would guide activity through most of the nineteenth century were set in the eighteenth. And, noted the Webbs, it 'passes imagination' to think how bad towns would have been without the commissions.[25]

The first three decades of the nineteenth century – the years of Napoleonic wars, Peterloo, factory agitation – saw continuation of these patterns, with establishment or enlargement of hospitals and dispensaries, the launching of public works projects both by rate-levying bodies and capitalist entrepreneurs. But increasingly these approaches to dealing with social ills were under stress. Growing towns, the coming of masses of unskilled workers, the widening cultural gap between these people and those who managed society, the rising militancy of the masses, the anti-Jacobinism that might be levelled at anyone who tried to accommodate them – all this overwhelmed the social fabric. Beyond this, the period was a hard one. Fighting Napoleon sapped the economy; there were frequent periods of dearth and outbreaks of urban (typhus) fever. At the end of the period came the first cholera epidemic. Arriving in Newcastle in 1831, and spreading throughout Britain, the cholera revealed both the inadequacy of means for controlling it – whether one saw these as sanitary works, means of isolating victims, or applicable medical skill – and the degree of distrust that had arisen between classes.[26]

While there was acknowledgement that problems of public health – understood to be problems of the condition of the working class – were truly public problems requiring coherent policy and on-going administration, there was bewilderment as to what the policy should be and what, exactly, its administrators could and should do. There were experiments: a quasi-public Board of Health made up of medical men was begun in Manchester in 1795 but it found itself unable to act in the centres of typhus, the new factories.[27] Under the auspices of the Privy Council, central boards of health were established in response to oubreaks of yellow fever in 1805/6 and cholera in 1831. Both were top-down efforts reflecting the consultation of the high-and-mighty of medicine by the high-and-mighty of politics. However energetically they might issue directives they were ill-positioned to see to their adoption.[28] In 1818 Parliament, following a select committee investigation, authorized establishment of local boards of health in

Irish cities to combat a typhus epidemic. The committee recognized the main cause of the fever as poverty but found it 'difficult to find an effectual remedy for poverty'. Although it called for relief from hearth and window taxes, it focused the public response on environmental nuisances – street-cleaning, fumigation, ventilation, and disinfection of infected houses. Among Irish medical men there was great difference of opinion as to whether this must be the extent of public involvement: some called for a public works employment programme, others for public distribution of food, fuel and clothing. Yet others insisted that such efforts remain the province of private charity and feared the pauperization of the poor.[29]

This experiment too, failed, yet the parliamentary discussions of this Irish fever epidemic do reveal the terms in which public health issues would be debated for most of the century. Should one combat disease by taking on the problem of poverty directly, coordinating relief and regulating employment? Could (and should) parliament guarantee the salubrity of towns and how far and on what grounds could public authorities interfere with rights of property? Public 'officers of health' were deemed necessary, but who would appoint them, oversee them, and what would be the scope of their activities?[30]

What we would now view as fundamental issues of social policy were thus arising in connection with matters of health. Such issues were especially troublesome to those seeking a science of efficient government, a set of axioms of political economy from which correct policy decisions could be deduced. Increasingly they were finding these principles incompatible with the public provision of many forms of social welfare. Concurrent with this agonizing over principles was a perceived crisis in the poor law – besides being expensive and inconsistent with the ideal of a free labour market, the old poor law undermined the character of its recipients, it was felt; it snuffed out confidence, ambition, prudence. A key concern in nineteenth century social policy would be that of the character of the poor; there were endless soul-searchings about the effects of charity, the distinction between the deserving and the undeserving poor.[31]

The outcome of this ideological conflict was the subdivision of the broad problem of wretchedness – poverty, disease, despair – into a number of separate though related problems, with quite different kinds of solutions: some of them reserved for voluntary charity, some for moral exhortation or education (often much the same thing), others the business of various professions or public bodies, and still others the business of no one at all. All this meant a narrowing and focusing of public health: the sphere of concern of the sanitarian in 1850 was significantly narrower than the sphere of concern of the humanitarian physician, the Lettsom or Haygarth, in 1770 or 1780.[32]

The issue of the effect on health of factory work provides a good example. The testimony of medical men as to the effect on children of long hours of work in hot, humid and dusty cotton mills was central in the campaign for factory acts.[33] In 1796 Thomas Percival argued that 'large factories are generally injurious to the constitution of those employed in them, even when no particular diseases prevail, from the close confinement which is enjoined, from the debilitating effects of hot or impure air, and from the want of the active exercises which nature points out as essential in childhood and youth, to invigorate the system, and to fit our species for the employments and for the duties of manhood.'[34] This concern for debilitation (a legacy of Cullen) was echoed by later medical men, yet under the factory acts the main role of Percival's successors – often, like P. H. Holland, committed to social and sanitary reform – would be certifying children as fit for work. Seeing a free market for labour as the only means through which the lives of the poor could be made better, these medical men allowed the work-place to be shunted off of the main line of public health.

We are fortunate to have a document that records the narrowing of that agenda in a single mind: *The Moral and Physical Condition of the Working Classes Employed in the Cotton Manufacture of Manchester* (1832), by Dr James Phillips Kay (later Kay-Shuttleworth), pupil of William Pulteney Alison of Edinburgh, yet confirmed political economist. Kay's pamphlet is full of tension. On the one hand, in good eighteenth century fashion he emphasized the law-like effect of the environment on the human constitution, physical, mental and moral: no one who understood 'that to drop a pebble on the surface of the world disturbs the planet' could fail to understand 'how, of equal necessity, events acting on the human spirit, in proportion to their novelty and power, disturb, for good or ill, the constitution of society.'[35] Cholera was co-extensive with degradation and vice, both indicator and result, Kay insisted, and factory work and slum living were the direct causes of degradation and vice – under 'the dull routine of a ceaseless drudgery' the 'grosser parts of our nature attain[ed] a rank development. To condemn a man to such severity of toil is, in some measure, to cultivate in him the habits of an animal.' Thus the factory led directly to the gin shop. Ideally, through prudence, the worker would rise in society, but all the while he was to be exercising prudence degradative forces would be accumulating. Though Kay wrote with great pathos about the lives destroyed by these forces, he was at a loss to see how they might be countered. He opposed factory acts, poor laws (a tax on capital), unions, feared working class activism, insisted the conditions of the work-place were a function of the state of trade. His solutions were minimal and often appear afterthoughts (police forces, housing regulations, moral suasion).[36]

Under the regime of political economy an issue such as improvement of the work-place, while it might remain a humanitarian issue, could not become a significant state-medical issue – notwithstanding periodic exposés of trades that systematically destroyed health. Shunted off the main line also would be such issues as child welfare, nutrition, matters of women's health (pregnancy, obstetrics, contraception), drunkenness, as well as particular diseases, like tuberculosis. Venereal diseases, mental illnesses, smallpox, and matters of food safety would hold an ambiguous status with respect to public health, each with an institution of its own. Housing would also occupy a marginal status.[37] For much of the rest of the century public health would be dominated by a focus on sensible filth – on whatever was dirty, messy, disgusting, degrading. Insofar as this carried with it a focus on health, this would be restricted largely to acute diseases (and only some of these) that might conceivably stem from exposure to filth.

Toward the end of his life Kay wrote that in the mid-1830s he had turned his attention to the 'arterial drainage' and water supply of towns as a means for improving the condition of society. Too busy to follow up the idea, he had turned it over to his friend Edwin Chadwick, then secretary of the Poor Law Commission.[38] As is well known, this 'sanitary idea' of water and drains was a key theme in Chadwick's 1842 *Report on the Sanitary Condition of the Labouring Population*, and the focus of the pioneering Public Health Act of 1848, and of Chadwick's brief career as member (and chief administrator) of the short-lived General Board of Health (Chadwick and his associates were purged in 1854, the Board was dissolved in 1858). Whatever the origins of Chadwick's preoccupation with water and sewers, it was his effort as indefatigable promoter that made 'public health' and 'sanitation' journalistic catchwords and that brought together a coalition that would sustain a remarkable sanitary activism for years to come. Chadwick's efforts also transformed what 'public health' was; he gave it the peculiar institutional and conceptual form it acquired in Britain. However critical they might be, his nineteenth-century successors were unable to reformulate it and continued to echo Chadwickian themes.[39]

With Chadwick we come to one of the most familiar periods in the history of state medicine. Yet even though key events of his career – the expulsion of medical men from leadership in the sanitary movement, the rise and fall of the General Board of Health, the great campaigns for small-bore sewers and sewage recycling, and the eclectic pragmatism of the medical men who ultimately succeeded him – are well known, there is much that is still obscure about that period and that career. As the pioneer of what have become basic amenities of civilization, Chadwick has, by-and-large, escaped critical scrutiny. He was also adept at projecting a consistent image of himself – as a discoverer of social reality who looked where no one else had, an empiricist who rejected conventions for experience, and the lonely leader of a party of virtue surrounded by the apathetic and corrupt. The effect of these assessments has been to make his rise and fall incomprehensible, and also to misrepresent (and underestimate) the ingeniousness of his achievement.[40] There is thus need to reassess Chadwick, as a social investigator, as a builder of political coalitions, finally as an ideologue and an administrator.

As an investigator, Chadwick has been seen as a pioneer in inductive social science. Eschewing the casuistry of political economy, he amassed sufficient data – on mortality, income, diet, environmental amenities – to test generalizations. These data, in Chadwick's view, demonstrated that diseases, caused chiefly by environmental filth, engendered destitution, burdening ratepayers with widows, orphans and the infirm. The compendium of evidence, from local poor law administrators (regional assistant commissioners and union medical officers) as well as from dispensary doctors, was indeed impressive, but Chadwick dealt with it not by generalizing but by extracting what fit his conclusions. In fact hard data were few and assessments of workers in the field varied greatly. Drainage and water problems were widely recognized, but several saw destitution as an indicator of the immorality of the poor, which better drains would do nothing to cure. Others, following eighteenth-century conventions, attributed disease to deprivation, and thus ultimately to the cyclicity of the new industrial economy. In short, the investigations (both for the *Sanitary Report* and for the Health of Towns Commission [1843–5]) disclosed the full range of problems of industrial towns. Chadwick, like Kay, denied that these problems were inherent to a free economy, but unlike Kay, who agonized over the implications of his economics, Chadwick suppressed heresy. Much relevant to public health never made it from local reports to the *Sanitary Report*.[41]

The view that disease was a function of environmental filth brought with it the expectation that prevention was a simple matter of installing high pressure water supplies, velocity-enhancing sewers, and sewage farms – a hydraulic system that would spirit away all evil. The effect of this new view was a redefinition of the problem. Matters of the health of individuals were subordinated to a concern with places and structures – pipes, streets, houses – which were presumed to reflect the condition of people, and presumed also to subsume and hence to obviate need for political, moral and economic considerations. The scope of this redefinition was remarkable indeed. One of the most shocking (to the investigators themselves) discoveries of the Health of Towns Commission was the revelation of widespread doping of small children and their consequent wasting into death. According to Chadwick's associate Lyon Playfair, the problem represented in the high mortality of opiated infants was not the availability of opiates, nor inadequate provisions for child care, nor poor diet, nor the economic conditions that made it impossible for working mothers to nurse, but lack of sewers. Emanations from filth made babies cross, inducing care-givers to quiet them with narcotics, claimed Playfair: with good sewers would come happy, quiet babies.[42]

Besides denaturing what might otherwise be an explosive social issue, the incident exemplifies the focusing of public health that was occurring in the early 1840s. Whether anyone really believed sewers would end the doping of children is questionable, but it is hard to deny that politically Chadwick's representation of the problem as one of infrastructure was remarkably astute. It succeeded for a number of reasons.

First, Chadwick forced the issues of preventive medicine and social regeneration upon two important constituencies where they had hitherto been peripheral. The first constituency was poor-law rate-payers and administrators. In insisting that sewers could eliminate much of the need for workhouses, Chadwick sought to put preventive medicine on the agenda of what was probably the most active of local government institutions in early nineteenth-century Britain. Though poor rates never did come to be used to finance sewers, the idea that investing in infrastructure was a prudent way of solving social problems (and lowering social costs) did stick.

The other constituency Chadwick embraced was that of the civic-minded improver: those active in improvement commissions and similar bodies who were working to make their environs prettier, safer, more efficient. Chadwick's system of local boards of health represented a rationalization of this *ad hoc* approach to local government; the Public Health Act gave a local board broad powers of municipal administration, even in matters (like street lighting) that had only the remotest connection to health. In many cases such commissions had been undertaking sanitary works, but bit by bit at great cost, having to return repeatedly to Parliament for permission to purchase lands or raise funds. By adopting the Public Health Act they could eliminate the vexation of going to Parliament, while its programme of long-term loans enabled them to undertake comprehensive systems of works instead of piecemeal improvements.[43] Over the years the boards of health did evolve into the basic units of English local government. This did mean, however, that local 'boards of health' might be only secondarily concerned with health. As (in many cases) the only effective institutions of local government, they were overwhelmed by day-to-day local administration and found street paving or widening more pressing than discovering disease (or even building sewers).[44]

Fusing public health with local government helped to transform the concept of health, and it changed what 'local government' was as well. On the one hand it was easy enough to equate 'public health' with whatever a local 'board of health' did and hence to see public health mainly in terms of municipal public works, not just sewers and waterworks, but broad, well-aired streets and parks, too. On the other, with 'public health' came legacies of eighteenth century philanthropy as well as more recent evangelism. Thus, to represent improvement as 'sanitary improvement' was to infuse it with righteousness; a newly flagged footpath, a length of drain, a sewage outfall works, was a contribution to the physical, mental and moral health of civilization and a sign manifest of the heroism of its builders. To be involved in such a crusade was holy, to oppose it sin. And even as 'local boards of health' evolved into 'local boards' and then into 'urban district councils', and as issues of social reform became submerged beneath the banality of administrative routine, the legacy of activist, utopian, even messianic sanitarianism never fully disappeared. It is intriguing to speculate how much the municipal gospel of the second half of the century reflected this odd marriage of municipal administration with the evangelism of domestic missionary movements and to wonder how close were the links between the new city-planning movement of the early twentieth-century and the utopian sanitarianism of Chadwick and his followers.[45]

Chadwick's focus on health as a matter of removing sensible filth appealed also to a third constituency, those outraged by the quality of the industrial environment. Lord Derby and others like him might know little about the long term effect of the exhalations of alkali works on health, but they did see damage to their estates and their trout streams. Although there was no lack of working-class environmentalism, the impact of pollution on the gentry surely facilitated legislation and public action. Here too, the uniting of enjoyment-of-property concerns with the life-and-death issues of epidemic fever and the emotional moral and social issues of uplift or squalor, gave the campaign against pollution a righteousness and immediacy it would otherwise have lacked.[46]

Chadwick's approach has often been seen as an application of the utilitarianism of Jeremy Bentham, whose secretary he had been during Bentham's last years. But just as Chadwick was no pure inductivist, so too the ideology in which he (and others) found warrant for sanitary improvement was far broader than utilitarianism. This was a view of nature and of the human place in it that rested on new science (mainly pathology and chemistry) but was as compatible with evangelism as Benthamism. In its loosest sense this ideology was one of environmental determinism and harmonious creation. From the eighteenth century came the view that the totality of environmental conditions determined (or at least significantly affected) the moral and physical condition of humans. From science – chiefly agricultural chemistry – came the idea that there was an ideal system of social ecology (set in natural law or ordained by God and outlined in the Levitical laws of hygiene). Such an outlook underlay the faith of Chadwick (and many others) that sewage farming *must* be profitable and salubrious, equally the belief that social, medical and moral problems were so interconnected that to solve one – that of filth – was to solve them all: drive out dirt and you drive out drunkenness, depravity and despair. It was inconceivable that nature (or God) meant things to be as they were, sanitarians insisted, surely new knowledge of the cycles of the elements of life and of the subtle effects of the environment on human well-being would make clear nature's rules for healthy living, for God was quite as much a rationalizer as Jeremy Bentham.[47]

Thus to see the early public health movement as solely an application of utilitarianism, e.g. simply as systematic investigation, analysis of alternatives, and rational response, misses much. It leaves out the utopianism, drawn from natural theology, leaves out Chadwick's shrewdness in liberating public health from the vagaries of charitable impulse (or the occasional exigencies of epidemics), and instead finding for it a central place on the agendas of those many people involved in raising and spending local rates. Likewise, seeing Chadwick as a centralist can easily misrepresent him. In comparison with continental traditions of central authority (and medical police) he was no centralist. His strategy relied on more-or-less traditional institutions of English local government, and as far as the Public

Health Act itself was concerned, with the exception of a few famous (but little-used) provisions for central government interference, it left local autonomy pretty much intact.[48] Chadwickianism – the coalition Chadwick established, his reformulation of 'public health' – characterized public health in Britain until the last two decades of the century.

Yet one should not overstress unity. Even in the late 1840s, at the height of Chadwick's power, there were, among the many who saw themselves as friends of sanitarianism, personal rivalries, ideological tensions, inter-professional conflicts, and technical and commercial controversies. While in its pamphlets the Health of Towns Association kept to the party line of the *Sanitary Report* (sewers not deprivation)[49] other short-lived sanitary and social reform organizations (e.g. the Christian Socialists) were unnecessarily alienated. Though he worked successfully with Lord Ashley (later Shaftesbury), Chadwick was unable to bring aboard the evangelical movement or the ordinary clergy.[50] Chadwick alienated the medical profession by his unwillingness to share power or to find a place in his scheme for doctors, by his promulgation of simplistic (and sensationalistic) aetiological theories, and by his snubbing of the many dispensary doctors who had committed their careers to public health.[51] William Farr, statistician to the Registrar General's Office, whose work was both empirically and theoretically important to the movement, was never fully incorporated into the movement, nor was R. A. Slaney, a Whig politician and champion of public health.[52]

Even without these allies Chadwick might have retained his position as administrator of the Public Health Act beyond 1854, but for his dogmatic insistence on inadequate technologies. Chadwick had staked his reputation, after all, on promises of the economy and efficiency of pipe sewers and sewage farms, and technical failure was accordingly a central element in his downfall. Not only did sewage irrigation prove marginal, but the cheap ceramic small-bore sewers he insisted on kept clogging and breaking and the soft water supplies he advocated were in some cases insufficient in quantity. To Chadwick and his engineers these were simply break-in problems typical of any new technology. They pushed ahead, increasingly losing the confidence of the local government agencies that were to take on the long-term debt. Some of the engineers Chadwick gathered around him were sycophants hoping to vault to the top of the profession by hitching their careers to him; as inspectors they were hypercritical of the plans of other engineers, as engineers-in-chief they often designed faulty works.[53] Here centralization was a problem, for it seemed

Chadwick would impose on towns untried schemes designed by inexperienced engineers that might prove far costlier than projected (and might, as in the case of river pollution due to water-carriage sewage, expose them to legal liabilities of unknown extent). Subsequent engineers and administrators of central agencies responsible for local public works (the Local Government Act Office from 1858 to 1871 and the Local Government Board thereafter) did not repeat the mistake. They saw their task as ensuring that plans were minimally satisfactory, not optimal, and tended to retard rather than encourage innovation.

On the demise of the General Board of Health in 1858 its responsibilities were divided. A Local Government Act Office, headed by John Lambert, took responsibility for sanctioning public works loans and for other routine matters of local administration. The new Privy Council medical department, headed by the London surgeon John Simon, took responsibility for the health of the nation. The split reflected the realization that not all matters of public health, particularly such predominantly medical matters as coordinating the national response to epidemics or administering vaccination could be subsumed into ordinary local government operations, no matter how energetic were the local boards of health. Yet it also reflected a view that innovation in health policy ought not to be encumbered by the routine of administration. The architect of this split was Simon, former medical officer of health for the City of London, who had become medical adviser to the General Board of Health after Chadwick's fall.

As with Chadwick, our view of Simon has been coloured by Simon's own presentation of his career, chiefly in his polemical *English Sanitary Institutions.*[54] He is known for bringing medicine and science into public health, thereby repudiating Chadwick's dogmatic equation of public health with sanitary engineering. Tactful and eloquent, he was far more successful than Chadwick in establishing a position in which he had access to the cabinet yet immunity from politics. Liberally interpreting the legislation that created his office, he sponsored comprehensive studies of health problems and pioneering biomedical research. In this view his resignation in 1876 is seen as unfortunate for public health; it represented the crushing of a politics of moral medicine by the amoral bureaucracy of poor law administration.[55] Yet Simon's career too needs reassessment; although important legislation was passed during his tenure (particularly with regard to vaccination and to the reorganization of local government law) many of Simon's initiatives were fruitless, and for reasons that had much to do with his personality and administrative style.

Simon did get off to a remarkable start. He did not repudiate Chadwick's anti-filth crusade, but did try to extend state medicine into such matters as occupational disease, housing, care of infants, consumption and malnutrition. The state's efforts were to be guided by a recognition of sources of excess mortality, mortality due to accidents of social organization.[56] Where Chadwick had used excess mortality as a rhetorical ornament, Simon saw a real epidemiological problem to be solved: not all excess mortality could be attributed to poor sewers, he suspected. On taking over as health chief he set his assistant, E. H. Greenhow, on an analysis of the causes of unnatural death. The resulting manifesto outlined the work he hoped to do in succeeding years. During the early 1860s his medical staff produced thorough, critical, often shocking reports on a variety of diseases and/or social problems – Edward Smith on nutrition, Julian Hunter on housing, W. A. Guy, William Bristowe and Smith on industrial diseases, Greenhow on infant diarrhoea.[57]

Yet their efforts were only marginally successful. Able to evoke outrage with a stroke of the pen, Simon, even more than Chadwick relied on revelation and righteousness to do the work of reform. This it could not do. Beyond the vast problem of gaining consent to interfere pervasively in the social and economic fabric was the overwhelming problem of just how things could be fixed – how could a legislator or administrator improve diet, for example, or make safer a trade that was inherently unsafe?[58] Simon's isolation from politics did not help; free to express opinion, he was also free to have it ignored. Yet Simon's personality was also an impediment. Where Chadwick, by temperament the administrator, had revelled in the minutiae of implementation (concerning himself, for example, with the design of kilns for firing sewer pipes) Simon was defiantly uninterested in such matters. During intense scrutiny by the Royal Commission on [London's] Water Supply in 1867–8, Simon was among the most vehement in condemning the existing supply from sewage-contaminated rivers, yet with regard to such questions as 'how pure was pure enough?' and 'how was one to know pure water?' he had little to offer and was only marginally involved.[59]

This elegant series of 'state-of-the-nation' reports having led nowhere, Simon turned in the late 1860s and early 1870s to establishing a scientific basis for public health. The research he sponsored varied greatly, from epidemiology to pathology. As an administrator of science Simon was not successful (nor were his successors); too often his investigators were too far removed – methodologically and conceptually – from the institutional research programmes of the continent.[60] Burdon Sanderson, in the early 1870s, tried to make sense of the role of microbes in disease, but without adequate means of culturing, isolating, or distinguishing microbes; Thudichum's search for the chemical signatures of certain diseases was uninformed by the new techniques and concepts of structural organic chemistry. It does not appear that Simon expected science to change preventive medicine significantly. To the end of his tenure as medical officer he remained a crusader against filth and doubted the specifity of diseases (and causes of diseases).[61] For Simon (to a degree for Chadwick too), science was authority. The aura of demonstrated knowledge complemented his eloquence; surely it would help to induce people to act.

Especially in the late 1870s and 1880s the content of that science itself seemed to militate towards government-by-experts. Breaking from the natural theology of earlier sanitarianism, Simon and many others – particularly materialists like John Tyndall, Edward Frankland, and T. H. Huxley – were envisioning a world full of hostile monads that only experts could perceive and control; public health depended on the expert, political authority had to be lodged in scientific authority. Not all sanitarians went along; many continued to follow Chadwick, Nightingale, and B. W. Richardson in believing that nature was basically good, and that all would be well if the public followed providential rules of hygiene, and that it was more important to continue a moral, humanitarian crusade than to master the intricacies of culturing typhoid bacilli. Tension was most visible with regard to vaccination and water-borne disease.[62] In most cases it did not explode into factional oppositions, for late-century public health was latitudinarian and there were multiple organizations and means of participation. At meetings of the Social Science Association (est. 1856), or its successor, the Sanitary Institute of Great Britain (est. 1877), one could revel in the enthusiasm of the sanitary crusade and hear much about ladies' sanitary associations or sanitary science for workingmen; in meetings of the Association of Municipal and Sanitary Engineers (est. 1873), or the Society of Public Analysts (1876), or the British Institute of Public Health (1893, membership restricted to holders of the diploma in public health) one could discuss technical minutiae with one's select colleagues. Many public health professionals were active in both sorts of groups.

In 1872 Simon, and many of his responsibilities, became part of the new Local Government Board, whose establishment effected the re-consolidation of local government administration with public health (poor law administration was thrown in as well). With greater powers to investigate and act, with loopholes and confusions eliminated, the LGB seemed in some ways a victory for those pushing for articulation and enforcement of national standards of health provision.[63] Indeed, medical men who had pushed for reform of health administration during the 1860s had envisioned such an agency as a veritable Ministry of Health, headed by a doctor-king (Simon).[64] Ironically, just as they succeeded in securing establishment of the bottom rank in this med-ocracy (in the mandatory appointment of medical officers of health to units of local government), its head was severed. Denied direct ministerial access, Simon felt unable to act independently and resigned the medical officership in 1876. Health, he recognized, had been subordinated to the administration of local government law; those in charge were preoccupied overseeing the conduct of elections, the assessment of rates, the accounting of expenditure, and the sanctioning of loans. Overwhelmed with paperwork, they insisted on routine; to tolerate independent action by staff members, however senior, was unthinkable.[65]

Simon's nineteenth century successors (Edward Seaton, George Buchanan, Richard Thorne Thorne), all former assistants, accepted that subordination. They were less visible and vocal than he, but probably no less effective. Certainly many of the epidemiological studies of outbreaks of disease done during the 1880s and 1890s were more rigorous than those of the 1860s and 1870s – the laboratory science, however, continued to be mediocre. Yet the political realities of the Local Government Board's existence – its struggle against other departments for funds and staff, the discomfort of important constituencies with elements of its structure and mission – did ensure that for the remainder of its existence it would never again aspire to medical activism.[66]

Yet a period of activism was beginning. Enthusiasm may have been lacking in central government, but a mass of newly hatched public health professionals, the most visible of whom were local medical officers of health, was finding much to do in individ-ual communities.[67] Notwithstanding the importance of Edwardian social legislation, a public health centred in local affairs was becoming predominant, and even national legislation was often following local initiative or confirming broad public opinion.[68] This new configuration would persist well into the twentieth century. As well as being geographically distinct from the earlier public health movement it was also, culturally, politically, and socially different.

Broadly speaking, preventive measures were concentrated less on the environment and more on the person; the vision underlying health reform came no longer from natural theology, more from socialism and eugenics; the old centres of activism – evangelical charity or technocratic Benthamism – gave way to the new centres of municipal socialism, town planning, and management of social welfare through hypothetico-deductive social (and biomedical) science. Finally, the discourse changed too, from one in which public health was a means of manipulating a threatening proletariat to one necessarily recognizant (and occasionally even expressive) of the new political power of that now-enfranchised proletariat.[69]

In some cases these changes can be traced to particular alterations in the physical, biological or political environment. Some problems that had seemed overwhelming no longer seemed so oppressive. With bacteriological studies of sand filtration confidence grew in the safety of water. With the new intermittent and contact filters the problem of sewage disposal, which had so vexed municipal governments for half a century, finally became manageable.[70] And if coal smoke still filled the air of the industrial city, a train at least allowed one – particularly the sort of 'one' likely to have the means to take legal action against it – to live further from the chimney. A new disease, diphtheria, could not easily be assimilated into the old filth paradigm of Chadwick, but had to be managed by means of a new paradigm of examination, isolation, and increasingly, decisive medical intervention. The new imperialism brought with it a broad constituency concerned for the health and size of the population, and led to interest in nutrition, working conditions, child and pre-natal care: in the old days of political economy, similar investigations of stature had failed to ignite that concern.[71]

If one seeks the broadest factors underlying these changes, two loom large: the extension of the franchise and the professionalization of public health. The impact of the newly empowered working classes is reflected in debates about the direction public health policy should take. Those who had been the objects of public action were (or at least were trying to become) its directors. For example, during its early years in the 1890s, the London County Council was besieged by petitions from workers' organizations insisting that it begin construction of sewage treatment works. A cleaner Thames was not their object, they wanted jobs. Where the Labour Party acquired control of municipal governments, as in the London suburb of West Ham, public health policy did change.[72] The public works that had formerly been undertaken to transform the physical, and ultimately the social and moral nature of the poor, were now undertaken to provide jobs. For those who needed them, jobs seemed more immediate than sewers; from our modern McKeownite perspective they may seem prescient in giving priority to food on the table over filth down the pipe. Even where Labour did not take full control, its influence was felt in the establishment of municipal 'works' departments, and in the return of housing to the public health agenda. Its impact is also manifested in the reconsideration of poor law policy, in the huge research programme established by Booth, Rowntree and the Webbs that would recognize multiple scenarios of pauperization, and make it impossible to perpetuate stereotypes of worthy widows or sturdy beggars, and make it possible to acknowledge cycles of capitalism as key sources of poverty.[73]

By no means, however, was this a people's public health. Some of what might seem a 'person-centredness' of the new public health reflected the agenda of germ-hunters, who were concerned with trapping their quarry not with facilitating a sense of well-being, or of imperialistic eugenists, for whom the populace was an object to be improved and rationalised. Public health continued to be characterized by strong conceptions of class division; as in the early nineteenth century, it remained one of the ways an 'us' dealt with a 'them'. This is especially evident in the perspective towards health issues in which women were centrally involved and in the response to tuberculosis.

The expanding electoral franchise did not until after the war take in women, and with regard to what was viewed as one of the most serious of the new public health problems, infant mortality, it was mainly women, either as wilful workers or ignorant housekeepers, who continued to be seen as the problem.[74] In programmes for inspection of schoolchildren, home visitation, education of new mothers, there remained ambiguity over whether the help given by the public health worker was support or accusation, encouragement or exhortation.[75] And as for tuberculosis, as F. B. Smith has shown, with greater concern about the disease came a host of new public health institutions, which in retrospect, seem much more concerned with regulation than prevention. Working-class consumptives (or those 'delicate' persons presumed to be at very early stages of consumption) were systematically sought out. Demands for reporting the disease might mean that their employment (and opportunities for subsequent employment) would be ended. Rules for the disinfection of personal items, for regulating contact with other family members, or for regular clinic attendence to receive medication overturned patterns of family life, and finally, consumptives might find themselves isolated and exploited in some sort of sheltered workshop. A quite different response – board games in Davos – existed for those better off.[76] Ultimately, the new programmes may have reified social distance quite as much as did the sewers of the Chadwickians.[77]

The second key characteristic of this new public health was the maturation and expansion of the professions of public health.[78] There had also been an enormous transformation in the personnel of public health. A small army of newly professionalized workers, including municipal engineers, sanitary engineers, water engineers, medical officers, sanitary inspectors, dispensary staff, reproduced in succeeding generations of members notions of the perpetuation of the profession through active engagement in public business. Increasingly they were no longer the hapless objects of factional patronage; instead their careers were shaped by their professions. Most clearly in municipal engineering, a professional career was a mobile one. One started as apprentice in one town, rose, as a position opened, to third assistant surveyor somewhere else, and moved on, picking up skills, to rise to a surveyorship, first of a small town, then perhaps of a larger town. And as institutions of local government grew, their management became too complicated for elected council members; the professional experts acquired greater freedom of action; more and more, the quality of social relations within a town, and the state of its environment would reflect their activity.[79] They alone had the special knowledge it took to convict food adulterers, inspect milk, trap drains, determine the safety of new construction, or discover carriers of deadly disease.

As Jane Lewis observes, British public health through much of the twentieth century has been hard to characterize. The maturation of the welfare state and the great changes in health policy that came with it did not transform public health in Britain; it remained an ill-unified amalgam of programmes and institutions, central and local, influenced by all manner of political, cultural and professional concerns, not all of them apparent. What has been absent is the utopianism of nineteenth-century public health, the notion of public health as a means of transforming society. If there have been philosophers of public health – new Chadwicks, Simons, or Nightingales – they have not been able to transform or even unify public health. The chief twentieth century candidate, 'social medicine', did not do that; it remained a concept mainly for theorists and idealists.[80] Modern institutions of public health, so busy keeping up with ordinary business in an era of budgetary constraint, can scarcely consider long-term goals, much less new concepts of health. Such considerations, as John Ashton has pointed out, are overdue.[81]

Notes

1. See for example Roy Acheson's representation of public health as 'an endeavour by any legitimate means that could be marshalled to ameliorate the circumstances of living in order to improve the health of the people'. R. Acheson, 'The British Diploma in Public Health: Birth and Adolesence', in E. Fee and R. M. Acheson (eds), *A History of Education in Public Health: Health that Mocks the Doctors' Rules* (Oxford: Oxford University Press, 1991), 55. W. Frazer, *A History of English Public Health, 1834–1939* (London: Balliere, Tindall, and Cox, 1950) remains a useful survey. Useful also are A. Wohl, *Endangered Lives: Public Health in Victorian Britain* (Cambridge, MA: Harvard University Press, 1983); F. B. Smith, *The People's Health, 1830–1910* (London: Croom Helm, 1980); and histories of the welfare state e.g. Derek Fraser, *The Evolution of the British Welfare State* (London: Macmillan, 1973).
2. This 'revolution in government' debate characterized scholarship in the 1860s and 1870s. Most new work on the growth of Victorian government is not structured around this dichotomy. See Roy MacLeod, 'Introduction' in Roy MacLeod (ed.), *Government and Expertise: Specialists, Administrators, and Professionals, 1860–1919* (Cambridge: Cambridge University Press, 1988), 1–24. Key papers in this debate are Oliver MacDonagh, 'The Nineteenth Century Revolution in Government: A Reappraisal', *Historical Journal,* i (1958), 52–67; S. E. Finer, 'The Transmission of Benthamite Ideas, 1820–1850', in G. Sutherland (ed.), *Studies in the Growth of Nineteenth Century Government* (Totowa, N.J.: Rowman and Littlefield, 1972), 11–32; Jennifer Hart, 'Nineteenth Century Social Reform: A Tory Interpretation of History', *Past and Present,* 31 (1965), 39–61.
3. Exemplifying this view is F. B. Smith, *The People's Health, 1830–1910.* Several works on cholera do so as well, especially Michael Durey, *The Return of the Plague: British Society and Cholera, 1831–2* (Dublin: Gill and McMillan, 1979). See also K. Figlio, 'The Historiography of Scientific Medicine: An Invitation to the Human Sciences', *Comparative Studies in Society and History,* xix (1977), 262–86; R. Cooter, 'Anticontagionism and History's Medical Record', in P. Wright and A. Treacher (eds), *The Problem of Medical Knowledge* (Edinburgh: Edinburgh University Press, 1982), 87–108; Ruth Richardson, *Death, Dissection, and the Destitute* (New York: Penguin, 1989).
4. On Scotland, for example, see R. A. Cage, *The Scottish Poor Law, 1745–1845* (Edinburgh: Scottish Academic Press, 1981); Thomas Ferguson, *The Dawn of Scottish Social Welfare: A Survey from Medieval Times to 1863* (London: Thomas Nelson, 1948); J. H. F. Brotherston, *Observations on the Early Public Health Movement in Scotland* (London: H. K. Lewis, 1952).

5. Much the same periodization, if with a different rationale, is used by Rosen, George Rosen, *A History of Public Health* (New York: MD Publications, 1958). Jane Lewis suggests we may be in a fourth formation, Lewis, *What Price Community Medicine? The Philosophy, Practice, and Politics of Public Health since 1919* (Brighton: Wheatsheaf Books, 1986), 11–12. The first and third of these formations are much less clear than the second, the standard public health of Chadwick and Simon, about which much has been written.
6. For a discussion of the nuances of various synonyms for 'public health' see R. Acheson and E. Fee, 'Introduction', in their *A History of Education in Public Health*, 8–12.
7. Both major biographies of Chadwick stress his role as innovator, R. A. Lewis, *Edwin Chadwick and the Public Health Movement, 1832–1854* (London: Longmans, Green, 1952); S. E. Finer, *The Life and Times of Sir Edwin Chadwick* (London: Methuen, 1952). M. W. Flinn provides an important introduction to Chadwick's *Report on an Inquiry into the Sanitary Condition of the Labouring Population of Great Britain (1842)* (Edinburgh: Edinburgh University Press, 1965).
8. Paul Slack, *The Impact of Plague in Tudor and Stuart England* (London: Routledge & Kegan Paul, 1985), 218–19. The efforts of pioneering demographers like Graunt and Petty were likewise isolated and uninfluential, Rosen, *History of Public Health,* 111–17.
9. Peter Mathias argues that the need for an effective military did lead to effective public health measures in garrisons and on ships, 'Swords into Plowshares: the Armed Forces, Medicine, and Public Health in the late 18th century', in J. M. Winter, (ed.), *War in Economic Development: Essays in Memory of David Joslin* (Cambridge: Cambridge University Press, 1975), 73–90. There were in fact remarkable efforts to improve military hygiene during the eighteenth century, Arnold Chaplin, *Medicine in England during the Reign of George III; the Fitzpatrick Lectures delivered at the Royal College of Physicians, 1917–18* (1919; reprint. New York: AMS Press, 1977), 75–106; N. Cantlie, *A History of the Army Medical Department* (Edinburgh and London: Churchill/Livingstone, 1973), Vol. 1; C. Lloyd and J. L. S. Coulter, *Medicine and the Navy 1200–1900,* Vol. III, 1714–1815 (Edinburgh and London: E. & S. Livingstone, 1961). Yet preventable diseases still killed large numbers of soldiers and sailors, John McNeill, 'The Ecological Basis of Warfare in the Caribbean, 1700–1804', in M. Utlee (ed.), *Adapting to Conditions: War and Society in the Eighteenth Century* (Tuscaloosa: University of Alabama Press, 1986), 26–42; Philip D. Curtin, *Death by Migration: Europe's Encounter with the Tropical World in the Nineteenth Century* (Cambridge: Cambridge University Press, 1989).
10. Thomas L. Haskell, 'Capitalism and the Origins of the Humanitarian Sensibility', *American Historical Review,* xc (1985), 339–61, 547–66. Complementing Haskell's analysis are Anne

Marcovich, 'Concerning the Continuity between the Image of Society and the Image of the Human Body – an Examination of the Work of the English Physician, J. C. Lettsom (1746–1815)', in P. Wright and A. Treacher (eds), *The Problem of Medical Knowledge*, 69–86 and Paul Langford, *Public Life and the Propertied Englishman, 1689–1798* (Oxford: Clarendon Press, 1991), 490–500. On eighteenth-century humanitarianism see David Owen, *English Philanthropy, 1660–1960* (Cambridge, Mass.: Belknap Press, 1964).

11. The most useful survey of these efforts remains M. C. Buer, *Health, Wealth, and Population in the Early Days of the Industrial Revolution* (London: Routledge, 1926). On medical aspects see J. V. Pickstone, 'Ferriar's Fever to Kay's Cholera: Disease and Social Structure in Cottonopolis', *History of Science*, xxii (1984), 401–19; *idem, Medicine and Industrial Society: A History of Hospital Development in Manchester and its Region, 1752–1946* (Manchester: Manchester University Press, 1985), 10–38; Francis M. Lobo, 'John Haygarth, Smallpox and Religious Dissent in Eighteenth-century England', in Andrew Cunningham and Roger French (eds), *The Medical Enlightenment of the Eighteenth Century* (Cambridge: Cambridge University Press, 1990), 217–53; Robert Kilpatrick, '"Living in the light": Dispensaries, Philanthrophy and Medical Reform in Late-Eighteenth-century London', in Cunningham & French (eds), *The Medical Enlightenment of the Eighteenth Century*, 254–80; Roy Porter, 'Cleaning up the Great Wen: Public Health in Eighteenth Century London', in W. F. Bynum and Roy Porter (eds), *Living and Dying in London, Medical History, Supplement 11,* (London: Wellcome Institute for the History of Medicine, 1991), 61–76. Rosen lists 16 provincial hospitals by 1760, 38 by 1800, and 114 by 1840. He lists 13 dispensaries in the provinces by 1798, 80 by 1840, *History of Public Health*, 148–9.
12. Buer, *Health, op. cit.* (note 11), 164–222.
13. Christopher Lawrence, 'Disciplining Disease: Scurvy, the Navy and Imperial Expansion 1750–1825', in D. Miller and P. Reill (eds), *Vision of an Empire,* in press. See also Dorothea Singer, 'Sir John Pringle and his Circle', *Annals of Science,* vi (1948), 127–80, 227–61.
14. C. Hamlin, 'Predisposing Causes and Public Health in Early Nineteenth Century Medical Thought', *Social History of Medicine*, v (1992), 43–70; J. V. Pickstone, 'Dearth, Dirt, and Epidemics: Rewriting the History of British "Public Health", 1780–1850', in Terence Ranger and Paul Slack (eds), *Epidemics and Ideas: Essays on the Historical Perception of Pestilence*, (Cambridge: Cambridge University Press, 1992), 125–48. W. F. Bynum, 'Cullen and the Study of Fevers in Britain', in W. F. Bynum and V. Nutton (eds), *Theories of Fever from Antiquity to the Enlightenment, Medical History Supplement 1* (London: Wellcome Trust, 1981); *idem*, 'Hospital, Disease, and Community: the London Fever Hospital, 1801–1850',

in Charles Rosenberg (ed.), *Healing and History: Essays for George Rosen* (New York: Science History, 1979), 97–115; Leonard Wilson, 'Fevers and Science in Early Nineteenth Century Medicine', *J. Hist. Med.*, xxxiii (1978), 386–407. See also James C. Riley, *The Eighteenth Century Campaign to Avoid Disease* (London: Macmillan, 1987).

15. John Mason Good, *A Dissertation on the Diseases of Prisons and Poor Houses* (London: C. Dilley, 1795), 25. On Good, an encyclopedist and evangelical socialist, see *DNB*, 22, 110–11.
16. Good, *Prisons and Poor Houses*, 44–53.
17. Lobo, 'Haygarth', 243–7.
18. For Alison, see his 'Observations on the Generation of Fever', in *Sanitary Condition of the Labouring Population, Scottish Local Reports*, PP, House of Lords, 1842, Vol. 28 (Irish University Press, Health series, Vol. 4); for Howard, see his *An Inquiry into the Morbid Effects of Deficiency of Food Chiefly with Reference to Their Occurrence Amongst the Destitute Poor* (London: Simpkin, Marshall, & Co., 1839); for Kay (later Kay-Shuttleworth) see his *The Moral and Physical Condition of the Working Classes Employed in the Cotton Manufacture in Manchester*, 2nd edn, (1832; reprint, New York: Augustus Kelley, 1970).
19. Rosen sees the somewhat earlier campaign against gin as equally prototypical, Rosen, *History of Public Health*, 138–9.
20. Robin Evans, *The Fabrication of Virtue: English Prison Architecture, 1750–1840* (Cambridge: Cambridge University Press, 1982); Michael Ignatieff, *A Just Measure of Pain: the Penetentiary in the Industrial Revolution* (New York: Pantheon, 1978). Margaret DeLacy, *Prison Reform in Lancashire, 1700–1850: A Study in Local Administration* (Stanford: Stanford University Press, 1986); cf. George Rosen, *A History of Public Health*, 143. As with the public health movement prison reformers might present their efforts as a rational response to an empirically demonstrated social problem, that of gaol fever, and particularly the legendary records of assize fevers, occasions in which the bringing of inmates into a court had set off gaol fever among the general public (and particularly the legal profession). But some of these cases were centuries old, and cannot be seen as the source of pressure for change. With new definitions of what was problematic and what was possible, modes of managing prisons that had long been acceptable were no longer satisfactory. For an exploration of the figurative implications of 'contagion' see Cooter, *op. cit.* (note 3).
21. See Boyd Hilton, *The Age of Atonement: the Influence of Evangelicalism on Social and Economic Thought, 1795–1865* (Oxford: Clarendon Press, 1988), 215–18. I am grateful to John Pickstone for bringing this work to my attention.
22. John Prest, *Liberty and Locality: Parliament, Permissive Legislation, and Ratepayers' Democracies in the Nineteenth Century* (Oxford:

Clarendon Press, 1990), 1–6; E. C. Jones and M. E. Falkus, 'Urban Improvement and the English Economy in the Seventeenth and Eighteenth Centuries', *Research in Economic History*, iv (1979), 193–223; S. Webb and B. Webb, *English Local Government: Statutory Authorities for Special Purposes* (London: Longmans, Green, & Co., 1922), 237–74; B. Keith-Lucas, *The Unreformed Local Government System* (London: Croom Helm 1980); Jesse Parfit, *The Health of A City: Oxford, 1770–1974* (Oxford: Amate Press, 1987); T.B. Dudley, *From Chaos to the Charter: A Complete History of Royal Leamington Spa* (1896; reprint. Leamington: Linaker, 1901); J. A. Hassan, 'The Growth and Impact of the British Water Industry in the Nineteenth Century', *Economic History Review*, 2nd ser., xxxviii (1985), 531–47.

23. S. Webb and B. Webb, *Statutory Authorities*, 274: 'Right down to the cholera epidemic of 1831–2 we find practically no suggestion that any work of town improvement should be undertaken on the ground that it would promote the public health.' See also Langford, *Public Life and the Propertied Englishmen*, 448–55.
24. E. P. Hennock, 'Urban Sanitary Reform a Generation before Chadwick?' *Economic History Review*, 2nd ser., x (1957), 113–20; cf. B. Keith-Lucas, 'Some Influences Affecting the Development of Sanitary Legislation in England', *Economic History Review*, vi (1953), 290–6.
25. S. and B. Webb, *Statutory Authorities*, 348.
26. Durey, *Return of the Plague;* Richardson, *Death, Dissection;* N. Longmate, *King Cholera – the Biography of a Disease* (London: Hamish Hamilton, 1968); R. J. Morris, *Cholera, 1832: the Social Response to an Epidemic* (New York: Holmes & Maier, 1976).
27. Pickstone, 'Ferriar's Fever to Kay's Cholera'; *idem, Medicine and Industrial Society*, 25–6.
28. C. Fraser Brockington, *Public Health in the Nineteenth Century* (Edinburgh: E. and S. Livingstone, 1965), 1–135.
29. F. Barker and J. Cheyne, *An Account of the Rise, Progress, and Decline of the Fever lately Epidemical in Ireland*, 2 vols, (London: Baldwin, Craddock & Joy, 1821), Vol. II, sections IV–V; Charles Creighton, *Epidemics in Britain, Vol. II, From the Extinction of the Plague to the Present Day* (Cambridge: the University Press, 1894), 267–8.
30. Barker & Cheyne, *op. cit.* (note 29), 1–8.
31. C. L. Mowat, *The Charity Organisation Society, 1869–1913: its Ideas and Work* (London: Methuen, 1961).
32. Pickstone, 'Dearth, Dirt'; Hamlin, 'Predisposing Causes'.
33. For medical testimony see Charles Wing, *Evils of the Factory System Demonstrated by Parliamentary Evidence* (1837; reprint. New York: Augustus Kelley, 1967); Robert Gray, 'Medical Men, Industrial Labour and the State in Britain, 1830–1850', *Social History*, xvi (1991), 19–43.
34. Quoted in Major Greenwood, *Some British Pioneers of Social*

Medicine (Freeport, N.Y.: Books For Libraries, 1948), 38–9.

35. James Phillips Kay-Shuttleworth, *The Moral and Physical Condition of the Working Classes Employed in the Cotton Manufacture of Manchester*, 4–5.
36. Kay-Shuttleworth, *op. cit.* (note 35), 15, 42–3, 45, 78, 91–7, 105–11. Shortly after the cholera, Kay suffered a nervous breakdown; he found moral solace eventually through a career as an educational reformer.
37. See, for example, F. B. Smith, *The Retreat of Tuberculosis, 1850–1950* (London: Croom Helm, 1988); Judith Walkowitz, *Prostitution and Victorian Society: Women, Class, and the State* (Cambridge: Cambridge University Press, 1980); Weindling, 'Linking Self Help and Medical Science: the Social History of Occupational Health', in Weindling (ed.), *The Social History of Occupational Health* (London: Croom Helm, 1985), 2–31; Ernst W. Stieb, with collaboration from Glenn Sonnedecker, *Drug Adulteration in Nineteenth Century Britain* (Madison: University of Wisconsin Press, 1959); A. Wohl, *The Eternal Slum: Housing and Social Policy in Victorian London* (London: Edward Arnold, 1977), 2–14; *idem*, *Endangered Lives*, chs 2, 10, 11. See also George Rosen, 'What is Social Medicine: A Genetic Analysis of the Concept?', *Bull. Hist. Med.*, xxi (1947), 686–8.
38. Frank Smith, *The Life and Work of Sir James Kay-Shuttleworth* (London: J. Murray, 1923), 33–4.
39. Major Greenwood, *Some British Pioneers of Social Medicine*, 86.
40. See note 4. Anthony Brundage, *England's 'Prussian Minister': Edwin Chadwick and the Politics of Government Growth, 1832–1854* (University Park, Pa.: Penn State University Press, 1988) has begun the job of giving a critical assessment of Chadwick.
41. Most interesting in this regard is the volume of *Scottish Local Reports*, PP (HL), 28, 1842 in which the overwhelming concerns were with issues of morality and poverty.
42. Playfair, 'Report on the Sanitary Conditions of the Large Towns in Lancashire', in *Health of Towns Commission, Second Report*, PP 1845, 18, (602), Appendix, pt 1, 67.
43. Wohl, *Endangered Lives*, ch. 4; Prest, *Liberty and Locality*.
44. V. D. Lipman, *Local Government Areas, 1834–1945* (Oxford: Blackwell, 1949).
45. E. P. Hennock's demonstration of the links between chapel-based networks and municipal government in Birmingham is suggestive in this regard, Hennock, *Fit and Proper Persons: Ideal and Reality in Nineteenth-Century Urban Government* (London: Edward Arnold, 1973). For links between the public health and town planning movements see A. Sutcliffe, 'Introduction: British Town Planning and the Historian', and Martin Hawtree, 'The Emergence of the Town Planning Profession', in A. Sutcliffe, (ed.), *British Town Planning: the*

Formative Years (Leicester: Leicester University Press, 1981), 2–14, 64–104; William Ashworth, *The Genesis of Modern British Town Planning: A Study in Economic and Social History of the Nineteenth and Twentieth Centuries* (London: Routledge, 1954). See also H. Finer, *English Local Government* (London: Methuen, 1933), 20–1.

46. Eric Ashby and Mary Anderson, *The Politics of Clean Air* (Oxford: Clarendon Press, 1981); Roy MacLeod, 'The Alkali Acts Administration, 1863–84: the Emergence of a Civil Scientist', *Victorian Studies*, ix (1965), 85–112; *idem*, 'Government and Resource Conservation: the Salmon Acts Administration, 1860–86', *J. British Studies*, vii (1968), 114–50; C. Hamlin, *What becomes of Pollution? Adversary Science and the Controversy on the Self-Purification of Rivers in Britain* (New York: Garland, 1987), 31–3.
47. C. Hamlin, 'Providence and Putrefaction: Victorian Sanitarians and the Natural Theology of Health and Disease', in Patrick Brantlinger (ed.), *Energy and Entropy: Essays from Victorian Studies* (Bloomington: Indiana University Press, 1989), 93–123; Graeme Davison, 'The City as a Natural System: Theories of Urban Society in Early Nineteenth-Century Britain', in D. Fraser and A. Sutcliffe (eds), *The Pursuit of Urban History* (London: Edward Arnold, 1983), 349–70; Hilton, *Age of Atonement.*
48. R. M. Gutchen, 'The Genesis of the Local Government Board', (Diss., Columbia University, 1966), 66–84, puts the case that state intervention was significant. See also Royston Lambert, 'Central and Local Relations in Mid-Victorian Britain: the Local Government Act Office, 1858–1871', *Victorian Studies*, vi (1962), 121–50. More recent writers have played down the extent of central government compulsion see Christine Bellamy, *Administering Central-Local Relations, 1871–1919: the Local Government Board in its Fiscal and Cultural Context* (Manchester: Manchester University Press, 1988); C. Hamlin, 'Muddling in Bumbledom: On the Enormity of Large Sanitary Improvements in Four British Towns, 1855–1885', *Victorian Studies*, xxxii (1988), 55–83.
49. Robert G. Peterson, 'The Health of Towns Association in Great Britain, 1844–1849', *Bull. Hist. Med.*, xxii (1948), 373–402.
50. G. Kitson Clark, *Churchmen and the Condition of England, 1832–1885: A Study in the Development of Social Ideas and Practice from the Old Regime to the Modern State* (London: Methuen, 1973); C. Kingsley, 'A Mad World, My Masters', in his *Sanitary and Social Lectures and Essays* (New York: Macmillan, 1889), 271–300.
51. On Chadwick's simplistic medical theories see Margaret Pelling, *Cholera, Fever, and English Medicine, 1825–1865* (Oxford: Oxford University Press, 1978).
52. John Eyler, *Victorian Social Medicine: the Ideas and Methods of William Farr* (Baltimore: Johns Hopkins University Press, 1979); Paul Richards, 'R. A. Slaney, the Industrial Town, and Early

Victorian Social Policy', *Social History,* iv (1979), 85–101.

53. C. Hamlin, 'Edwin Chadwick and the Engineers, 1842–1854: Systems and Anti Systems in the Pipe-and-Brick Sewers War', *Technology and Culture,* xxxiii (1992), 680–709.
54. Most scholarship follows Royston Lambert's excellent, if partisan biography, *Sir John Simon, 1816–1904, and English Social Administration* (London: McGibbon & Kee, 1963).
55. Roy MacLeod, 'The Frustration of State Medicine, 1880–1899', *Medical History,* xi (1967), 15–40; Jeanne L. Brand, 'John Simon and the Local Government Board Bureaucrats, 1871–6', *Bull. Hist. Med.,* xxxvii (1963), 184–94; Lambert, *Sir John Simon,* 547–77.
56. Simon, 'Papers relating to the Sanitary State of the People of England', in Simon, *Public Health Reports,* 2 vols, edited by E. Seaton (London: Churchill/Sanitary Institute, 1887), I, 427–88.
57. Brockington, *Public Health in the Nineteenth Century,* 194–231; Rosen, 'What is Social Medicine?', 693–6.
58. Cf. Greenhow, 'Proceedings in Reference to the Diarrhoeal Districts of England', in *Second Report of the Medical Officer of the Privy Council,* PP, 1860, 22 [2736], 57–160. Greenhow, studying infant diarrhoea, found it widely attributed to poor child care, and thus to the employment of mothers. Yet, like Playfair, this cause, because it was not a preventable cause, was reduced in status to an 'aggravating cause', losing precedence to the old Chadwickian problem of general filth.
59. *Royal Commission on Water Supply,* PP, 1868–9, 33, [4169], *Evidence,* 2810–38, 7127–34. For Simon's disinterest in details see his testimony to the Royal Sanitary Commission, *First Report,* PP, 1868–9, 32, [4128], *Evidence,* 2004.
60. Much the same could be said for British sanitary science in general. See John Eyler, 'The Conversion of Angus Smith: the changing role of Chemistry and Biology in Sanitary Science, 1850–1880', *Bull. Hist. Med.,* liv (1980), 216–24.
61. Simon, 'Filth Diseases and their Prevention', in Medical Officer of the Privy Council and the Local Government Board, *Annual Report to the Local Government Board,* n.s. 1, PP 1874, 31, [1066], 9–43.
62. D. Porter and R. Porter, 'The Politics of Prevention: Anti-Vaccinationism and Public Health in Nineteenth-Century England', *Medical History,* xxxii (1988), 231–52; Hamlin, *What Becomes of Pollution?,* ch. 8; Lloyd Stevenson, 'Science down the Drain – on the Hostility of certain Sanitarians to Animal Experimentation, Bacteriology, and Immunology', *Bull. Hist. Med.,* xxix (1953), 1–26; Charles Rosenberg, 'Florence Nightingale on Contagion: the Hospital as a Moral Universe', in Rosenberg (ed.), *Health and Healing: Essays for George Rosen* (New York: Science History, 1979), 116–36.
63. Jeanne L. Brand, *Doctors and the State: The British Medical Profession and Government Action in Public Health, 1870–1912* (Baltimore: Johns Hopkins University Press, 1965), 7–21; Bellamy, *Administering*

Central-Local Relations, 111–23.

64. See Steven J. Novak, 'Professionalism and Bureaucracy: English Doctors and the Victorian Public Health Administration', *Social History*, vi (1973), 440–62.
65. Bellamy, *Administering Central-Local Relations*, 123–4, 136–8.
66. *Ibid.*, Roy MacLeod, *Treasury Control and Social Administration: A Study of Establishment Growth at the Local Government Board, 1871–1905*, Occasional Papers in Social Adminstration, 23 (London: Bell, 1968); Brand, *Doctors and the State*, 81–2.
67. Dorothy Watkins, 'The English Revolution in Social Medicine, 1889–1911', (Ph.D. Thesis University of London, 1984), especially 23.
68. Bellamy, *Administering Central-Local Relations*, 198–209, 220, 223–4.
69. But see David Armstrong, *The Political Anatomy of the Body: Medical Knowledge in Britain in the Twentieth Century* (Cambridge: Cambridge University Press, 1983), 10–18; H. Finer, *English Local Government*, 11–12
70. C. Hamlin, *A Science of Impurity*, ch. 9; *idem*, *What becomes of Pollution?*, ch. 10.
71. Bernard Semmel, *Imperialism and Social Reform: English Social-Imperial Thought, 1895–1914* (New York: Doubleday, 1971). Cf. Wing, *Evils of the Factory System*, lxxi–xci.
72. Greater London Record Office, *LCC Main Drainage Agenda Papers*, November/December 1892; J. W. Marriott, 'London over the Border: A Study of West Ham during Active Growth, 1840–1910', (Ph.D. Thesis, Cambridge University, 1984), 154–79; N. H. Buck, 'Class Structure and Local Government Activity in West Ham, 1886–1914', (Ph.D Thesis, University Kent, Canterbury, 1980), 347–8.
73. A. M. McBriar, *An Edwardian Mixed-Doubles: the Bosanquets Versus the Webbs: a Study in British Social Policy, 1890–1929* (Oxford: Clarendon Press, 1987).
74. Deborah Dwork, *War is Good for Babies and other Young Children: A History of the Infant and Child Welfare Movement in England, 1898–1918* (London: Tavistock, 1987); B. Harrison, '"Some of them Gets Lead Poisoned": Occupational Lead Exposure in Women, 1880–1914', *Social History of Medicine*, ii (1989), 171–95.
75. C. Davies, 'The Health Visitor as Mother's Friend: A Woman's Place in Public Health, 1900–1914', *Social History of Medicine*, i (1988), 39–59.
76. F. B. Smith, *The Retreat of Tuberculosis, 1850–1950* (London: Croom Helm, 1988).
77. Armstrong, *Political Anatomy*, especially 36–7; Patricia Garside, 'Unhealthy Areas': Town Planning, Eugenics, and the Slums, 1890–1945', *Planning Perspectives*, iii (1988), 24–46; Dorothy Porter '"Enemies of the Race": Biologism, Environmentalism, and Public Health in Edwardian England', *Victorian Studies*, xxxiv (1991), 160–78.

78. This is a central theme of Harold Perkin, *The Rise of Professional Society: England Since 1880* (London: Routledge, 1989).
79. Finer, *English Local Government,* 222–3. A superb study of local government bureaucracy is G. C. Clifton, 'The Staff of the Metropolitan Board of Works, 1855 – 1889: the Development of Professional Local Government Bureaucracy', (Ph.D Thesis, London School of Economics, 1986).
80. Lewis, 'The Public's Health: Philosophy and Practice in Britain in the Twentieth Century', in E. Fee and R. Acheson, *A History of Education in Public Health,* 195–229; *idem, What Price Community Medicine?,* 2–3; C. Webster, 'The Origins of Social Medicine in Britain', *Bull. Soc. for the Social History of Medicine,* 38 (June 1986), 52–5; D. Porter, 'What was Social Medicine? A Historiography of the Concept (or George Rosen revisited)', *Bull. Soc. for the Social History of Medicine,* 38, (1986), 47–51.
81. J. Ashton and Howard Seymour, *The New Public Health: the Liverpool Experience* (Milton Keynes: Open University Press, 1988); J. Ashton and J. Ubido, 'The Healthy City and the Ecological Idea', *Social History of Medicine,* iv (1991), 173–80.

4

The People's Health: Public Health Policies in Sweden

Karin Johannisson

In current comparative research on the welfare state, the Scandinavian experience is often referred to. Among the Scandinavian countries Sweden is widely regarded as the foremost example, characterized by harmonious cooperation between major agents such as the state, private enterprise and trade unions. Community spirit is strong, having grown out of deep historical roots, resulting in an ability to join around well-defined goals in the name of a collective good. Since the sixteenth century, Sweden has been characterized by ethnic and religious homogeneity, a paternalistic state working through a well-organized bureaucracy and a state church – with priests, doctors and administrators acting as civil servants – and, since the nineteenth century, the dissemination of ideology and ideas about welfare policy to the average man through the Adult Education Movements.

In this context, i.e. the population considered as the main capital of the state, public health has been on the agenda for two hundred years. In post-war Sweden the highly set goals seemed to be within reach. The standard of living was raised to a level at which class distinctions were diminishing, and the public health-care system was operating through a network of medical services accessible to everyone at little or no expense. Even if this vision is being severely challenged in the 1990s, with ill health again increasing, especially along class lines, the Swedish health-care system rose within a welfare model characteristically named the People's Home.

It is striking that the concept of public health, by definition, seems to be associated with problems related to urbanization and industrialization. But in a country as thinly inhabited as Sweden, this process did not start on a grand scale, until the late nineteenth century. The fact that a programme for public health was elaborated more than hundred years earlier in Sweden points to the need for a more precise definition of the concept, one which encompasses all centralized activities aimed at improving the health conditions of a population.

Mercantilistic Health Policies

The history of public health in Sweden begins in the second half of the eighteenth century. Mercantilist ideas and policies had a strong hold on the Parliament. A unique era in Swedish medical politics opened up. Population growth was the focus of the debate, following basic mercantilist principles about the exploitation of natural resources by means of a large labour force and the concomitant attempt to strengthen the economic power of the state. From this point of departure, attempts were made in the 1740s to ascertain the number of inhabitants in the country, resulting in the establishment, by an Act of 1748, of national registration, on a parochial basis, of population and vital statistics. The system (*Tabellverket,* predecessor to the National Central Bureau of Statistics) from this point forward supplied pioneering demographic statistics. In 1752 the first shocking figure on the size of the population was presented: just over 2 million people inhabited Sweden (including Finland). For a small country on the periphery of Europe, trying to uphold its interests on the international market, these figures were deemed so embarrassing that a governmental decision was taken classifying them as highly secret. Strategies were devised to increase the population. There was great optimism about the rate at which this increase might run: ten, twenty, even thirty million, an optimism based on exaggerated hopes for Sweden's natural resources, fuelled by old myths about Sweden as the chosen land bulging with dormant riches.

As the natural resources were already present, the real need thus entailed increasing the number of productive labourers. There seemed to be three courses of action: 1. encouraging immigration, 2. stimulating the birth rate, and 3. helping the existing population to survive through better health and health services. In the latter case the efforts, logically enough, were to be focused on lowering infant mortality and combating the devastating diseases that killed the youngest and most productive, i.e. the epidemics.

In a sanguine programme presented by mercantilistic scientists and economists, and enthusiastically supported by political power – represented by the leading party of the Parliament (*Riksdag*) – all three methods were discussed. Although, at first, the discussion was dominated by bold speculations on how to stimulate immigration and the birth rate respectively, it soon focused on public health measures.

Here, too, the optimism was unlimited. When, in 1752, the Parliament asked the *Collegium Medicum* (forerunner to the National Board of Health) to comment on the figures regarding the causes of death statistics presented by *Tabellverket,* the reply radiated an assurance that was typical of the time.

Thus the *Collegium* considered that of the 7,191 people who had died of smallpox and measles, 'at least 6,000 could have been spared by sensible care and appropriate medicine'; of the 4,054 dying of fevers, 3,000 people 'could have been saved'; of the 3,112 who succumbed by dysentery, 2,000 could have been restored to health; of the 1,704 victims of ague at least 1,000 surely could have regained their health; of the 651 women who died in childbirth 400 could have been saved if midwives had been available: 2,816 people had died of whooping cough, and of those 2,000 probably could have regained their health, and so on. This made the potential rate of recovery nearly 75 per cent!

In the 1750s to 1770s the *Collegium Medicum* delivered a series of reports to the Parliament, presenting data and analyses of public health issues. These reports explicitly underline state interest as the primary purpose of health care (this argument, it is true, could also be used for infrastructural, professional and political reasons). Thus, in 1756, there was a comment to the effect that at least 17,000 of the 50,000 who died each year could be cured if there were more medical officers and health services. It was pointed out that not only were labour force and taxes thereby lost, but tens of thousands of unborn children, i.e. potential workers, were wasted.

With the need to save labour force for the state as the starting-point, a comprehensive programme for medical and health care was enforced. The first hospital (*Serafimerlasarettet*), intended explicitly for curable patients, was opened in Stockholm in 1752 and only a few decades later, there were already 20 of its kind distributed throughout the country. Local financing and, to some extent, state subsidies based on a system of luxury taxation on theatres, operas, lotteries, wines etc., were to pay for setting up these hospitals. This type of financial support through public contribution was controversial when, in 1815 by parliamentary decision, a special charge was to be paid by every citizen to finance the care of patients afflicted with venereal disease. In 1873, this surcharge was changed into a general health care taxation.

Royal decrees of 1763 and 1766 regulated public assistance for the sick, poor and disabled, thus splitting up the traditional hospital institution and, from then on, submitting medical care to central control, under which:

- The role of *Serafimerlasarettet* as a prototype for institutions reserved for the curable was confirmed.
- State hospitals were formally reserved for 'the dangerous and dreadful' (i.e. the mentally ill). Those falling under this category were considered incurable and to be placed in custody.
- Parishes and local communities were supposed to set up poorhouses for the old, the poor and those who were incapable of taking care of themselves, but still neither totally helpless nor dangerous.

Simultaneously, an impressive programme for health care was enforced: each district should have its own publicly employed medical officer and midwife, drugs be distributed to the poor from local depots, and the necessary hospital care offered free of charge; parish priests, bell-ringers and midwives would be mobilized in prevention campaigns on personal hygiene, epidemics, venereal disease, infant care and breast-feeding. Smallpox vaccination was introduced and made compulsory in 1815, making Sweden the most progressive European country in this respect. Further, health education was to be propagated by the production of cheap, advice literature and by systematic use of the almanacs (a splendid means of communication since they were in every man's house).

Though not conducted systematically, and not including public sanitation reforms, it was a grandiose and radical programme. It is noteworthy that it came very close to the medical reforms to be presented by the Comité de méndicité and Comité de salubrité of the French revolution – but from standpoints that were ideologically and politically very different. Thus within the Swedish programme, health care was indeed considered to be an obligation of the state, but for the sake of state interest itself, while the concept of health care as a social right seems to presuppose the modern concept of citizenship elaborated by the revolution.

One more thing made the Swedish health programme progressive: the systematized use of a state church and a publicly employed clergy serving as mediators between political power, local government and the individual. The priests played an important role not only in religious matters, but in collecting population data, handling basic medical care, determining causes of death, and distributing general information, thereby caring for and controlling the bodies as well as the souls of the weak.

In the last decade of the eighteenth century mercantilist policy had declined. This led to a void in medical policy. The ideas of the medical police system elaborated by Johann Peter Frank were propagated at the University of Uppsala by Anders Berch, professor of political economy, but without any implementations in practice. Influences of the French Enlightenment and revolution were generally weak, with a few exceptions leaving no noticeable traces on medical debate. As a state-supported political programme preventive medicine was dropped.

The Nineteenth Century: Proletarization, Moralizing, Cholera

A challenging question is: to what extent did the preventive programme of the eighteenth century contribute to improving the health of the population? The decline in mortality during the nineteenth century was one of the most radical changes in the country's demographic history. The general death rate began to drop dramatically from about 1810 onwards, and in no year thereafter did deaths exceed births. The population grew at a steadily increasing rate, almost doubling between 1750 and 1850, reaching 5.2 million by 1900. Practically the entire decline in deaths was due to a reduction in infant mortality. From a level of 20 per cent during the eighteenth century, the rate had dropped to about 8.5 per cent by the year 1900.

This decline must be analysed as a continuous social process, wherein medical innovation played a less important role than did better nutrition, an overall higher standard of living, and improved communication with the medical establishment.

The relationship between institutional medicine and a population thinly spread over a large area was a crucial point. Low population density and modest urbanization levels (15.1 per cent in 1880) implied that very few ever saw a publicly employed district medical officer, making private practice economically feasible only in larger cities. The rural population-to-doctor ratio stayed above 40,000 until the 1830s, while urban rates hovered somewhere below 1,500.

The scarcity of doctors caused eighteenth-century medical policy to remain in the hands of government, with little or no influence exercised by the medical profession. The *Collegium Medicum* was only marginally involved in the activities establishing a general public health programme; publicly-employed hospital and district physicians were expected to represent state interests. Consequently, the medical profession was hardly prestigious, an evaluation confirmed by the many complaints made by the district doctors in their annual reports to the *Collegium Medicum.* These reports, which were compiled and handed over to Parliament, constitute a most valuable source of material for the history of Swedish medicine. Here we find, among other things, the disease panorama described and analysed as well as the available drugs and therapeutic techniques, reports on life styles, nutrition, drinking, housing, climatological data etc.

The reports also contain important information about popular attitudes towards academic medicine, attitudes dominated by scepticism and an unwillingness to see a doctor when ill. First of all, there were religious reasons: disease was sent by God or fate, and curable only by them or death; second, if disease was the result of supernatural power, why should one trust a doctor operating from naturalistic premises; third, the medical officer represented governmental authorities, while the people were more confined to local patriarchalism and hierarchies, preferring capable folk-practitioners from their own stratum of society; fourth, people tended to be suspicious of the seemingly arbitrary drugs and therapeutics used by the doctors, preferring the traditional, 'visual' methods of empiricist healers.

These attitudes towards disease, causes of disease and cures against disease, however, were (as is all health behaviour) class-related, as was health itself. In the urban, secularized and bourgeois groups attitudes towards the body, disease, cures and doctors were very different. These groups relied upon private city practitioners from their own social stratum, sharing the same cultural milieu. Whereas the towns may have already had a doctor-dominated health care system from the late eighteenth century onwards, this was not the case in rural areas until the late nineteenth or early twentieth century.

Throughout the nineteenth century the balance of power among the medical actors was shifting. In 1813, the *Collegium Medicum* was transformed from a professional union into a central governmental authority (the National Board of Health, in 1968 the National Board of Health and Welfare). This meant that the medical profession was gradually transformed from a humble civil service – squeezed between governmental demands for rapid and explicit results on the one hand, and suspicion on the part of those expected to be cured on the other – into a distinguished profession which worked in close cooperation with, but not subordinate to governmental policy. In the last decades of the century, imbued with ideas stemming from evolutionism, social hygiene and the theories of degeneration and genetic inheritance, the medical profession took on the role of a key player in politics, an expert not only in matters of medicine, but in matters of society as well. 'The physician has to take over the old role of the priests', opined one representative. And this must be done in a way that may not always seem attractive to the individual, but in the name of all of society and its future. All aspects of human life, the private and the public, the physical and the moral, must be integrated in the physician's observations, ruminations and activities .

The disease panorama of the nineteenth century was, as in all of Europe, dominated by epidemics and infectious diseases: the brutal spectrum of children's diseases, malaria, dysentery, cholera, typhoid fever, pneumonia, pleuritis. Venereal disease, arthritis and alcoholism were also reported to be great problems. Pulmonary tuberculosis was increasing dramatically in the northern parts of Sweden during the latter half of the century, reaching a peak around 1900, and not to be pressed back until the second and third decades of the twentieth century. Among the everyday scourges, melancholia, gastric catarrh, chlorosis and ache were specially mentioned.

These patterns of disease can be followed through the annual reports published from the 1850s onwards by the National Board of Health, complemented by statistics on mortality and morbidity, hospital register figures and military statistics. Thus, of the 18-year-old boys who enlisted in the middle of the century (Sweden has had a compulsory military service system since 1812) about 40 per cent were rejected for varying reasons related to disease and disability.

Prevention was given no priority during these decades before the breakthrough of bacteriology. Of course there were the old health programmes extolling the virtues of personal health, but this was a programme directed towards the privileged, not the general population. Emphasizing individual responsibility, however, allowed the doctors to moralize a great deal, supplying an immediate explanation for the poor health conditions of a growing proletariat: the main cause was 'poor health behaviour', i.e. poor dietary habits, alcohol and coffee abuse, immorality, parental negligence of infants, failure to consult a doctor when ill, etc.

The low priority given to prevention led to the successive consolidation and expansion of the acute-care model. By the turn of the century, there were approximately 21,000 hospital beds in Sweden. The network of district and city practitioners, midwives and hospitals was steadily growing. In 1850, there were 400 physicians, by 1880 the number had increased to 555 and, by 1900, to 1,131. (The 1880 figures, however, still suggest only 1.22 active physicians per 10,000 population.)

In 1834, Sweden was struck by the cholera pandemic. Only a few weeks before sermons had been held in churches throughout the country, humbly thanking God for saving Sweden from this horrifying enemy. The panic grew as the contagion spread, and many cities were struck by a dreadful mortality. The quarantine decree of 1770 was strengthened, and sanitary cordons erected along coasts and main road lines. Pointing, however, to the interruptions to trade and commercial interests, together with epidemiological ineffectiveness, a bill on temporary mitigation was forced through by the Parliament in 1854.

The preventive measures directed towards the individual were at first rigid, leaning on central and local authorities for their enforcement, and discussing compulsory isolation of the victims. With increasing awareness, however, that custody did more to spread than to strangle the contagion, the preventive programme turned to the temporary dispensaries for providing information, medical advice and arranging hospital transportation. Hospital care was to be voluntary. In Sweden, as in other countries, cholera attacks and the social response to cholera, manifested inherent class antagonisms as well as suspicion towards the authorities who might knowingly spread the contagion in order to reduce society's most despised groups.

The Emergence of the Modern State: Hygiene, Sanitation, Eugenics

Cholera most brutally attacked in the slums. The urbanization process was slow in Sweden, but accelerated during the last decades of the nineteenth century when Sweden underwent tremendous changes of industrialization and modernization, transforming the country from a backward agrarian society into a modern industrial state. The 1880s has been characterized as the era in which the features of modern social life began to appear in Sweden, but also in which the price of industrialization was already visible. In the larger cities working-class areas grew along with filth, poverty and poor health. The sanitation problems were enormous.

At the same time bacteriology had started its triumphant march, having been introduced into Swedish academic medicine in the 1870s. The institutionalization of public health began in 1867, when a bill was voted in Parliament proposing the establishment of a professorship in public health. The argument was simple: 'as our doctors cannot cure the diseases, we must try to control their causes'.

The first Public Health Act of 1874 was followed by the establishment of local Boards of Health; they were to be responsible for sanitation, sewage, water supply, etc., and by the help of a so-called health police (local sanitary inspectors and medical officers), the enforcement of their provisions and instructions. Furthermore, the rural and urban doctors were urged to control 'those factors harmfully effecting public health: 1. lack of fresh air; 2. lack of fresh water; 3. insufficient or unfit food; 4. negligence of personal hygiene; 5. unfit housing and clothing; 6. alcohol abuse, immorality; 7. negligence of seeing a doctor when ill'. The number of local Boards of Health multiplied rapidly, and at the end of the nineteenth century they were all connected in an efficient network, which reported regularly to the National Board of Health.

In 1876, the first professor of public health *(Allmän hälsovårdslära)* was appointed to the Karolinska Institute, the medical school of Stockholm. In 1899, a special section for hygiene within the Swedish Medical Association was opened and, in 1907, the National Laboratory for Bacteriology (*Statens bakteriologiska laboratorium*) was opened, followed a few years later by the State Medical Institute (*Statsmedicinska anstalten*).

The results of this mobilization were impressive. By the turn of the century infant mortality had declined dramatically (but was still high: nearly 10 per cent among legitimate, and 17 per cent among illegitimate children), and the infectious diseases were on the retreat (but still represented the major cause of death).

Population growth had been strong and, in the latter part of the nineteenth century, generated a new 'population debate'. If the problem of depopulation dominated eighteenth-century policies, now the opposite problem was at the forefront. In Sweden, as in most European countries, Thomas Malthus' thesis seemed brutally confirmed by increasing proletarization and its attendant problems of malnutrition, ill-health, and symptoms of 'degeneration' such as alcoholism, venereal disease and tuberculosis. The problem was indeed complicated, a question not only of quantity, but of quality as well. A country undergoing great changes and modernization, while trying to hold its own in international competition, depended greatly upon strong, healthy and loyal citizens. Within political and medical debate the viewpoint was maintained that loss of the poor and miserable could be overlooked, or even encouraged.

A first alternative was to liberalize emigration. Sweden, like most European countries in the middle of the nineteenth century, abolished the emigration restrictions which were introduced in the mercantilistic era of the eighteenth century. The effect was radical. Between the late 1860s and the start of the First World War, one million people emigrated, most of them rural workers, resulting in a loss of one-fifth of Sweden's population.

A second alternative was to reduce population growth by contraception. But to traditional values, stamped by conservative family and sexual ideals, this solution seemed not only controversial, but questionable even with respect to long-term utilitarian strategies.

Wouldn't contraceptives result in fewer children among the 'better' social groups, whereas the proletarians would go on multiplying unrestrainedly? Following an intense, politically volatile debate in Parliament, and with strong support by the National Board of Health, information about and distribution of contraceptives were forbidden by a law code of 1910 (revoked in 1938).

A third way was to improve the population with respect to quality, by taking action on questions of social hygiene, thereby combating, at their very roots, the main causes of disease and ill-health, deficiency and undesirable genetic inheritance and, at the same time, opening up a new programme for health education.

The hygiene movement of the early twentieth century is most interesting. Inspired by a mixture of political, scientific and moral interests it was to act as a guideline for a whole social project: to allow Sweden to leave filth, ignorance and backwardness behind, and to rise like a Phoenix as a modern state. Thus the concept of people's health (*Folkhälsa*) became a major metaphor not only for health, but for a national striving for strength, efficiency and rationality.

This interest in hygiene and health was associated, in various ways, with the social changes taking place on a national level, but also with trends on the scientific and pseudoscientific international scene, such as Social Darwinism, eugenics, ideas regarding degeneration and inheritance, and a growing concern about the implications of demographic stagnation.

From the political and ideological points of view, there was an entire set of arguments for the value of improving national health by systematized action. The humanitarian and egalitarian motives (that is equal access to health care) were there of course, but they were, by far, outweighed by rational arguments such as *first* the need for an effective labour force and high quality reproduction (combined with exaggerated fears of foreign infiltration and Asian crowds swelling across the Swedish borders), and *second* by the fear of the economic strain that care for large numbers of 'deficient' would put on public assistance. Further, hygiene could be used as an instrument to handle class antagonism and restore order and social harmony in a society undergoing great social upheaval.

All these arguments were elaborated in a huge array of medical literature on hygiene and health education. The role of the medical profession was central to this movement, the close cooperation between governmental and medical authority so characteristic of Sweden here being actualized. The exchange was reciprocal: the state needed a new type of expertise to watch over an ever more complex society; the physician strengthened his professional identity by expanding into new social areas. Thus, the early twentieth century saw a wave of medicalization, integrating in the medical sphere a whole set of everyday life experience (sexuality, criminality, the vicious child).

Interesting patterns related to class, race and gender can be discerned in the 'ideological' disease panorama of the period. The diseases considered to be the most severe threats to society were – not unexpectedly – tuberculosis, venereal disease and alcoholism, social scourges believed to flourish in the slums, and from these morally feckless margins of society to be spread into the 'better' classes. This was a tricky issue in public health debate, some medical representatives harshly opposing environmentalist public health, maintaining that this did nothing more than to multiply the most miserable groups of society by helping them to survive.

The main focus, however, was not on these groups, but on the population as a whole with the productive labourers and diligent middle class in the centre. Investigations considering children, mothers and soldiers were quoted by doctors and politicians to prove that standards of health were poor, pointing to an explosive increase of caries and a decreasing capacity for breast-feeding as the signs of a progressive degeneration.

In addition to this, a whole panorama of so-called cultural diseases was pointed to, i.e. diseases related to the problems that industrialization, urbanization and modern life might bring down upon the urban middle and upper class individual, such as neurasthenia, hysteria, chlorosis, mental illness and a general, wide-spread ill-health among bourgeois and upper-class women. Thus a situation was depicted, predominantly by the medical profession, where illness was a most severe threat to the future of the nation, rationalizing resolute engagement from state authorities in close cooperation with the doctor–experts.

At the same time, innovative actions were taken to beat those diseases considered to be the most severe threats to society: tuberculosis, venereal disease and alcoholism. Interestingly enough, this meant different strategies with different actors at the centre, thus comprising a complex system of medical initiative.

The war against tuberculosis was started in the early twentieth century through private and medical organizations, whereas venereal disease was fought by means of extreme authority, introducing the regulation of prostitution as a main strategy, including a system of police supervision, custody, enforced labour and compulsory care. Regarding alcoholism, the preventive strategies were connected to the Temperance Movement and integrated into a broader system of the Adult Education Movements relying on anti-authoritarian co-operation with working class representatives. Not until the 1920s and 1930s were these public health concerns systematically to be submitted to central control.

The relation – and contradiction – between state and individual interests was to be a crucial point in the public health campaign of the early twentieth century. This was especially visible in the strategies discussed to eliminate the 'deficient' from the total of the population: contraception, sterilization, confinement and restrictive marriage laws (i.e. compulsory health control before marriage). Among these four possible ways the latter was deemed the best. In 1915 a new marriage law was introduced prohibiting the mentally ill, deficient and epileptics from marriage.

Eugenics was on the agenda since the turn of the century, and was gaining increasing support not only from politicians and the medical establishment, but from all groups engaged in the hygiene movement. In 1922, by parliamentary decision and with royal confirmation, a National Institute for Eugenics was opened in Uppsala, initiated by the physician and anthropologist Herman Lundborg, and supported by a range of medical professors and representatives from all political parties, among these Hjalmar Branting, future Prime Minister of the first Social Democrat government.

In the 1930s

As long as hygiene meant mere sanitation reforms, it was a politically uncontroversial strategy. But demanding individual mobilization as well, made the project more complicated. The concept of social hygiene, elaborated by Alfred Grotjahn, implied that disease should not be identified as biological entities, but as social processes, moving throughout society, dependent upon individual behaviour and social relations. In the public health debates of the 1920s and 1930s this was to be increasingly stressed: 'Bad habits have to be rectified, the ignorant must be informed, the irresponsible be awakened. What is needed is a comprehensive, politically organized propaganda campaign of education that is intense and demanding.' With these words, the programme was formulated in the 1930s by such leading Social Democrat ideologists as Alva and Gunnar Myrdal.

During the preceding decade, new paradigms had found their way, largely among doctors and public health politicians. A shift from a medical to a social perspective, from a biological to a sociological view of man, from disease to potential disease was visible. A new type of experts moved into the centre of the public health debate: the psychologists, psychiatrists, criminologists and sexologists. Within the social hygiene debate, the interest was focused on defining the borders with regard to health and disease, normality and abnormality. New psychiatric concepts such as psychopathy, anomaly, abnormality and social and mental depravity were introduced, linking medical and social control together in a confusing network. With these types of diagnostic constructions, social sanctions such as separation, confinement and sterilization seemed to be legitimized. In 1934, the first sterilization law was introduced; in 1941 it was strengthened. Up until 1975, when the law was revoked, 60,000 individuals, of which 90 per cent were women, and following in each case a decision by the National Board of Health, would be sterilized in Sweden on eugenic, medical and social indications. The opposition to this eugenic programme was amazingly weak.

At the same time, deterministic approaches to physical, mental and social disability as tied to inheritance, paradoxically enough, were combined with a strong optimism and confidence in preventive measures, i.e. the possibility of tracing potential disease-carriers and, by prevention and care, protecting them from future illness.

Thus initiatives were taken in the fields of infant and school health care. Studies done in 1928/9 described only 5.36 per cent (!) of the children as 'healthy'. Weakness, low weight, tuberculosis, spinal defects, malformation due to rickets, infections, psychoneuroses and caries were found to be the destroyers of the future health of the population.

Another strategy was to find formal and informal tools for information campaigns and disease prevention among the population as a whole. In 1919, the Society for Public Health was founded; a few years later the Mental Health Movement was introduced, modelled on the Mental Hygiene Movement in the United States, and forensic and child-psychiatry were established. During these years, the public health debate was kept alive within the discourse of social hygiene, meaning that state interest took precedence over individual interest.

In the early 1930s, a new type of initiative in the field of social medicine was taken by radical, socially oriented physicians such as Gunnar Inghe and Gustav Jonsson, stressing (though Inghe was a great admirer of Alfred Grotjahn) a perspective of understanding more than that of paternalistic control. The first pioneering works conducted by this perspective, dealt with illegal abortion and the health of smelting workers. 'Investigations of this type were not welcomed in all circles', Inghe commented, pointing to the tension between two perspectives on social hygiene; the old one, which focused on state interest and associated concepts of inferiority, deficiency and biological inheritance and the new perspective, which looked at the interests of the individual and emphasized concepts of environment, 'life chances' and social inheritance.

Studies undertaken by the National Trust for Social Work (*Centralförbundet for socialt arbete*), an association for voluntary social reform undertakings, confirmed, that for large groups in society, the needs were still numerous: people lived in overcrowded and damp housing and suffered from malnutrition, tuberculosis and a wide range of infectious diseases. The average standard of living was still miserable. War, the depression and unemployment were hollowing out the possibility of welfare growth.

Public Health and the Modern State

In 1931/2, the need reached a peak: 161,000 unemployed, and behind these figures were the families who were underfed, anaemic, coughing. The crisis forced a change, which was to be represented by the Social Democrats coming to power in 1932. Now public health was integrated into an all-encompassing political project: the building of the modern welfare state.

By now demographic stagnation seemed to be an undeniable fact. Birth-rates had been dropping since the beginning of the century, exposing Sweden as having the lowest birth-rate in all of Europe. In *Kris i befolkningsfrågan* (1934), from its very first day, a best-seller, the situation was described by Alva and Gunnar Myrdal fatefully, in terms of a slow, national suicide. This meant that a powerful counter-attack was called for. Measures were to be taken immediately to stimulate birth-rate as well as to reform the general prevention system, medical care, health care, child care and maternity care.

To change the population issue from an abstract state and power interest into a programme for social reform was a brilliant move. How was society to be built so that it encouraged individuals to strengthen their zest for life, keep strong and healthy, and enhance their fertility?

The political reaction was strong, supported by changes in the parliamentary power structure, introduced in 1917, which concentrated the power into an elected government. A huge number of bills were presented to Parliament in 1935, demanding immediate initiatives. In response to this, the Social Democratic government appointed a Population Committee which, in short time, presented a set of reports discussing, and proposing solutions to the qualitative as well as the quantitative aspects of the public health issue. Thus reports were presented on sterilization, issues of sexuality, abortion, child and maternity care, nutrition, housing, health insurance, dental care, health checks of school-age children etc. With amazing swiftness they were followed by a great spate of legislation and funding, based on the principle of equal access.

About the same time (1938), a so-called National Institute for Public Health (*Statens Institut for Folkhälsan*) was established, initiated by the National Board of Health and financially supported by the Rockefeller Foundation. The task was defined as occupational health, hygienic supervision of food and housing, and health information. Behind the institutionalization, an interesting struggle for power can be noted between the National Board of Health, who wanted to keep the public health problem a strict medical issue, and the Ministry for Social Affairs, who demanded that public health be integrated into a broader context of social and political solutions.

This government activism was especially significant because the balance of political power engendered an increasing commitment to socialized medicine. As director of the National Board of Health between 1935 and 1952, the prominent socialist physician, Axel Höjer, made great efforts toward socializing medicine, backed up by the Social Democrats who have maintained a stable government since 1932.

The socialization of the public health, outpacing the medicalization which characterized the early twentieth century, carried with it an important focus on prevention and health care. In 1943, Höjer was instructed by the Ministry for Social Affairs to consider a comprehensive analysis of the Swedish health care delivery system. In his report Höjer stressed first that all health care services needed by the individual should be offered free of charge, and second that it should be the duty of the community to deliver this by means of an extended and regulated organization, including and coordinating public health, medical care and preventive medicine. A main principle was the presentation of a general plan, featuring a network of health centres, either at the hospitals or outside, to offer preventive as well as curative treatment.

The Höjer Report was massively criticized from many quarters, the critique from the Swedish Medical Association being particularly strong. There were several reasons for this. The report focused quite intensely on sensitive issues of manpower supply, remuneration and speciality rules, impinging on the core interests of the medical profession; furthermore the main point of prevention seemed provocative.

Consequently the Report did not lead to immediate legislation and administrative reforms. Certain of its principles and proposals however, are still basic and of focal interest today: 1. The principle of access to all kinds of health services as an individual right and a governmental responsibility, with all services provided at little or no expense by public institutions and a publicly employed corps of professionals. 2. County council responsibility for comprehensive planning and delivery of health services, including outpatient care as well as preventive medicine .

Since then, the ideology of prevention has been striving for confirmation and resources, whereas clinical medicine is partly supported by a primary health care system (*vårdcentraler*), which handles roughly 35 per cent of all outpatient visits. In 1992, by a governmental decision, a new Institute for Public Health was established. The focus is set on prevention and health education, the aim, once again, on convincing economic and medical policy makers as well as the individual that in the long-run, it is wiser to alleviate the conditions which cause diseases than to treat them when already having come into existence.

Conclusion

The great spate of public health legislation did not occur until the 1930s when it was initiated and later carried through, by the Social Democratic government. By this time, medical policy making was integrated into the scope of public welfare, characterized by great optimism about the possibility of creating social harmony by rational means. Health could be, and indeed had to be created, planned and taught. Universal access to medical care, health information and a reasonable occupational environment, was believed to entail equal access to good health; thus class distinctions in respect to health would be eliminated. This means that the Swedish public health programme, ideologically, was constructed within a strongly egalitarian context, proceeding from an image of man as essentially rational.

Public health policies were guided by strong governmental involvement, embracing the medical profession itself. It is generally acknowledged that the status of the medical profession is reduced in proportion to the degree of state intervention. In Sweden, this is not the case – though 85 per cent of the physicians are publicly employed – mainly because of an historical tradition, in which the central authority acknowledged its need for physicians to supervise the health of a nation, characterized by low population density and modest urbanization levels by giving these doctors social security and prestige in return. Compared to the other Scandinavian countries however, the Swedish medical profession has been generally quiescent on issues such as health insurance, financing systems and challenges to the private sector.

The ultimate purposes of modern Sweden's public health policy were manifold. The need for productive and reproductive labourers was explicitly mentioned by Höjer as the director of the National Board of Health; an efficient and equally distributed health care system was the base for an optimal productive output in a country trying to adapt its economy to an international market.

Of course, there were other considerations, most notably, the possibility of overcoming class distinctions. After all the Swedish term for public health is the people's health (*Folkhälsa*), suggesting a scope not limited by differences of class, gender, income and influence. It's no coincidence that the demand for governmental health intervention increased in times of intensified class conflict (for example around the 'big strike' of 1909, or in the 1930s).

Another purpose was the cultivation of the people through general education and popular guidance, an idea rooted in the nineteenth-century educational tradition typical of the Scandinavian countries. In the case of medicine and hygiene, the demand for general education could be supported by scientific, politically neutral arguments, thereby allowing for the effective and relatively uncontroversial creation of a consensus on specific norms and values adapted to the requirements of a changed social economy. In this respect, a most important collaboration was established in the 1940s between political authority, the medical associations and the Adult Education Movements, resulting in a set of health campaigns, which emphasized the relationship between health and state obligation, but also between health and individual responsibility. Realised within a strongly egalitarian ideology, the motto 'Equal health care for all' made Sweden a model of efficient health care.

Bibliography

1. Gunnar Broberg and Mattias Tydén, 'Eugenics in Sweden: Efficient Care', in Gunnar Broberg, Bent Hansen and Niels Roll-Hansen (eds), *Eugenics in Scandinavia* (forthcoming).
2. Rolf Å. Gustafsson, *Traditionernas ok: Den svenska hälso- och sjukvårdens organisering i historie-sociologiskt perspektiv* (Stockholm: Esselte studium, 1987).
3. Arnold J. Heidenheimer and Nils Elvander (eds), *The Shaping of the Swedish Health System* (London: Croom Helm, 1980).
4. Axel Höjer, *Den öppna läkarvården i riket* (SOU, Stockholm, 1948).

5. Karin Johannisson, 'Folkhälsa: Det svenska projektet - 1900talets första decennier', *Lychnos,* 1991.
6. *Idem,* 'Why Cure the Sick? Population Policy and Health Programs Within 18th Century Swedish Mercantilism', in Anders Brändström and Lars-Göran Tedebrand (eds), *Society, Health and Population During the Demographic Transition* (Stockholm: Almqvist & Wiksell International, 1988).
7. Sven E. Olsson, *Social Policy and Welfare State in Sweden* (Lund: Arkiv, 1990).
8. Eva Palmblad, *Medicinen som samhällslära* (Göteborg: Daidalos, 1989).

5

The Expert and the State in Russian Public Health: Continuities and Changes Across the Revolutionary Divide

Susan Gross Solomon

For comments on an earlier draft of this paper, the author wishes to thank John F. Hutchinson (Simon Fraser University) and Mark B. Adams (University of Pennsylvania). The support of the Hannah Institute for the History of Medicine and the Spencer Foundation is gratefully acknowledged.

Introduction

The comparativist who approaches the English-language studies of public health in Russia, both before and after the Revolution of 1917, will invariably be struck by the emphasis on the relation of physicians to the state.

Among those who study pre-revolutionary Russian public health, that relation has been the centre of attention, not only when the subject was the development of the medical profession itself,[1] but also in research on more specialized subjects such as the struggle against epidemics,[2] the efforts at famine relief,[3] the treatment of mental illness,[4] and the campaign against prostitution.[5]

This scholarly focus is understandable. The Russian medical profession developed within the rigid confines of the state's bureaucratic structure. As early as the mid seventeenth century, all medical education was subsidized and supervised by the state. Graduating physicians were expected to repay the state for their education by working as government employees in the armed forces, in state-owned mines, in prisons, or in provincial towns.[6] The duties of Russian physicians to the state as enshrined in the Medical Statute of 1857[7] were so extensive that all doctors – even those in private practice[8] – were effectively public employees or, as one historian has put it, 'servants of the state'.[9]

For their part, Russian physicians made a series of demands upon the tsarist state, foremost among which was the demand for recognition of their expertise on matters of public health. Most often, the effort to secure recognition led physicians to seek increased autonomy from the state in the conduct of their professional duties; but from time to time, the quest for recognition led physicians to seek closer involvement with the state in the design or the administration of public health programmes.[10]

Russian physicians may have been united in the view that their expertise warranted official recognition, but they did not concur about the type of expertise that was of paramount value. Within the medical community, there were heated debates over whether public health ought to be a narrow discipline concentrating on specific aspects of disease or a broad field whose purview was illness as a whole.[11] There were also disagreements about whether the solution to the pressing problems of public health lay in social reform, sanitary science, or the laboratory science of bacteriology.[12]

In Western research on Soviet public health, we find the familiar emphasis on the relation of physicians and the state that characterized scholarly research on the pre-1917 period.[13] With good reason. After the Bolsheviks assumed power, not only did the education, training and licensing of the physician remain under the control of the state[14] but, now for the first time, health administration was centralized under the newly-formed Commissariat of Public Health of the Russian Republic,[15] physicians were integrated into a state-controlled union which brought together all medical workers,[16] and the duties of the physicians to the state were vastly increased and spelled out in minute detail.[17] Although some private medical practice continued to be tolerated throughout the 1920s,[18] over all, after 1917, the involvement of the state in the professional activities of physicians increased exponentially.

The fact that the overarching problematic – the relationship of public health experts and the state – remained relevant across the revolutionary divide had a discernible impact on Western scholarhip. Western historians who studied the development of Soviet public health readily acknowledged the Bolshevik innovations in the delivery of health care – the commitment to deliver free, universal and high-quality medical care accessible to all.[19] But when it came to the familiar issue of the relation of the medical profession to the state, they tended to look at the same groups that had been prominent before 1917 – the bacteriologists, the epidemiologists and the sanitarians. This paper will argue that, in doing so, they overlooked the emergence of a new group of public health experts – the social hygienists.

And yet, social hygienists were hardly from a marginal group in Soviet public health. According to its architects, the success of the Bolshevik 'revolution' in public health depended upon the emergence of a physician 'who would be as much at home in sociology as in biology, as much interested in preventing illness as in curing it'.[20] In the formation of this physician–researcher, the pivotal discipline was social hygiene (*sotsial'naia gigiena*), a field which borrowed and adapted elements both of German *soziale medizin* of the first two decades of this century and of pre-revolutionary Russian community medicine.

However much it owed to the German and Russian traditions in public health, Soviet social hygiene was a distinctive field. From the early 1920s, when it was first institutionalized as a separate field in the medical schools and in specially designed research institutions, until the end of that decade, social hygiene occupied a special position in public health. It was social hygienists who articulated the officially accepted view that disease was primarily a social phenomenon; it was social hygienists who were entrusted with the task of spearheading the drive for preventive medicine in the medical schools; it was to social hygienists that the state turned for serious research and expert advice on a range of social problems deemed threatening to public well-being. Finally, of all the fields of public health, it was social hygiene that was closest to the centre of power. The first Commissar of Public Health, N. A. Semashko, considered himself a social hygienist: he argued strenuously for the acceptance of the field in public health and even wrote the first Soviet textbook on the subject.[21]

The pivotal role of social hygiene in Soviet public health not only brought a new group of experts to prominence, it also broadened the scope and orientation of public health itself. In commissioning physicians to do research on issues of public health, the state medicalized a series of issues that had previously been treated as questions of law and order. In giving the mandates for the study of these issues to social hygienists, the state signalled its willingness to entertain the view that the solution to those health problems lay in social reform.

This paper will be devoted to examining the role played by social hygiene in Soviet public health in the first decade and a half after the Bolsheviks took power. Such an examination is indispensable for a full picture of the continuities and changes in public health in revolutionary Russia. A study of Soviet social hygiene, however, requires extensive historical retrieval. In present-day Western writing on Soviet public health, there is almost no mention of the vibrant field of social hygiene that flowered in the first decade and a half after the revolution.[22] For understandable reasons. Like so many other innovative intellectual enterprises in post-revolutionary Soviet public health, social hygiene was swamped by the events of the late 1920s.[23] To complicate the process of historical retrieval further, the laudatory accounts of the achievements of Soviet social hygiene written by English-speaking travellers and fellow-travellers who visited Russia during the 1920s and 1930s have been all been forgotten, dismissed by many as ideology.[24] To be sure, there are a half-dozen accounts of social hygiene written by Soviet scholars in the 1970s, but those accounts ignore the very dimensions of the story that are of greatest relevance to the problem of public health experts and the state – namely, the struggle of Soviet social hygienists for recognition both from the government agencies responsible for public health and from physicians specializing in other areas of medicine and public health.[25]

Apart from its interest for students of Russian public health, the story of Soviet social hygiene speaks directly to those who study social medicine across cultures. According to conventional wisdom, in most countries the sociological approach to public health reform was eclipsed by the advent of bacteriology and epidemiology.[26] In the case of Soviet social hygiene, we have a sociological approach to public health protected and patronized by a state that was committed both to far-reaching social change and to the advance of medical science. To what extent were these commitments seen as contradictory by those who made policy for public health?[27] And what was the impact on the development of Soviet social hygiene of the dual commitments of its patron? Further, in the story of Soviet social hygiene we have an instance of scientific expertise being commissioned by a state which endorsed the principles of scientific management and yet feared technocracy. To what extent did the fact that the public health experts possessed 'correct' political credentials mitigate the state's apprehensions about technocracy? At what point did 'credentialism' become insufficient? The purpose of this paper will be not so much to provide definitive answers as to argue for the importance of posing these questions.

Public Health Physicians and the State under the Tsars

A canvass of Western scholarly literature on Russian public health written during the last three decades reveals not only shared research agendas, but also a set of commonly-held intellectual assumptions that animated those agendas. The pioneering historical study of the development of Russian public health was Nancy Frieden's *Russian*

Physicians in an Era of Reform and Revolution, 1865–1905.[28] The focus of Frieden's book was the Pirogov Society of Russian Physicians – the first nation-wide Russian medical association founded in 1885.[29] Tracing the evolution of that Society from its creation until the revolution of 1905, Frieden told the story of what she termed the 'transformation of physicians from state servants in low to middling positions enjoying slight social prestige' to proud professionals.[30] That transformation was fraught with struggle, for the tsarist state severely constrained the functioning of physicians while at the same time only reluctantly acknowledging their expertise in matters of public health.

On the troubled relation of Russian physicians to the state, there are two theses in Frieden's book. The strong thesis argues that, although Russian physicians were public employees, they sought the very type of professional autonomy from the state enjoyed by their colleagues in Western Europe.[31] The autocracy prevented physicians from achieving Western-style professionalization and therefore, so runs the argument, some physicians deliberately chose to do health work in the *zemstvos,* the local self-governing institutions that had been established in 1864 to carry out a variety of functions relating to the economic and welfare needs of provinces and districts.[32] Physicians opted for the *zemstvos* in the expectation that in this setting they would be able to design an occupational pattern that would be less subject to the controls of the central administration. This expectation made eminent sense given the increasing devolution of jurisdiction over public health to these local institutions by the central authorities from the 1860s on.[33] According to Frieden, the physicians' wager on the *zemstvos* turned out to have been well-placed. 'In pursuing their professional goals within the *zemstvos,* Russian physicians actually emulated the pattern of professionalization of physicians in Western Europe.'[34]

A more nuanced – and in my view more interesting – variant of this thesis emerged in the Epilogue to Frieden's book. Here the author described community physicians as somewhat ambivalent about the state's proper role in medical reform. 'Ambivalence toward the state modified the physicians' efforts for professional autonomy. Dependent on the state for guidance and rewards, they knew that their most realistic approach to productive work was to enlist the state as an ally in reform... The "we-they" antipathy of the intelligentsia towards the bureaucracy was not the automatic response of most physicians, who did not necessarily regard state service as a form of co-optation.'[35] Indeed, according to Frieden the community physicians had a strong orientation to public service. It was only the government's failure to give physicians the right or the opportunity to use their expertise that moved many from reformism to political radicalism.[36]

Frieden's work put two closely related aspects of the relationship between Russian physicians and the state squarely on the agenda of Western researchers. The first of these was the pattern of professionalization of Russian physicians. The second was the role of physicians in politics. A third issue – the changing face of public health expertise – was discussed, but not, as we shall see, within the compass of the relationship between physicians and the state.

A – Russian Physicians as Medical Professionals

In his fine doctoral dissertation on the Pirogov Society in the turbulent period 1917 to 1920, Peter Krug raised important questions about the aspirations and self-image of the Russian public health physician. In contrast to Frieden, in the Russian physician of the period 1880–1917, Krug saw neither a failed private practitioner nor a government servitor, but rather a distinct type of professional.[37] As he put it, 'As a result of their professional interest in public employment, the physicians dominating the Pirogov Society and the Russian public health movement never sought the type of professional organization created by physicians in Western Europe and North America....'[38] Krug's reading of the records of meetings of the Pirogov Society persuaded him that the Society members were primarily interested not in autonomy from the state, but in 'the active promotion of public medicine, constantly seeking to expand the scope of activity of public physicians in the process, in order to justify the increase of public expenditures necessary for the support of public medical programs.'[39] Although he did not say so explicitly, Krug's view of the Pirogov physician as a distinct type of medical professional suggested an attitude towards government closest to that described in Frieden's more nuanced thesis.

In his authoritative treatment of the politics of Russian public health from 1890 to 1918, John F. Hutchinson deepened the discussion by examining the issue of Russian medical professionalization from an interactive perspective. Hutchinson began from the fact that among Russian physicians there was a diversity of approaches and goals which defied 'the attempts by Pirogov physicians of one view or another to enforce visions of unity on one another.....' The failure of Russian physicians to develop as a corporate group, he argued, was as much a function of internal divisions within the medical profession as it was a result of the opposition of the autocracy. 'With Russian physicians battling each other, and refusing to understand one another's point of view, it was easy for the tsarist regime to withhold the corporate status which physicians had achieved in other countries.'[40]

B – Russian Physicians as Political Actors

Frieden's work also spawned inquiry into the involvement of community physicians in politics. In explaining the radicalization of Russian physicians in 1905, she had argued that it was only the refusal of the tsarist regime to acknowledge physicians' expertise which ultimately drove them to political action. In this view of Russian physicians as political *malgré eux* Krug essentially concurred. Indeed, he went further, suggesting that the public health physicians were inclined to cooperate with whatever state would give them the authority and deference they so ardently desired. Thus it was that in the turbulent years 1917–20, a substantial wing of the leadership of the Pirogov Society leadership went over to the Bolsheviks.[41] To Krug there was nothing anomalous in this. In contrast to others, he argued that the Pirogov opposition to the Bolsheviks had never been based on ideological grounds;[42] it stemmed rather from the physicians' fear of losing some of the control over the health institutions that they had gained under the provisional government.[43] Apprehensions on this point proved groundless, for the Bolshevik leadership proved willing to employ and defer to physicians who had been associated with the Pirogov Society. And thus, far from enjoying less deference and authority than they had under the tsarist, and even the Provisional, governments, Pirogov physicians found their status enhanced after 1917.

As part of making his case on this point, Krug furnished evidence that the Pirogov Society continued to survive into the middle of the 1920s.[44] From this he went on to suggest that there was nothing inherently out-moded about the Pirogov physicians in the new conditions. While he admitted that by mid-decade the leadership of the Pirogovtsy had moved away from the Society, Krug explained that the physicians had simply 'turned their attention to newer organizations, which, enjoying the use of public resources, appeared to have offered greater opportunity for research and experimentation'.[45]

On this last point, John Hutchinson parted company with Krug. While he acknowledged that the Pirogov Society survived 1917 and that its journal continued – albeit with an interruption – to publish until 1922, Hutchinson submitted that the former Pirogovtsy who went over to the Bolsheviks were not espousing the approach to public health that was characteristic of the Society a decade earlier.

Indeed, in Hutchinson's view, the ideology of *zemstvo* medicine (which he defined as consisting of a few homilies such as central government is bad, local government is good; private practice is wicked, public practice is noble[46]) did not survive the Bolshevik revolution. It was not the Bolsheviks who killed *zemstvo* medicine, however; *zemstvo* medicine was dead long before 1917. In a tightly reasoned and persuasive article, Hutchinson submitted that it was the war, with its demand for centralized activity in health care delivery and research that spelled the death-knell of *zemstvo* medicine.[47]

In essence, Hutchinson's explanation of the eclipse of community medicine rested on a modernization argument. In Hutchinson's view, a modern public health effort required centralized medical administration. His writings bespeak support for proponents of the creation of a centralized health administration for Russia: S. P. Botkin (1887), G. E. Rein (1914) and Z. P. Solov'ev, the architect of the Russian Commissariat of Public Health founded in 1918.[48] For Hutchinson, the question of the most effective administration of public health was intimately related both to the profile of professionals working in public health and to the content of public health itself.[49] Because many of the advances in medical science (particularly in the area of bacteriology) required the support of a centralized health administration and infrastructure, it seemed logical that progressive public health physicians would want to work with a centralized health administration. And indeed, looking at the historical record, Hutchinson discovered substantial support among pre-revolutionary Russian physicians for the centralization of medical administration. As he put it, he found 'pioneers of medical innovation who sought more rather than less state control over physicians and reformers who had already turned a deaf ear to the evangelists of local autonomy before 1917'.[50] The finding that not all the physicians saw the state as the 'other' was genuinely revisionist in its implications, for it challenged the conventional portrait of the community physician as the foe of centralized administration and of state intervention.

One of the most important contributions of Hutchinson's history of Russian public health lay in putting the question of the relations between power and expertise from the vantage point of the state. According to him, the dilemma for the state was to give deference to the medical experts without at the same time losing control of public health. In 1914, Rein had proposed to solve the problem with a tacit contract: the state would grant authority and expertise to the medical profession, and then only its academic wing, on the understanding that it would keep its house in order. In what was almost an aside,

Hutchinson claimed that this kind of bargain was essentially that struck by the newly founded Commissariat of Public Health formed in 1918.[51]

C – The Russian Public Health Physician as Expert

In the Western literature, the demand by Russian physicians for recognition of their expertise emerges as a leitmotif of their relations with the tsarist state between 1865 and 1917. While the demand for recognition may have been a constant, the bases upon which physicians laid claim to expertise underwent substantial change during that period.

For the half century that preceded the revolution of 1917, the core of teaching and research in Russian public health was the field of general hygiene (*obshchaia gigiena*) which had become a separate subject of study in Russian medical schools in the late 1860s.[52] In the period 1870–90, general hygiene was a broad, umbrella field. Indeed, those who spoke on behalf of general hygiene in this period were reluctant to confine their field to any single set of concerns or to particular methodologies; on the contrary, they took pride in the claim that general hygiene embraced all systematic study of public health. Looking at the content of the Russian courses in general hygiene throughout the 1870s and into the 1880s, we find the emphasis on environmental sanitation that was characteristic of public health teaching in many countries at the time.[53] Public health physicians stressed the impact on health of environmental factors (air, water, climate) and made proposals for sanitary reform. Gradually, under the influence of F. F. Erisman who began to teach hygiene at Moscow University in 1882, they became interested in the relationship between disease and social (read 'economic') factors.[54] To understand the latter relationship, they relied on empirical and statistical evidence.[55]

But Erisman's prototypical physician was not to be a detached social analyst; his mission was to be close to the people. According to Frieden, for most of this period, the Russian public health physician claimed authority on the basis of his service to the people.[56] Part of the service ethic of physicians included doing public health education. For the Pirogov physician, the basis of the educational effort was always prevention. Suspicious of the efficacy of curative medicine in dealing with the infectious diseases and epidemics that ravaged Russia,[57] the community physician looked first and foremost to preventive medicine.

By the early twentieth century, Frieden noted, the limitations of physicians' claims to status on the basis of service to society had been revealed. At that point, Russian physicians began to claim authority on the basis of their scientific expertise, much as their colleagues in the West had done at an earlier period.[58] But the invocation of scientific expertise as the basis for the claim to authority tended to divide, rather than unify, the Russian medical profession. Specialists in experimental medicine and the leading figures at the St Petersburg Military-Medical Academy, who were located close to the centres of power and scientific knowledge, achieved recognition first. Community physicians, based as they were in the rural sector, were on the periphery both politically and scientifically.[59] As Hutchinson put it, 'The St. Petersburg medical establishment was always ready to provide promotion, rewards and honors for medical scientists whose work was more theoretical than practical... physicians and scientists interested in the social and environmental aspects of disease and in the prevention of disease through social change could make little headway in the capital city.'[60]

To add to his disadvantages in the quest for recognition, the community physician was a confirmed generalist in an age of specialism. His claim to authority had always rested on the breadth of his knowledge, rather than on his specialization in any one area of public health.[61] Even the sanitary physicians who began to function in the sanitary executive commissions that had been set up in the wake of the cholera epidemic of 1892/3 were not regarded as specialists in public health.[62] Their task was to complement the work of the ordinary *zemstvo* physician by using the raw data collected from the clinic to analyse morbidity and mortality in the region. As Hutchinson put it, the sanitary physician was functioning 'not only as a hygienist, but also as a statistician, topographer, anthropologist and even ethnographer'.[63] For the purposes of the argument of this paper, it is important to note that until well after the turn of the century, the collection of social data about illness was seen not as a specialized function, but rather one that could be carried out by rank-and-file *zemstvo* physicians.

Between 1880 and 1910, the right of the broad generalist to speak on behalf of all of public health was challenged not once, but several times, by different groups of specialists. Three of those challenges are of particular relevance to the story being told here. To begin with, in the late 1880s, when the bacteriological revolution began to spread in Russia, some bacteriologists led by Mechnikov made bold to take over public health using the argument that successes in the laboratory had made obsolete the traditional preoccupation of general hygienists with sanitary and social reforms.[64] *Zemstvo* physicians reacted to these attempts with hostility on the grounds that the rush to the laboratory might undermine the long-standing efforts to reduce poverty and improve hygiene education. The antipathy to bacteriology in Russia is reminiscent of the reactions of some sanitarians in England and, to a lesser extent, America. But in Russia the hostility to bacteriology was compounded by the apprehension of physicians that their employment in the *zemstvos* would be threatened by the scientific advances.[65] The efforts of bacteriologists in the late 1880s to take over public health failed, but by the end of the century, bacteriology had been established in Russia as a separate discipline in the medical schools and in specialized research institutions.[66] Thanks to the political acumen of the bacteriologist Gabrichevskii, a compromise was reached with community physicians according to which 'hygiene would remain a subject of medical education and sanitary reform an appropriate field of applied knowledge'.[67] By 1902, bacteriology was accepted by the Pirogov Society; three years later bacteriologists and sanitarians were working together first to fight cholera and then to oppose the tsarist regime.

A decade later, there was a second challenge to the authority of the public health generalist, this one issued by champions of a new type of sanitary physician whose competence lay in the area of hydrographics and sanitary engineering. The new sanitary physician, proposed by A. N. Sysin, was 'neither the sociologist–statistician–topographer of the Pirogov tradition nor the experimental hygienist at home in the laboratory; instead he was a technical specialist who ... pooled his expertise to fulfil grand schemes of public works'.[68] According to Hutchinson, 'it was precisely this professional exclusive aspect of sanitary engineering that the traditionalists most feared. Their ideal sanitary physician was in constant contact with the people, meeting them as healer, adviser, confidant'.[69] But in the ranks of 'younger sanitary physicians who were dissatisfied with the constraints imposed by the traditional emphasis on sociological and statistical research', there was substantial support for Sysin's sanitary engineer.[70]

Third, at the end of the first decade of the twentieth century, the claims of general hygienists were challenged from yet another direction – this time by public health physicians interested in the social factors which affected the occurrence of disease. These physicians urged both the creation of a separate course in community medicine (*obshchestvennaia meditsina*) which would pay more attention to social aspects of health and the establishment of a research centre that would study social dimensions of public health.[71] At the XI Pirogov Congress in 1910, there was even a proposal to mount a separate course on 'community medicine' for medical students.[72] In part because of the First World War, little came of the proposal. While the champions of 'community medicine' (*obshchestvennaia meditsina*) had some success in introducing courses containing material on social factors into economic and technical institutes, they were unable to penetrate the hide-bound medical faculties.[73]

But institutional resistance was not the sole reason for the defeat of proponents of community medicine. In fairness it must be said that community physicians often lacked a clear idea of what they meant by 'social factors': the courses they proposed were often grab-bags of those aspects of public health (administrative as well as social) that did not fit neatly under the old rubric of 'general hygiene'. Indeed, writing in 1913, V. Ia. Kanel, one of the most insightful and critical proponents of social medicine, explained the problem with rare acuity. He argued that for real progress to be made in forging a social medicine in Russia, not only would social hygiene have to break away from general hygiene and set itself up as an independent field, but sociological thinking would have to mature to the point where it could enrich social hygiene.[74]

Some linguistic clarification is in order here. With the exception of Kanel, in using the term 'doctor–sociologist' (*vrach-sotsiolog*) to characterize a physician, community physicians rarely had in mind a practitioner of systematic sociology whose scientific focus (whether theoretical or empirical) was the relationship between disease and the social fabric. Among community physicians, what earned a doctor the designation 'sociological' was first and foremost his proximity to the people. Indeed, in the discourse of most spokesmen for community medicine in the late tsarist period, the term *'sotsiolog'* was often loosely used as a synonym for a social worker, social welfare worker, or social activist.[75] This usage, we may note, was very much in tune with the orientation of pre-revolutionary Russian sociology. In the words of the leading Western interpreter of that sociology, 'its strength was primarily in articulating the social consciousness and the social conscience of the intelligentsia'.[76]

In the literature on the development of public health systems in Western Europe, the reliance on social reform, social work and sanitary measures to alleviate the causes of disease has generally been portrayed as characteristic of traditional public health, while bacteriology and sanitary engineering have been hailed as the hallmarks of a modern scientific approach to public health.[77] This set of characterizations was never subjected to serious scrutiny by scholars whose subject is pre-revolutionary Russian public health. For understandable reasons. By the end of the first decade of the twentieth century, the field of bacteriology had been institutionalized for some two decades in Russia and a new type of sanitary science was just emerging. At the same point in time, the social approach to disease (read 'community medicine') was labouring under serious handicaps. Not only was it encountering resistance in the established institutions, but its proponents did not have a clear idea of its content. In addition, it seemed to be the province of old-style 'do-gooders' or reformers, many of whom had gone on record as resisting the claims of biological or sanitary science. In short, to many community medicine seemed like little more than 'a science of social assistance'.[78]

As we move into the Soviet period, the fields of bacteriology and sanitary science – by all accounts the cutting edge of Russian public health – continued their development. Their persistence across the revolutionary divide shaped the perception by Western scholars of the ecology of fields in public health. Indeed, in a curious way, the unbroken development of these fields worked against the discovery by our historians of the emergence of a new field of science in Soviet public health – namely, the science of social hygiene which was dedicated first and foremost to studying in a systematic way the impact of social factors on disease.

Public Health Expertise and the Soviet State

The doom-and-gloom scenarios, so widespread in Russian medical circles in 1917, about the impending loss of influence by physicians under the Soviet regime proved grossly exaggerated.[79] Western historical research reveals that, almost as soon as they came to power, the Bolsheviks consulted physicians, took advantage of their services, and involved them in the administration of public health at every level.[80] Indeed, far from attempting to destroy the medical profession, the new regime recognized the unique expertise of physicians and supported the movement for higher qualifications for doctors.[81] Most important, with Lenin in the lead, the Bolsheviks courted 'bourgeois' medical specialists. As Peter Krug put it, by spring of 1919, the schism between the Pirogov Society and the Soviet government had been largely healed 'through common recognition of the principle that physicians should play the leading role in public health affairs'.[82]

What kind of expertise was most desired by the new regime? Given the serious public health problems which beset the country in the wake of the revolution, the new regime understandably turned first to specialists in the handling of epidemics and famine.[83] This was not merely a fire-fighting action: in fact, after the health crises of the immediate post-revolutionary period had abated somewhat, work in epidemiology intensified. At the end of the decade, this field was institutionalized as a separate discipline in the medical schools – formal acknowledgement of its achievements and importance.[84]

But the leading figures in Soviet public health were also committed to forging new disciplines. A canvass of the waves of reform of the medical school curriculum which punctuated the 1920s shows clearly that, while experimental medicine continued to be seen as indispensable for the 'physician of the future', the framework for the activity of that physician was now seen as sociological. As A. V. Mol'kov, the intellectual leader of the social hygienists put it, medicine 'in its modern conception, while not tearing itself away from its biological grounding and its natural science basis, is by its nature and its goals a sociological problem'.[85]

In 1924, the new vision was fleshed out in an official call to the medical schools to produce physicians with:

> 1. a serious natural science preparation, as familiar with physico-chemical and biological sciences as with the laws underlying the biological processes;
>
> 2. enough social science background to comprehend the social environment;
>
> 3. materialist thinking without which it is impossible to understand the relationship of an organism to its environment;
>
> 4. the ability to examine the patient in relation to his work life and lifestyle;
>
> 5. the ability to study the occupational and social conditions which give rise to illness and not only to cure the illness, but to suggest ways to prevent it.[86]

This new type of physician was envisaged not as a specialist, but as a generalist. But then, the 1920s were the heyday of universalism in Soviet medical education. All medical students took the same course of study; specialization was postponed until after graduation from medical school.[87] In all likelihood, the commitment to 'encyclopaedic' knowledge was a reaction both against the minute gradations in the status of physicians that had prevailed under tsarism and against what many critics viewed as the tendency of modern medicine to become increasingly abstract, divorced from the population.[88]

The commitment to universalism was not only deeply felt, it was widely held. Indeed, it was not merely the established medical faculties that were charged with preparing the new type of physician; a 1926 decree of the Council of People's Commissars called for the standardization of the medical curriculum across the Russian Republic (RSFSR).[89]

The curriculum, which was mandatory for all students, reflected the new socio-biological approach to public health.[90] A course on social science was linked to the course on general biology, giving a 'synthesis of natural and social sciences'. In the last three years of the five-year course of study, the number of hours devoted to hygiene was increased significantly. The hygiene disciplines were required to stress 'the interaction of external and social factors on the health of the whole population and of separate groups'.[91] All teaching from the third year on had to proceed under the slogan of the 'synthesis of curative and preventive medicine'. The clinics were to be 'steeped in social prophylactic content' and linked directly to economic life. The new emphasis on the social approach to public health was the more striking because it was enshrined in a curriculum whose goals were both to increase the requirements for medical study[92] and to modernize the course of study to reflect advances in medical science.[93]

Social Hygiene as a Science of Public Health

The heart of the new approach to public health was the field of social hygiene. As A. V. Mol'kov was to put it later, "The reform of medical education was in the air from the very first days after the revolution, and it was translated into practice with the introduction into the new system of a new discipline – social hygiene.'[94] The new discipline was defined by its spokesman as 'the study of the influence of economic and social factors on the health of the population and on the ways to improve that health.'[95]

Although the field of social hygiene was a creature of the post-revolutionary period, the discipline itself had roots in existing traditions of public health. In their stress of the importance of preventive medicine, social hygienists drew upon the pre-revolutionary tradition of community medicine. In defining their approach to health and disease and in laying out the research agenda of their field, Soviet social hygienists adapted a great deal from German *soziale medizin* of the first two decades of this century.[96] To indicate lines of intellectual filiation is not, however, to minimize novelty. The distinctive feature of post-revolutionary Soviet social hygiene was the primacy it gave to social factors in explaining the occurrence and spread of disease. For Soviet social hygienists, social factors were not additional variables to be included alongside other factors in the explanation of disease; social factors were the heart of the explanation.

The revolution of 1917 set in motion the process of institutionalizing social hygiene in Soviet public health. In 1920, the First All-Russian Session on Medical Education which met in Moscow put forward a suggestion to introduce a course on social hygiene into the medical curriculum.[97] In 1922, less than two full years later, with the patronage of the Commissar of Public Health, N. A. Semashko, the first department of social hygiene was opened for the medical faculties of the three Moscow medical faculties.[98] Within five years, there were 15 such departments throughout the Russian Republic.[99] In 1923, with social hygiene still taking form as a distinctive discipline, a new research institution, the State Institute for Social hygiene (henceforth referred to by its Russian acronym GISG) was founded to coordinate and conduct research on problems in social hygiene.[100]

Of the Western historians of Russian public health mentioned earlier, only Peter Krug dealt in any detail with social hygiene as a field of Russian public health.[101] And in his writings, Krug consistently took the position that social hygiene was not unique to the Soviet period; it had deep roots in *zemstvo* medicine. In an article published in 1976, he used the term 'social hygiene' to refer to the sociological approach to disease which rose to prominence in Europe in the mid nineteenth century, in the period between the dominance of the climatic theory and the germ theories of disease. In Krug's view, *zemstvo* physicians were far more comfortable with the sociological approach than with the biological approach to disease.[102] In a paper delivered in 1980, Krug located social hygiene even further back in Russian history: he submitted that whereas the term 'social hygiene' was not used in Russia until the years immediately preceding the First World War, the core concepts of social hygiene appeared in Russia as early as the 1870s under such rubrics as social medicine *(sotsial'naia meditsina)*, public medicine *(obshchestvennaia meditsina)* or public hygiene *(obshchestvennaia gigiena)*. Among the core concepts of social hygiene Krug included:

1. the conviction that physicians should play a large role in public policy;
2. the contempt for a narrow role that was based either on therapeutics or sanitary engineering;
3. a firm belief in preventive medicine including the sociological study of statistics;
4. an intense missionary zeal.[103]

In drawing a straight line between the social activism of Russian community medicine of the 1870s and Soviet social hygiene, Krug was giving the familiar Russian spin to the notion of the 'sociological' approach to health and disease, that is, he was equating 'sociology' with social work.

In his dissertation, Krug asserted a connection between the 'social hygiene' of the *zemstvo* physicians and the Soviet field of social hygiene on different grounds. He presented social hygiene as 'one of the points of contact' between the Pirogovtsy and the Bolsheviks after 1917. Both Bolshevik and Pirogov physicians 'drew their deep interest in social hygiene from the same theoretical background: the view that the health of various groups within the population was determined by the influence of external factors, particularly socio-economic and that the improvement of external conditions would lead to lower disease and death rates'. For the Bolshevik physicians, so ran the argument, 'such an outlook was clearly linked to Marxist ideology; for the Pirogovtsy, it evolved as an essential part of the *zemstvo* medical tradition, with its populist underpinnings'.[104] In focusing on the fit between social hygiene on the one hand and the ideologies of both Marxism and populism on the other, Krug played down the scientific content of social hygiene.

It is the argument of this paper that there is much more to Soviet social hygiene than the core identified by Krug. To be specific, this paper argues that in the 1920s Soviet social hygiene was developing into a science with its own theoretical starting point and problems, its own research agenda and its own methodology. While there may have been specific points of resemblance and even some intellectual filiations between Soviet social hygiene and pre-revolutionary Russian community medicine, as a self-contained discipline with its own priorities and perspectives, social hygiene was unique to the Soviet period.

The issue of the scientific status of social hygiene was at the heart of the debates about the field's legitimacy in the 1920s. Spokesmen for general hygiene, keen to retain their field's long-standing hegemony in public health, insisted that for all its pretensions, the 'new' social hygiene was nothing more than an intellectual approach. Social hygienists, for their part, defended the differentiation of their field from general hygiene on the grounds that the social questions they treated were of such importance that the creation of a separate discipline devoted to those questions was warranted; at the same time, they insisted that their field qualified as a science.[105] The intensity with which the scientific status of social hygiene was debated testifies to the cachet which the term 'science' enjoyed for those who studied social, as well as natural, phenomena.

If we take seriously the claims of the leading spokesmen for Soviet social hygiene in the 1920s, we must examine the field not only for signs of statistically-oriented work on problems of public health, but also for evidence of embryonic social science research on questions of health and society. For the scholar, the assessment of the claims of Soviet social hygiene to scientific status is not a simple matter. The literature on social science in its nascent stages is better developed for some countries than for others. To be specific, for France, Germany, Britain and the United States, there is a rich scholarly literature on the two 'sources of sociology': social theory and empirical social research which flourished under the umbrella of such fields as geography, agricultural economics, medicine, and law.[106] Students of pre-revolutionary Russian intellectual history have written about the strong tradition of social statistics gathering[107] and about the rich vein of social thought.[108] The forcible truncation of academic sociology (both theoretical and empirical) in the early 1920s[109] understandably forestalled inquiry into the subsequent development of empirical social research in the Soviet Union. And yet historical examinations of such fields as law and rural studies have shown beyond any doubt that empirical social research continued to exist throughout much of the 1920s in Soviet government institutions and specialized institutes.[110] It is alongside such social research that the work of Soviet social hygienists must ultimately be judged.

From the beginning, Soviet social hygiene was intended to be both a descriptive and prescriptive science.[111] Its practitioners were to examine the social conditions within which disease occurred and spread and to propose social measures which would contribute to the all-important goal of preventing disease. To what extent did social hygiene fulfil this mandate?

First, Soviet social hygiene had developed a distinctive approach to the study of health and disease. It is worth noting that in contrast to the usual pattern of institutionalization of scientific specialities, Soviet social hygiene was established as a teaching field in the medical schools and as a field of inquiry in specialized research institutions before its content was hammered out.[112] The core of the social hygienists' approach was the belief in the primacy of social factors in the aetiology of disease. While they did not deny the biological underpinnings of disease, social hygienists began from the assumption that illness was primarily a social phenomenon, best understood in its societal context. This position, we should note, put social hygienists in the centre of what was a spirited discussion among Soviet physicians over the causes of disease. At one end of the spectrum were those who insisted on the significance of purely biological factors; at the other end were those who argued for a strictly sociological approach to disease.[113]

The middle ground was not easy to stake out. As a 'hybrid field' social hygiene drew upon elements of both natural and social science.[114] On one side, the field was flanked by bacteriology which had been institutionalized as a laboratory science in the late 1880s and by epidemiology which was making increasing efforts to be experimental in the 1920s.[115] On the other side, it was flanked by an empirical sociology that was still in its nascent stages. In contrast to psychology and anthropology which had been well established in Russia for some time, sociology was just beginning to make its way in the period 1917–20. Beginning in 1918 in St Petersburg, new courses in sociology were set up and new institutes opened; according to some authoritative accounts, there were even sociological manuscripts in progress.[116] By 1921, however, the empirical study of society had ceased to exist under the rubric of sociology,[117] thus depriving social hygienists for the remainder of the decade of a developed sociology on whose emergence V. Ia. Kanel had correctly placed so much importance.

In elaborating their approach to health and disease, social hygienists adapted the focus on the social factors which had been developed by such German proponents of social medicine of the first two decades of the twentieth century as Alfred Grotjahn, Benno Chajes and Alfons Fischer. Significantly, the Soviet social hygienists celebrated their connection with the Germans, seeing no contradiction between acknowledging an intellectual debt and asserting the 'novelty' of their field (Semashko called the field 'the offspring of October'.[118] The Soviet textbooks on social hygiene made extensive reference to German research on the social factors influencing disease.[119]

In addition to the cachet they enjoyed as a result of their connections with German social medicine, Soviet social hygienists profited from the fact that their socio-biological approach to disease fit well both with the official commitment to social change (as exemplified for example, in the project to create the 'New Soviet Man'[120]) and with the nurturist premises broadly accepted in Soviet society at the time.[121]

Second, social hygienists had a clearly defined research agenda for their field. Though that agenda was continually expanding, it was animated by firm principles of inclusion and exclusion. Whereas proponents of Russian community medicine, who had agitated in 1910 for a more social approach to disease, tended to include under the rubric of 'community medicine' all things that did not strictly belong in general hygiene,[122] Soviet social hygienists treated general hygiene as the residual category, casting out from the social basket all public health problems that were not either social diseases (e.g., alcoholism, prostitution, narcotics, venereal disease) or diseases whose social aetiology was the centre of study.

In 1926–7, when the field of social hygiene was at its height, its research agenda embraced a striking array of problems: population (birth, death and migration), consumption (nutrition), social disease (alcoholism, narcotics and venereal disease), sexual life (sex education and prostitution), work (industrial accidents and women's work) and collective life (housing, education and leisure).[123] Research on some of these questions (e.g., alcoholism, narcotics, prostitution, venereal disease, industrial accidents) was initiated in response to government mandates; but work on other topics (e.g., nutrition, birth and death, questions of leisure, sexology) was pursued as part of the struggle of social hygienists for turf within public health.

Third, throughout the decade, Soviet social hygienists were engaged in refining research methodologies appropriate to their subject matter. The methodological work was high-priority for social hygienists: the *kabinety* of the State Institute for Social Hygiene (GISG) were organized on a methodological basis; and in 1924 a separate Methodological Council of the Scientific Institutes of the Commissariat of Public Health was established under the aegis of GISG.[124]

In identifying and refining a set of methodologies appropriate to their field, social hygienists were, therefore, venturing into uncharted waters. To be sure, social hygienists were engaged in the collection of medical statistics; indeed, many of the leading social hygienists worked at various levels in the statistical agencies formulating programmes for data collection.[125] But among its leading proponents, the field of social hygiene was seen as requiring much more than the collection of social statistics on health.[126] Indeed, throughout the 1920s, social hygienists were applying and refining a variety of other methods: anthropometry,[127] demography,[128] structured questionnaires,[129] social surveys,[130] and anamnesis.[131] So diverse were the methodological interests of researchers that within GISG a special bureau was opened to coordinate research methods.[132]

How did Soviet social hygienists regard their science? Several elliptical – indeed almost shorthand – statements by the Commissar of Public Health, Nikolai Semashko, provide important clues. First, to the outside observer, the descriptive work of Soviet social hygienists bore an interesting resemblance to the early social-problems sociology of the Chicago school.[133] But it was not nearly as benign. Indeed, as Semashko put it in 1927, the essence of Soviet social hygiene was its 'social sting' *(zhalo)* which came from the analysis of the social factors contributing to disease. That critical edge, he insisted, was invariably absent from social medicine in capitalist countries.[134]

Second, taking a leaf from the book of the German social hygienist A. Kisskalt, Semashko declared that Soviet social hygiene was the 'hygiene of the underprivileged'.[135] This dictum should not be taken to mean that Soviet social hygienists concentrated exclusively on correlating disease and the factor of social class. As one might expect, Soviet social hygienists did examine the connections between the incidence of disease and social class, but they also explored the connections between illness and such factors as the degree of urbanization, place of residence (geographical location), culture and sub-culture; time use (budget studies), occupational patterns and family situation.[136] The result of their efforts was empirical social research which gave real content to the term 'physician–sociologist' *(vrach-sotsiolog).*

Third, Semashko declared that social hygiene was 'its own type of political literacy in the medical schools'.[137] By this he appears to have meant that the field was politically correct both in the sense that it stressed the importance of social reform[138] and that it was espoused by Bolsheviks.[139] Indeed, with a few notable exceptions, all of the Soviet social hygienists enjoyed unimpeachable credentials as Bolsheviks; some could even boast credentials as 'old Bolsheviks'[140] Semashko's formulation – pithy though it was – glossed over the hard questions. Were the correct political credentials indispensable for the recognition of expertise? Who determined the 'correctness' of political credentials? And what happened when politically correct experts disagreed in their analysis and recommendations? The answers to these questions would be hammered out in the course of the 1920s.

Social Hygiene as Spearhead of Preventive Medicine

As described by Semashko in 1922, the physician of the future was to be concerned as much with prevention as with cure. The commitment to prevent disease had been an integral part of pre-revolutionary community medicine, but Soviet social hygienists intensified that commitment, putting prophylaxis at the heart of the new medicine.[141]

But what field should be at the basis of the preventive effort? By mid-decade, social hygiene had assumed the leadership of the 'prophylactic' departments *(kafedry)* in the medical schools, having successfully challenged the long-standing hegemony of general (for this period read 'experimental') hygiene. Intriguingly, the ball was so firmly in the court of the social hygienists that the struggle was fought out on the question of which field (general or social hygiene) had the right to pronounce authoritatively on the social factors influencing disease![142] In 1926, the position of social hygiene among the prophylactic disciplines was further bolstered in the Plan for Higher Medical Education which made mandatory a common curriculum for all medical schools. In that curriculum the number of hours devoted to social hygiene was increased, and the methodological aspect of social hygiene were taught separately from the substantive aspects.[143]

Nor was the influence of social hygiene in the medical schools confined to the prophylactic disciplines. In 1924, Z. P. Soloviev, the Deputy Commissar of Public Health, called for the inclusion of the preventive emphasis in the teaching of clinical subjects.[144] In effect this was a mandate to integrate the clinical and preventive disciplines. The logic behind this mandate was clear: to have a single department in the medical school devoted to preventive medicine while the rest 'did as they pleased' would not advance the cause of prevention.[145] Until the second half of the decade, the commitment to 'integration' remained a formal one. But the 1926 Plan decreed that clinics, in which students received part of their training, were to be infused with a 'social prophylactic emphasis'.[146]

What did 'social prophylaxis' mean? Although the term was never defined precisely (despite being bandied about with alarming frequency), at the minimum it implied that the key to preventing illness lay in social measures.[147] This having been said, the emphasis on social prophylaxis did not mean that the traditional fields of bacteriology, epidemiology and sanitary science were to be de-emphasized. On the contrary, from 1920 on, physicians of these profiles met with great frequency to review their progress in combating a variety of scourges – typhus, the plague, hunger, to name but a few.[148] Out of these meetings came not only a variety of important measures to combat epidemics, but also an increased sense of professional solidarity.

In much the same way, emphasis was also placed in this period on producing a cohort of qualified sanitary physicians.[149] After graduation from medical school and three years of medical practice, physicians were entitled to apply for 'up-grading' *(usovershenstvovanie).* The first post-revolutionary refresher courses were organized under the aegis of the Commissariat of Health's section on sanitary epidemiology. As of 1922, in Moscow the academic part of the refresher courses was given in the Sanitary-Hygiene Institute of the State Institute for Public

Health (GINZ); in Leningrad, interested physicians applied to the Institute for Up-Grading of Physicians. The course of training for the sanitary physician was divided into two parts: the first part consisted of refresher courses in bacteriology, epidemiology, hygiene and sanitation; the second part involved being seconded to various sanitary agencies for work.[150]

In a curious sense, there was a dual status system at work here. The epidemiologists, bacteriologists and sanitary physicians, working as they were in public health institutions, were actively engaged in preventing illness. Semashko himself called the sanitary doctor 'the pioneer of prophylactics throughout and everywhere'.[151] According to official ideology, however, the key to prophylaxis was its social character. The distribution of institutional prestige, however, cut in the opposite direction. The State Institute for Public Health (GINZ), the place of choice in Moscow for refresher courses in bacteriology, epidemiology and sanitary science was recognized as the premier research institution of the Commissariat of Public Health, while the State Institute for Social Hygiene (GISG) – the bastion of social prophylactic ideology – enjoyed considerably less prestige.[152]

Denouement: The Challenge to Social Expertise

Beginning in 1928, the goal of preventing illness came under serious review. In part, the review was prompted by budgetary problems associated with the adoption of the policy of rapid industrialization. Unlike in Germany and France, where the onset of industrialization was the catalyst for the development of social, and particularly industrial, hygiene,[153] in Soviet Russia, industrialization was sponsored and directed by the state which, in order to achieve heightened rates of economic growth, deflected resources from other sectors of the economy, among them health care. Given the reduction in the budgets for public health[154] and a corresponding shortfall in the total allocations for the medical schools, it is hardly surprising that the new *kafedry* of preventive medicine fared less well than the more established *kafedry* of curative medicine. But it was also the case that by the end of the 1920s, there was a notable lack of enthusiasm for preventive medicine – both among teachers in the medical schools and among medical students. One medical school professor is reported to have told students, 'We are here to teach you so that you can earn a living, not be sanitary doctors!'[155]

In the new climate, social prophylaxis came under particular attack. How is this to be explained? By the end of the decade, technocracy had become a burning issue in official circles. The well-worn Soviet question *Kto kogo* (Who whom?) usually applied to political issues was being raised *vis-à-vis* the state's relation with experts. In 1928 VARNITSO, a Marxist ideological organization that sought to enlist members of the scientific-technical intelligentsia was formed.[156] The attack on the bourgeois specialists set in motion by the trial of the Shakhty engineers in April 1928 spilled over into a more pervasive assault on all experts who espoused technocratic views.[157]

In a climate of general distrust of technocratic views, social hygiene was understandably seen as threatening. The social hygienists' approach to social diagnosis implicitly indicted a regime which, if it had not created the social conditions which made for illness, at the very least had allowed those conditions to persist. Even more to the point, followed to its logical conclusion, the social hygienists' approach to prophylaxis suggested that social-economic reform held the key to the improvement of public health. By the late 1920s, the regime was formulating its own design for rapid change – a design which gave little quarter to socio-economic improvement. Small wonder that the regime regarded with suspicion the claims to authority over public health advanced by social hygienists who had their own agenda.

The first indicator of the attack on social prophylaxis came in the restructuring of the medical schools in 1930. In early 1930 Semashko was removed from his post as Commissar of Public Health allegedly 'in accordance with his request'.[158] Within six months of Semashko's 'reassignment' the medical institutes were divided into three faculties: the 'curative-prophylactic' faculty which prepared specialists in surgery, therapy and dentistry; the 'sanitary-prophylactic' faculty which prepared specialists in general sanitation, communal living, industrial sanitation, as well as physician– epidemiologists; and the faculty of 'protection of mothers and children' which prepared specialists in maternity and infant care.[159] The division of the medical school into faculties was accompanied by a reduction in the length of the course of study. But that reduction fell differentially: as of 1930, sanitary-prophylactic faculties, to which physicians interested in social hygiene were directed, required only three and a half years to complete, whereas the other two faculties required four years.

Not long after education in social hygiene was attacked, the research work of social hygienists came under attack. In late 1930, GISG was converted into the Institute of Organization of Health Care and Hygiene; its top priorities were administrative – practical health care and organization.[160] To the extent that it endured at all after that point, social research on health and disease was conducted by statisticians.

How did social hygienists respond to the attack? Instead of fighting back, social hygienists switched course. For example, in October 1930 when prevention was under fire, A. V. Mol'kov – one of the leading spokesmen for social hygiene throughout the 1920s and the Director of GISG – took the unusual step of trying to disaggregate social hygiene and prevention. He argued that the real 'prophylactization' of clinical teaching required the divorce of the prophylactic emphasis from 'special' (read social hygiene) departments and its insertion into the clinical departments.[161] Had Mol'kov's statement been issued in the period 1925–9 when the *kafedry* of social hygiene were spearheading the drive for integration, it might have gone unnoticed; issued as it was in 1930, when the *kafedry* of social hygiene were under attack, the statement suggests that in order to save prevention (a goal to which Mol'kov had been committed long before 1917),[162] he was willing to sever it from social hygiene, the field he had helped to define.

What were the implications of the attack on social hygiene for the goals which social hygienists had been pursuing since the beginning of the decade? The division of medical education into three separate streams spelled the death knell to the effort to integrate preventive and curative medicine. To be sure, the term 'prophylactic' was applied both to the curative faculty and to the sanitary faculty, but the prophylaxis to which it referred differed remarkably from that which social hygienists had advocated throughout the previous decade. The prophylaxis of 1930 was embedded in practical work; indeed, it seems to have been exemplified in the work of the polyclinics.

Equally important, with specialization the by-word of the day, the social hygienists' original dream of training physicians with broad social horizons as well as deep scientific culture fell by the wayside. As of 1930, the archetypical public health doctor became the sanitary physician. But the sanitary physician of the early 1930s was less well steeped in biology than was a graduate of either of the other two faculties. And he was less well trained in sociology than the social hygienists had urged. Indeed, the new sanitary physician was to be an expert in sanitary technology, not in social criticism.[163] Lest the prohibition against technocracy be lost on the audience, a 1930 article called for the production of 'social engineers' whose mandate was to work in the technique of industrial safety and sanitary technique![164] By 1931, the metaphor had changed again: there were repeated calls to phase out the 'doctor–craftsman' in favour of the 'doctor–organizer–social–activist' whose strong suit was his ability to understand Marxist ideology.[165]

Within the space of a decade, then, the profile of the ideal public health physician underwent drastic change. In the official designs for the future, the socially conscious physician supported by the state whose mandate was to diagnose the social causes of illness and recommend social remedies was displaced by the sanitary scientist doing technical work marked out for him by those who commissioned his work.[166]

There is a terrible irony here. Whereas Semashko had once remarked that in the bourgeois nations the social hygienist was prevented from being critical, the same fate now befell the Soviet social hygienist. Whereas Semashko had once celebrated the *zhalo* (sting) of Soviet social hygiene, that sting now became the point of vulnerability of the field.

Conclusion

The case of Soviet social hygiene raises some intriguing issues about public health expertise and the state. First, from the point of view of the physicians, there is the question of the impact of official recognition upon the functioning of experts. Historians of Russian public health have documented a half century of striving by Russian physicians for official recognition of their expertise on matters of public health. The development of public health in the Soviet period suggests that recognition did not come without its costs. The increased recognition – indeed, the reliance – by the Commissariat of Public Health on social hygiene expertise brought with it more, rather than less, state intervention in professional activity. What turned out to matter was not the brute fact of experts' recognition by the state, but the nature of the state (in this case autocratic) which enlisted the expertise of physicians!

Then there is the question of the attitude of the state to public health expertise. In a recent thought-provoking piece, Dorothy and Roy Porter surveyed the range of forms which social medicine had taken in Germany, France and Britain. According to the authors, despite some variation, all instances of social medicine 'depended on' a state whose actions in public health were scientifically-informed and technocratically-determined. To social medicine thus defined, the authors juxtaposed socialist medicine. In cases of socialist medicine, the state is seen as 'a political, rather than technical, entity'. Socialist medicine 'looks for the causes of health and sickness in the economic relations of production and the social relations of class and seeks prevention through changing the political relations of power'.[167]

Was Soviet social hygiene a form of social medicine or of socialist medicine? This paper suggests that, in terms of its content, Soviet social hygiene straddled the line between these two ideal types. Its analysis of the aetiology of disease tended to be closer to the 'socialist' type, although social hygiene researchers looked for the causes of disease not only in social class factors, but in a variety of other factors as well.

The Porters' distinction directs us to look not only at the type of social knowledge about health and disease that was being provided by experts, but also at the attitude of the state towards experts and expertise. The paper has documented a change in the profile of the ideal public health physician from the socially-involved 'doctor–sociologist' (whose mandate was as much to diagnose society itself as to diagnose illness) to the sanitary physician (whose mandate was to follow directives). The nature of the change suggests that, while initially the state may have sought scientific information about public health, by 1930, it was unwilling to give credence to the claims to authority over Russia's pressing health problems launched by any group on the basis of its scientific research. By 1930, in the Porters' terms, the Soviet state behaved much more like a political, than like a technocratic entity. The behaviour of the Stalinist state towards its experts is particularly significant because in Soviet Russia, the state was the major patron (and addressee) for public health science.

The case of Soviet social hygiene raises not only the question of expert-state relations, but also the issue of the role of social medicine in public health. In the case at hand, bacteriology and epidemiology co-existed not with social reformism of the old type, but with scientifically-based social medicine which urged the importance of social change as the key to the improvement of public health. It is important to note that the social hygienist's stress on social reform was not an instance of do-goodism that refused to die, an anachronistic belief that refused to be eclipsed. Rather, the social hygienists' commitment to 'scientific' social change mirrored the commitment of the regime, a commitment which was used to legitimate the seizure of power in 1917.

The fact that Soviet public health in the 1920s accommodated strong commitments both to medical science (bacteriology, epidemiology and sanitary science) and to social reform (in the sense advocated by social hygienists) may well prompt the rethinking of conventional wisdom on the development of public health. This having been said, we may note that, at the end of the 1920s, the co-existence of these two orientations in public health apparently challenged the Soviet state which resolved the issue in favour of an apolitical medical science.

Notes

1. See Nancy Frieden, 'Physicians in Pre-Revolutionary Russia: Professionals or Servants of the State?', *Bulletin of the History of Medicine,* 49 (1975), 20– 9; *idem,* 'The Russian Cholera Epidemic, 1892–1893, and Medical Professionalization', *Journal of Social History,* 10 (1977), 538–59; Peter F. Krug, 'The Debate over the Delivery of Health Care in Rural Russia', *Bulletin of the History of Medicine,* 50 (1976), 226–41; Samuel Ramer, 'Who was the Russian Feldsher?' *Bulletin of the History of Medicine,* 50 (1976), 213–25. John T. Alexander, *Bubonic Plague in Early Modern Russia: Public Health and Urban Disaster* (Baltimore: 1980); Nancy Frieden, *Russian Physicians in an Era of Reform and Revolution, 1856–1905* (Princeton: 1981); John F. Hutchinson, 'Society, Corporation or Union? Russian Physicians and the Struggle for Professional Unity (1890–1913)', *Jahrbücher für Geschichte Osteuropas,* 30 (1982), 37–53; *idem,* 'Tsarist Russia and the Bacteriological Revolution', *Journal of the History of Medicine and Allied Sciences,* 40 (1985), 220–39; *idem, Politics and Public Health in Revolutionary Russia 1890–1918* (Baltimore: 1990).
2. Alexander, *op. cit.* (note 1), Frieden, 'The Russian Cholera Epidemic'.
3. Richard G. Robbins, Jr., *Famine in Russia, 1891–1892: The Imperial Government Responds to a Crisis* (New York: 1975).
4. Julie V. Brown, 'Psychiatrists and the State in Late Imperial Russia', in A. Scull and S. Cohen (eds), *Social Control and the State* (New York: 1983), 267–87; *idem,* 'Revolution and Psychosis: The Mixing of Science and Politics in Russian Psychiatric Medicine, 1905–1913', *The Russian Review,* 46 (1987), 283–302.
5. Laurie Bernstein, 'Yellow Tickets and State-Licensed Brothels: The Tsarist Government and the Regulation of Urban Prostitution', in Susan Gross Solomon and John F. Hutchinson (eds), *Health and Society in Revolutionary Russia* (Bloomington, In.: 1990), 45–65.
6. Frieden, 'Physicians in Pre-Revolutionary Russia', 20–1.
7. For a description of the Medical Statute, which set out formally the duties of physicians and the criminal penalties they could incur for failure to fail to fulfil those duties, see *ibid.,* 25.
8. According to data that covered 9/10 of the medical profession, in 1889, the percentage of physicians in private practice in Russia was 26.3; in 1903, that percentage had risen to 33.3. See Frieden, *Russian Physicians,* 211. It was well known that even public physicians engaged in small amounts of private practice to supplement their

modest incomes. See Hutchinson, *Politics and Public Health,* 58–9.

9. Frieden, ' Physicians in Pre-Revolutionary Russia'.
10. This point is made in John F. Hutchinson, 'Politics and Medical Professionalization after 1905', in Harley Balzer (ed.), *Professions in Russia at the End of the Old Regime* (Cornell University Press) forthcoming.
11. Similar sorts of debates occurred in the United States in the early decades of this century. See Elizabeth Fee, 'Competition for the First School of Hygiene and Public Health', *Bulletin of the History of Medicine,* 57 (1983), 339–63.
12. These debates are familiar in the history of public health. For an analysis of their occurrence in England, see Lloyd G. Stevenson, 'Science Down the Drain', *Bulletin of the History of Medicine,* 29 (1955), 1–26.
13. See Krug, 'Russian Public Physicians'; Neil B. Weissman, 'Origins of Soviet Health Administration', *Narkomzdrav,* 1918–1928, in Solomon & Hutchinson (eds), *Health and Society,* 97–120; Sally Ewing, 'The Science and Politics of Soviet Insurance Medicine', *ibid.,* 69–96; Samuel C. Ramer, 'Feldshers and Rural Health Care in the Early Soviet Period', *ibid.,* 121–46; Susan Gross Solomon, 'The Limits of Government Patronage of Science: Social Hygiene and the Soviet State, 1920–1930', *Social History of Medicine* (October, 1990), 405–35; Christopher Williams, 'War, Revolution and Medicine: Petrograd Doctors, 1917–1920', Paper presented to the Study Group on the Russian Revolution, Lincoln College, Oxford, 4–6 January, 1991.
14. Susan Gross Solomon, 'Social Hygiene in Soviet Medical Education, 1922–1930', *Journal of the History of Medicine and Allied Sciences,* 45 (1990), no. 4, 607–43. Compare this to the description of pre-revolutionary education in medicine as found in M. D. Grmek, 'Les Bases Historiques de L'Enseignement Medical en Russie', *I-re partie, Episteme,* anno IV, n. 2 aprile - giugno (1970), 131–45; II Partie, *ibid.,* no. 4 dicembre (1970), 334–56.
15. A. I. Nesterenko, *Kak byl obrazovan Narodnyi kommissariat zdravookhranenie RSFSR: Iz istorii Sovetskogo zdravookhraneniia (oktiabr' 1917 g.– iul. 1918 g.)* (Moscow: 1965); Weissman, *op. cit.* (note 13).
16. In the revolutionary days in 1917, a variety of medical unions were created. See Hutchinson, *Politics and Public Health,* 181–8. By early 1918, most of the medical unions which had been set up in the wake of February 1917 had been brought under the umbrella of the new Medical Workers Union *(Vsemediksantrud).* See Williams, 'War, Revolution, and Medicine', 15.
17. See G. Karanovich and S. Cherniak, *Professional'nye prava i obiazannosti meditsinskogo rabotnika* (Moscow: 1927). The vast number of physicians' obligations to the state described here in minute

detail should be compared against those set forth in the much slimmer book, L. Valerianov, *Prava i obiazannosti vrachei* (St Petersburg: 1913).

18. For the extent of that private practice and some indications of the complex of problems which the government faced in dealing with it, see P. M. Gubinskii, 'Meditsina gosudarstvennaia i chastnaia', *Vestnik sovremennoi meditsiny,* no. 5 (1928), 302–5; L. Bronshtein, 'O chastnom kapitale v dele zdravookhraneniia', *Voprosy zdravookhraneniia* no. 2 (1930), 1–3.
19. The principles of the new Soviet medicine were articulated by the first Commissar of Public Health, N. A. Semashko, in June of 1918 in a speech entitled 'Fundamental Tasks of Soviet Medicine on the Local Level'. For a description, see Weissman, *op. cit.* (note 13), 97.
20. N. A. Semashko, 'Sotsial'naia gigiena, ee sushchnost, metod i znachenie', *Sotsial'naia gigiena (*1922), 1, 8.
21. See N. A. Semashko, *Nauka o zdorovye obshchestva: Sotsial'naia gigiena* (Moscow: 1921). N. A. Semashko (b. 1874), one of the most prominent Bolshevik physicians, began his involvement with Marxism in 1893. Arrested for Marxist activities, he emigrated to Switzerland in 1906, where he developed a close relation with Lenin. In April of 1917, he returned with Lenin to Russia, In July 1918, Semashko was named first Commissar of Public Health. See the entry on Semashko in *Bol'shaia Sovetskaia Entsiklopediia,* Vol. 50 (1944), 738. For a discussion of the limits on Semashko's ability to protect social hygiene, see Solomon, 'The Limits of Government Patronage of Science'.
22. See, for example, Vicente Navarro, *Social Security and Medicine in the USSR: A Marxist Critique* (London: 1977); Michael Ryan, *The Organization of Soviet Medical Care* (Oxford: 1978); William Knaus, *Inside Russian Medicine: An American Doctor's First Hand Report* (New York: 1981); Michael Kaser, *Health Care in the Soviet Union and Eastern Europe* (London: 1976); Christopher Davis and Murray Feshbach, 'Rising Infant Mortality in the USSR in the 1970s', Bureau of the Census, US Department of Commerce (Washington, D.C.: 1980).
23. To be sure, the 'Great Break' of 1928–31 affected not only medicine, but almost all fields of science and the arts. For essays on the impact of the events of the late 1920s on Soviet intellectual and cultural life, see Sheila Fitzpatrick, *Cultural Revolution in Russia* (Bloomington, In.: 1980).
24. For example, Horsley Gantt, *A Medical Review of Soviet Russia* (London: 1928); Arthur Newsholme and John Kingsbury, *Red Medicine: Socialized Health in Soviet Russia* (London: 1934); Henry Sigerist, *Socialized Medicine in Soviet Russia* (New York: 1937). The clear exception to the pattern of neglect is Henry Sigerist whose work and thought have recently been revived.
25. See, for example, I. V. Vengrova and Iu. A. Shilinis, *Sotsial'naia*

gigiena v SSSR (Moscow: 1976); E. Ia. Belitskaia, *Problemy sotsial'noi gigieny* (Leningrad: 1970).

26. This point is made in Elizabeth Fee and Dorothy Porter, 'Public health, preventive medicine, and professionalization: Britain and the United States in the nineteenth century', in Elizabeth Fee and Roy M. Acheson, *A History of Education in Public Health: Health that Mocks the Doctors' Rules* (Oxford: Oxford University Press, 1991), 33.
27. A similar puzzle is presented by the simultaneous support of the Russian Commissariat of Public Health for 'hereditarian' eugenics and 'environmentalist' social hygiene. Mark Adams has argued that this situation is anomalous only if one thinks of the Commissariat of Health as having been created 'from the top down' to implement a specific policy line. He contends that the Commissariat was built up 'from below' on the basis of its contacts and dealings with various medical specialities. See Mark B. Adams, 'Eugenics as Social Medicine in Revolutionary Russia: Prophets, Patrons and the Dialectics of Discipline-Building', in Solomon & Hutchinson, *op. cit.* (note 5), 200–1.
28. Frieden, *Russian Physicians.*
29. The Pirogov society (officially the Society of Russian Physicians in Memory of N. I Pirogov) was not the first medical society in Russia, but it was the first nation-wide society. See *ibid.,* 118–22.
30. *Ibid.,* 5.
31. According to Frieden, Pirogov physicians compared their lot unfavourably with that of physicians in England and France. Hutchinson argues that for Pirogov physicians there was one criterion according to which the success of all systems of public health was measured – namely, the degree to which the delivery of health care was independent of state control. With this yardstick in mind, the Pirogov physicians hailed England as the ideal and denigrated France because of the excessive centralization of its government. In Hutchinson's view these perceptions were 'selective and distorted'. See Hutchinson, *Politics and Public Health,* 73–4.
32. The *zemstvos* were introduced at the time of the emancipation of the serfs and the great reforms. See Kermit Mackenzie, '*Zemstvo* Organization and Role within the Administrative Structure', in Terence Emmons and Wayne Vucinich (eds), *The Zemstvo in Russia: An Experiment in Local Self-Government* (Cambridge: 1982), 31–78. The *zemstvos* provided medical services free of charge to the three-quarters of Russia's population who lived in the countryside. For a discussion of the *zemstvo* work in public health, see Samuel C. Ramer, 'The *Zemstvo* and Public Health', in *ibid.* 279–314.
33. In the 1860s, there was a dual public health structure in the provinces: the gubernatorial authorities had jurisdiction over major health issues, while the *zemstvos* supervised secondary problems. A series of epidemics in the 1870s demonstrated the superiority of the

zemstvo approach to health care and, as a result, the central government shifted more medical power to the *zemstvos.* See Nancy M. Frieden, 'The Politics of Zemstvo Medicine', *ibid.*, 318. The treatment of health work by the central administration was far from typical; in many cases, the period after 1865 saw the effort by the centre to recapture authority from the *zemstvos.*

34. Frieden, *Russian Physicians*, 28. Frieden admitted that initially for physicians work in the *zemstvos* was much like work in government service, but she insisted that the cholera epidemic of 1892/3 provided *zemstvo* physicians with new opportunities. Almost overnight, physicians found themselves being granted new authority, new powers. Frieden, 'The Russian Cholera Epidemic',550.
35. *Ibid.*, 314.
36. The enhanced powers granted to physicians during the cholera epidemic of 1892/3 were not enshrined in law and, therefore, almost as soon as the worse effects of the epidemic were over Russian physicians were once again relegated to their former position as government servitors. See Frieden, 'The Russian Cholera Epidemic'.
37. Krug, *op. cit.* (note 13).
38. *Ibid.*, 283.
39. *Ibid.*, 284.
40. Hutchinson, 'Society, Corporation, or Union?', 52. Hutchinson explained that, to the extent it included the rights of professionals to establish limits on their obligations to society, the idea of corporate autonomy for physicians was opposed both by the autocracy and by radical physicians.
41. For Krug the cooperation between the community physicians and the new state began in the period 1918–20. Community physicians were given some control over the struggle against the epidemics ravaging Russia. At the same time, the Bolsheviks also turned aside some of the claims to legitimacy made by the *feldsher*s (paramedics). On both of these issues, the Bolsheviks lined up with community medicine.
42. Krug made a similar point about the Pirogovtsy and the tsarist state. He argued that the Pirogovtsy never opposed the idea of a centralized medical bureaucracy *per se;* they were hostile to the St Petersburg medical establishment and to the leaders of the prestigious Military Medical Academy only because they had been excluded from these circles.
43. Krug, *op. cit.* (note 13), 286 ff. Hutchinson disagreed with Krug on this point. He argued that the Pirogovtsy had achieved comparatively little during the time of the Provisional Government.
44. Here Krug's target was the Soviet historian of medicine/activist M. Barsukov who portrayed the Pirogovtsy as saboteurs whose doom was sealed by the Bolsheviks. *Ibid.*, 297–311.
45. *Ibid.*, 273.
46. Hutchinson, *Politics and Public Health,* 73.

47. John F. Hutchinson, 'Who Killed Cock Robin? An Inquiry into the Death of Zemstvo Medicine', in Solomon & Hutchinson (eds), *Health and Society,* 3–26. Hutchinson claimed that, as early as 1910, spokesmen for *zemstvo* medicine were having a hard time trying to maintain the traditional ideology. *Ibid.*, 12.
48. This attitude is clear in Hutchinson's article, 'Politics and Medical Professionalization'.
49. See Hutchinson, *Politics and Public Health,* xvi–xvii.
50. *Ibid.*, xix–xx.
51. *Ibid.*, 199–202.
52. In the first half of the nineteenth century, public health was regarded as an administrative ('medical police') concern, the rudiments of which were communicated to students in courses on legal medicine.
53. This orientation was typical of the field of public health elsewhere in the same period. See Jane Lewis, 'The public's health: philosophy and practice in Britain in the twentieth century', in Fee & Acheson, *op. cit.* (note 26), 198.
54. In his discussion of the epidemiology of the nineteenth century Ackerknecht identified three types of theories: the physico-chemical or geographical (including the miasmists and tellurists); the biological (the bacteriologists and parasitists) and the sociological. Ackerknecht admitted that the 'sociological' approach often gave greatest weight to economic factors, but he justified his use of the label 'sociological' on the grounds that he wished to contrast that approach with biological theories. See Erwin Ackerknecht, 'Anti-contagionism between 1821 and 1867', *Bulletin for the History of Medicine,* 22 (1948), 592–3.
55. Frieden, *Russian Physicians,* 80. There was a long history of statistical study of mortality in Russia, dating back to the eighteenth century.
56. *Ibid.*, 313–15.
57. *Ibid.*, 140.
58. *Ibid.*, Epilogue.
59. Hutchinson, 'Tsarist Russia and the Bacteriological Revolution', 427.
60. Hutchinson, *Politics and Public Health,* 22.
61. *Ibid.*, 62. 'Diagnostician, therapist, surgeon, ophthalmologist, and sometimes midwife as well, the *zemstvo uchastok* physician was idealized in the publications of the Pirogov society as a heroic jack of all trades'. *Ibid.*, 61. Not only was the Pirogov physician a generalist in practice, but, as Hutchinson put it, 'The ideology of community medicine discouraged specialization.'
62. It is important to note that the Sanitary Executive Commissions which began to function in the 1890s were composed primarily of physicians; after 1904, the sanitary commissions were dominated by non-medical administrators. See Frieden, *Russian Physicians,* 284, 287.
63. Hutchinson, *Politics and Public Health,* 61.

64. These attempts are described in Hutchinson, 'Tsarist Russia and the Bacteriological Revolution'.
65. *Ibid.*, 430.
66. L. Ia. Shkorokhodov, *Materialy po istorii meditsinskoi mikrobiologii v dorevoliutsionnoi Rossii* (Moscow: 1948), 200 ff.
67. *Ibid.*, 432.
68. Hutchinson, *Politics and Public Health,* 70. Aleksei Nikolaevich Sysin (b. 1879) was the director of the Nizhni-Novgorod sanitary bureau and a rising member of the Pirogov Society before the revolution of 1917. After the Bolsheviks took power, he was head of the sanitary-epidemiological section of the Russian Commissariat of Public Health from 1918–31. See the entry on Sysin in *Bol'shaia meditsinskaia entsiklopediia,* 5 (1935), 239–40.
69. Hutchinson, *Politics and Public Health,* 70.
70. *Ibid.*, 66.
71. For a history of the efforts to set up a course on community medicine, see Z. G. Frenkel, *Obshchestvennaia meditsina i sotsial'naia gigiena* (Leningrad: 1926), 9–31; for the projected research centre, see N. F. Gamaleia, 'K voprosu o Ministerstv'e Narodnago Zdraviia', *Gigiena i sanitariia,* I (1910), 1–32.
72. Mol'kov declared that while these proposals were interesting, it was difficult to identify their underlying principles. See Mol'kov, 'K voprosu o peresmotre', 24.
73. See Solomon, *op. cit.* (note 14).
74. V. Ia. Kanel, 'Sotsial'naia meditsina, ee sushchnost' i znachenie'. *Obshchestvennyi vrach* (1913), 439 ff.
75. For a sense of the relation between 'sociology' and 'doing good' in the evolution of British social science, see Philip Abrams, *The Origins of British Sociology, 1834–1914* (Chicago: 1968); Lawrence Goldman, 'Statistics and the Science of Society in Early Victorian Britain; An Intellectual Context for the General Register Office', *Social History of Medicine,* Vol. 4, no. 3 (December, 1991), 415–35.
76. Alexander Vucinich, *Social Thought in Tsarist Russia: The Quest for a General Science of Society, 1861–1917* (Chicago: 1976), 243.
77. 'Bacteriology thus became an ideological marker, sharply differentiating the "old" public health, mainly the province of untrained amateurs, from the "new" public health, which belonged to scientifically trained professionals. Fee & Porter, *op. cit.* (note 26), 33.
78. I owe this term to Dorothy Porter.
79. For a discussion of the early apprehensions of the physicians about their likely treatment at the hands of the Soviet regime, see Mark G. Field, 'The Hybrid Profession: Soviet Medicine', in Anthony Jones (ed.), *Professions and the State: Expertise and Autonomy in the Soviet Union and Eastern Europe* (Philadelphia: 1991).
80. For the overlap in personnel between the Pirogov Society and the new Russian Commissariat of Public Health, see Krug, 'Russian

Public Physicians', 229–67.

81. The premium placed by the Bolsheviks on improving the qualifications of physicians was evident in their treatment of the bid by the *feldshers* for status equal to that of physicians. For a detailed analysis, see Ramer, *op. cit.* (note 13), 121–45; Krug, 'Russian Public Physicians', 229–67.
82. *Ibid.*, 220.
83. For as detailed discussion of the role of anti-epidemic work in forging links between the Pirogov physicians and the new regime, see *ibid.*, 190–3. See also Hutchinson, *Politics and Public Health,* 187.
84. I owe this chronology to Daniel P. Todes.
85. A. V. Mol'kov, 'K voprosu o peresmotre obshchego plana prepodavaniia gigienicheskikh distsiplin v vysshei medskole', *Sotsial'naia gigiena* no. 2 25. A. V. Molkov (1870–1947) was the head of the Pirogov Society's Commission on the Spread of Hygiene Education (1900–18). He then became the Director of the State Museum for Social Hygiene (1918–22) and the Director of the State Institute for Social Hygiene (1923–30). For a biography, see A. P. Shishkin, 'A. V. Mol'kov—organizator i rukovoditel' instituta sotsial'noi gigieny Narkomzdrava RSFSR', *Sovetskoe zdravookhranenie,* 1970, no. 10, 64–8.
86. I. S. Ruzheinikov, 'Reforma vysshego meditsinskogo obrazovaniia', *Biulleten' Narkomzdrava* (1924), no. 11, 27. This description of the physician of the future continued to be sounded until the end of the decade.
87. Specialization was reserved for refresher courses. For the history and development of the net of refresher courses for medical students, see M. G. Savchenko, *Ocherk razvitiia sistemy povysheniia kvalifikatsii vrachebnykh kadrov v SSSR* (Kishinev: 1967).
88. A. V. Mol'kov decried the increasing specialization of late tsarism as the epitome of the move away from 'encyclopedism'. See Mol'kov, 'K voprosu o peresmotre', 4.
89. 'Meditsinskoe obrazovanii', *Bol'shaia meditsinskaia entsiklopediia,* (1936), XVII, 667.
90. The socio-biological approach was not unique to social hygiene. There were a variety of hybrid fields in Russian from the early twentieth century on. See Mark B. Adams, 'The Soviet Nature-Nurture Debate', in Loren R. Graham (ed.), *Science and the Soviet Social Order* (Cambridge, Mass.: 1990), 97–8.
91. Karanovich and Cherniak, *Professional'nye prava,* 194/5.
92. The interest in raising medical qualifications was clear from the directive of the Council of People's Commissars. See 'O podniatii kvalifikatsii okanchivaiushchikh vuzov', cited in *ibid.*, 196.
93. The new curriculum was divided into two parts – preparatory and specialized. In the preparatory section, the basic courses were biology, physiology and biochemistry. Botany and zoology were incorporated

into general biology. Pharmacy and pharmacology were eliminated; and the number of hours devoted to morphological disciplines was reduced by over 33 per cent. New languages and military sciences were introduced as compulsory. In the specialized section, the *kafedra* of general pathology became pathological physiology; the courses on medical diagnostics and semiotics were united in a *kafedra* of propadeutics of internal diseases. To that *kafedra* an independent course on physical methods of treatment was attached. *Ibid.*

94. A. V. Mol'kov, 'Predislovie', in A. V. Mol'kov (ed.), *Sotsial'naia gigiena* (Moscow: 1927), 7.
95. Semashko, 'Sotsial'naia gigiena, ee sushchnost', 8.
96. Their particular favourites were Alfred Grotjahn, Benno Chajes and Alfons Fischer. It is interesting to note that while the Soviets greatly admired Grotjahn, with few exceptions, they did not share his enthusiasm for eugenics.
97. A. N. Sysin, 'K voprosu o programme prepodavaniia gigieny na meditsinskikh fakul'tetakh', *Sotsial'naia gigiena* I (1922), 19–20.
98. M. S. Brodskii, 'K istorii partiinikh Bolshevistskikh organizatsii vysshei meditsinskoi shkole', *Sovetskoe zdravookhranenie* (1963), no. 9, 63.
99. Vengrova and Shilinis, *Sotsial'naia gigiena v SSSR*, 122–3.
100. *Ibid.*
101. John Hutchinson mentioned Gamaleia's proposal of 1910 to create a Ministry of Public Health with a State Institute of Social Hygiene as its research arm. Hutchinson, *Politics and Public Health*, 75. A description of the scope of the proposed Institute suggests that to Gamaleia 'social hygiene' was a field that concerned itself with questions of sanitation, sanitary technology, sanitary legislation.
102. Krug, 'The Debate Over the Delivery of Health Care'.
103. Peter Krug, 'Social Hygienists and Medical Education: A Century of Debate', Paper presented at the convention of the American Association for the Advancement of Slavic Studies, Philadelphia, 7 November, 1980, 7.
104. Krug, 'Russian Public Physicians', 197–8.
105. That debate has been analysed in detail in Solomon, *op. cit.* (note 14).
106. Anthony Oberschall, *Empirical Social Research in Germany, 1848–1914* (The Hague: 1965); Suzanne Schad, *Empirical Social Research in Weimar Germany* (The Hague: 1972); Terry N. Clark, *The French University and the Emergence of the Social Sciences* (Cambridge, Mass.: 1973); David Elesh, 'The Manchester Statistical Society: A Case Study of Discontinuity in the History of Empirical Social Research', in Anthony Oberschall (ed.), *The Establishment of Empirical Sociology: Studies in Continuity, Discontinuity and Institutionalization* (New York: 1972), 31–72; See M. J. Cullen, *The Statistical Movement in Early Victorian Britain: The Founding of Empirical Social Research* (London: 1975); Dorothy Ross, *The Origins*

of American Social Science (Cambridge: 1991).

107. For the development of statistical science in pre-revolutionary Russia, see A. A. Kaufman, *Statisticheskaia nauka v Rossii. teoriia i metodologiia, 1806–1917* (Moscow: 1922). For an English language discussion of some of this work, see Robert E. Johnson, 'Liberal Professionals and Professional Liberals:The *Zemstvo* Statisticians and Their Work', in Emmons & Vucinich *op. cit.* (note 32), 343–64.
108. Vucinich, *op. cit.* (note 76).
109. Elizabeth Ann Weinberg, *The Development of Sociology in the Soviet Union* (London: 1974), ch. 1.
110. See Louise B. Shelley, *Soviet Criminology: Its Birth and Demise* (Philadelphia: 1977); Susan Gross Solomon, *The Soviet Agrarian Debate: A Controversy in Social Science, 1923–1930* (Boulder, Co.: 1978).
111. Social hygienists had little compunction about combining description and prescription in their science.
112. The fact that social hygiene was institutionalized before its substance had been defined was usual. For a discussion of the implications of this pattern of development for the content of the field, see Solomon, *op. cit.* (note 13).
113. For the spectrum of views on this issue, see L. A. Mamedova, 'Nekotorye teoreticheskie voprosy meditsinskoi nauki v gody stanovlenie sovetskoi vlasti', *Sovetskoe zdravookhranenie (1988)* no. 2, 62–6. Among Soviet social hygienists there were of course regional variations in the precise mix of social and biological factors considered. See Solomon, 'Social Hygiene and Soviet Public health', in Solomon & Hutchinson, *op. cit.* (note 5), 181–3.
114. I owe the conception of such fields to Mark B. Adams.
115. O. G. Birger, 'Eksperimental'naia epidemiologiia', *Gigiena i epidemiologiia* (1925) no. 5, 56–67. For paeans of praise to the accomplishments of this field, see V. A. Liubarskii, 'Dostizhenie v oblasti mikrobiologii i epidemiologii v gody 1917–1927 v SSSR', *Vestnik sovremennoi meditisiny* (1928) no. 2, 90–8.
116. Pitirim Sorokin, 'Sostoianie russkoi sotsiologii za 1918–1922g.g.', *Novaia russkaia kniga* (1922) no. 10, (oktiabr), 7–10.
117. See V. I Klushin, 'Sotsiologiia v petrogradskom universitete (1920–1924)', *Vestnik Leningradskogo universitete* (1964) no. 5, 70–81.
118. N. A. Semashko, 'K desiatiletiiu Oktabria', *Sotsial'naia gigiena 1927,* no. 10, 3.
119. See *Sotsial'naia gigiena* edited by A. V. Mol'kov, *et al.* (Moscow: 1927). This was the first Soviet textbook in social hygiene. It contained numerous references to the research described in *Handwörterbuch der sozialen Hygiene* edited by Alfred Grotjahn and J. Kaup (1912–13).
120. Raymond Bauer, *The New Man in Soviet Society* (Cambridge, Mass.:1952). For an interesting interpretation of the period, see

Richard Stites, *Revolutionary Dreams: Utopian Vision and Experimental Life in the Russian Revolution* (Oxford: 1989).

121. For a fine discussion of this point, see Adams, *op. cit.* (note 90).
122. For an excellent description of these early attempts to broaden the notion of general hygiene, see Frenkel, *Obshchestvennaia meditsina.*
123. For a discussion of the social hygiene research agenda, see Solomon, *op. cit.* (note 113), 185–9.
124. A. P. Shishkin, 'Sotsial'no-gigienicheskaia napravlennost' deiatel'nosti nauchno-issledovatel'skikh institutov narodnogo kommissariata zdravookhraneniia RSFSR v 20–30-e gody', *Sovetskoe zdravookhrannenie,* (1978), no. 7, 69.
125. F. D. Markuzon, *Ocherki po istorii po sanitarnoi statistike v dorevoliutsionnoi Rossii i v SSSR* (Moscow: 1961). Some public health physicians who had been active in public health before the Revolution (for example, Bogoslovskii and P. P. Kurkin) were working with the data on mortality and morbidity. Note also that some social hygienists had an active interest in statistical methods. See G. A. Batkis, 'Ocherki po statisticheskoi metodologii', *Sotsial'naia gigiena,* 12–13 (1928), 19–35.
126. E. Iakovenko, 'O predmete i zadachakh sotsial'noi gigieny', *Sotsial'naia gigiena,* 2 (1923), 12. Iakovenko said it was not just new numbers that social medicine would adduce using the sociological method, but the reality hiding behind the numbers.
127. M. A. Koldobskii, 'O nektorykh metodakh otsenki fizicheskogo razvitiia', *Sotsial'naia gigiena,* 7 (1926), 90–112; V. V. Bunak, 'O rabote ekspertnoi kommissii po standardizatsii antropometricheskoi instrumentov', *ibid.*, Prilozhenie.
128. P. I. Kurkin, 'Ocherk genealogicheskoi statistike', *ibid.*, 38–91. See also G. A. Batkis, 'K voprosu o vychislenii srednogo vozrasta po statisticheskikh i demograficheskikh issledovaniakh', *Sotsial'naia gigiena,* 12–13 (1928), 82–9. In 1929, a demographic bulletin was put out by the statistical department of GISG. 'Demograficheskii biulleten', *Sotsial'naia gigiena* (1929) 2, 99–103.
129. For example, see A. V. Mol'kov, 'Opyt podkhoda k izucheniiu problema pola', *Sotsial'naia gigiena,* 6 (1925), 36–8. Also, L. S. Gurvich, 'K voprosu o vyrabotke ratsional'nykh metodov obsledovaniia polovoi zhizni', *Sotsial'naia gigiena,* 7 (1926), 30–54.
130. See A. V. Mol'kov, 'Alkogolizm, kak problema izucheniia', *Gigiena i epidemiologiia,* (1926), no. 7–8, 37–46. Also see, 'Ob organizatsii nauchno-issledovatel'skikh rabot v oblasti izucheniia alkogolizma kak sotsial'no-gigienicheskoi problemy', *Sotsial'naia gigiena,* 7 (1926), 5–12.
131. One important area in which anamnesis (medical case histories) was used was research on abortions. See M. Magid and M. Wenkovsky, 'Zur statistik des illegalen abortus', *Archiv für soziale Hygiene und Demographie,* Neue Folge, Bd. VI (1931), 427.

132. A. V. Mol'kov, 'Tezisy ob organizatsii ob'edinnennogo konsultatsionnogo biuro sots-gigienich. uchrezhdenii NKZ po metodike sotsial'no-gigienicheskikh issledovanii', *Sotsial'naia gigiena* 3–4 (1924), 166–72.
133. For a discussion of Chicago sociology of that same period, see Robert E. L. Faris, *Chicago Sociology, 1920–1932* (San Francisco: 1967); Jerzy Szacki, *History of Sociological Thought* (Westport, Conn.: 1977), 436–64. For an indication of the place of social problems research in the total agenda of the Chicago school, see Lester R. Kurtz, *Evaluating Chicago Sociology* Chicago, (1984), 80–4.
134. Semashko, 'K desiatiletiiu oktabria', 4. The introduction by the editor to the first issue of *Sotsial'naia gigiena* also charged that the tsarist regime had tried to marginalize all attempts to introduce social hygiene measures. 'Ot redaktsii', *Sotsial'naia gigiena,* 1 (1922), 3.
135. Semashko, 'Sotsial'naia gigiena, ee sushchnost', 10.
136. Social hygiene research on alcoholism gives an excellent indication of the range of social variables that social hygienists took into account in studying the impact of society on illness. See Susan Gross Solomon, 'David and Goliath: The Rivalry of Social Hygienists and Psychiatrists for Authority over the *Bytovoi* Alcoholic', *Soviet Studies,* Vol. XLI, no. 2 (April 1989), 254–75.
137. Semashko, 'Sotsial'naia gigiena, ee sushchnost', 10.
138. In 1927, Semashko had said that social hygiene would never be successful unless it was grounded in socio–economic conditions. Semashko, 'K desiatiletiiu oktabria', 5. This position was not new. Four years earlier Semashko had made it clear that improvement in health would come only through broad social measures. N. A. Semashko, 'Ocherednye zadachy sotsial'noi gigieny v Rossii', *Sotsial'naia gigiena,* 2 (1923), 7.
139. Semashko, 'Sotsial'naia gigiena, ee sushchnost', 10. In this context Semashko remarked that in Germany the field that approximated Soviet social hygiene most closely was also promoted by socialists.
140. All but one of the members of the core group of social hygienists had engaged in 'revolutionary activities' against the tsarist regime; most social hygienists had Marxist credentials of one stripe or another; a few had even joined the Bolshevik Party before 1917. For detailed biographies, see Solomon, *op. cit.* (note 13), 417–18.
141. It is clear that the Soviets intended to put real teeth into their commitment to prevention. For example, Mol'kov complained that even after 1917, when prevention had acquired a real place in public health, the teaching of hygiene at I and II Moscow Universities remained the same as it had been a quarter century earlier. See Mol'kov, 'K voprosu o peresmotre', 21.
142. The triumph occurred at the First All-Union Meeting of the Representatives of Prophylactic Departments of the RSFSR held in April of 1925. See Solomon, *op. cit.* (note 14).

143. *Meditsinskoe obrazovanie: uchebnye plany meditsinskikh vuzov i programmy neklinicheskikh ditsiplin* (Moscow: 1927).
144. Cited in G. Dembo, 'O reformakh i reforme v meditsinskom obrazovanii', *Voprosy zdravookhraneniia* (1929), no. 12, 41.
145. This argument was spelled out clearly in A. Shapshev, 'Podgotovka sovremennogo vracha v VUZe', *Vestnik sovremennoi meditsiny* (1929), no. 18, 960–1.
146. V. M. Bronner, 'Perspektivy vysshego meditsinskogo obrazovaniia. Tezisy doklada', *Biulleten' Gusa,* (1927), no. 11, 11.
147. Until the end of the 1920s, there was a minority view which interpreted social prophylaxis as essentially social work. For a view of the new Soviet doctor as social worker, see S. A. Gurvich, 'Evoliutsiia lichnosti vracha', *Moskovskii meditsinskii zhurnal* (1928), no. 10–11, 13.
148. For an indication of the frequency of those meetings and the wide range of topics discussed there, see I. S. Blokh, 'S'ezdy bakteriologov, epidemiologov, i sanitarnykh vrachei za desiat let', *Gigiena i epidemiologiia* (1927), no. 10, 76–82.
149. Complaints about the quality of the sanitary physicians being produced continued to punctuate the 1920s. For example, see Ia. M. Stanislavskii, 'Itogi II Soveshchaniia institutov po usovershenstvovaniiu vrachei (28 iuniia - iiulia 1928 g)', *Profilakticheskaia meditsina* (1928), no. 8, 125–33.
150. Prior to the revolution, sanitary physicians were trained in the Bacteriological Institute in St Petersburg under Diatroptov (1909–10). Later three-month courses were established in St Petersburg in the Clinical Laboratory of Professor G. V. Khlopin, and in Moscow in the medical faculty of Moscow University under Professor Orlov. *Spravochnik sanitarnogo vracha* edited by N. K. Ignatov, V. A, Lazarev and S. I. Slonevskii (Moscow: 1928), 448–9.
151. N. A. Semashko, 'Sanitarnoe delo i desiatiletiie Oktiabr'skoi revoliutsii', *Gigiena i epidemiologiia* (1927), no. 10, 7.
152. See the rank ordering of institutions at the end of *Spravochnik sanitarnogo vracha.*
153. George Rosen, *A History of Public Health* (New York, 1958), 233–90.
154. See Christopher M. Davis, 'Economics of Soviet Public Health, 1928–1932,' in Solomon and Hutchinson *op. cit.* (note 5), 146–172.
155. 'Izbrannye stenogrammy zasedanii', *Sotsial'naia gigiena,* (1928), no. 12–13, 239. As I have argued elsewhere, a considerable segment of the medical profession had never been persuaded of the virtues of preventive medicine. Solomon, *op. cit.* (note 14).
156. Kendall E.Bailes, *Technology and Society under Lenin and Stalin* (Princeton, N.J.: 1978) 70, 131–2.
157. For a first-rate discussion of the issue of technocracy in Soviet political life, see Bailes, *op. cit.* (note 156). See also Kendall E. Bailes, 'The Politics of Technology', *American Historical Review* (April 1974), 445–69.

158. 'Ob osvobozhdenii N. A. Semashko ot obiazonnosti Narkomzdrava RSFSR', *Voprosy zdravookhraneniia* (1930), no. 5, 85.
159. The decree reorganizing medical education was passed in June of 1930 by the Council of People's Commissars of the Russian Federated Republic. See 'Meditsinskoe obrazovanie', *Bol'shaia meditsinskaia entsiklopediia* (1936) XVII, 667.
160. Vengrova and Shilinis, *Sotsial'naia gigiena,* 170.
161. A. V. Mol'kov, 'Kak profilaktizirovat' klinicheskoe prepodavanie', *Na fronte zdravookhranenie* (1930), no. 10, 23.
162. See Mol'kov's pre-revolutionary work on dwelling space and nutrition, A. V. Mol'kov, *Zhilishche, ego znachenie i ustroistvo. Mery k' uluchsheniiu zhilishch* (Moscow: 1909); A. V. Mol'kov, *Pishcha, eia znachenie dlia zdorov'ia pitaniia trudiashchiikhsia* (Moscow: 1910).
163. 'Iz deiatel'nost' biuro profilakticheskikh kafedr', *Sotsial'naia gigiena,* (1930), 1–2, 4.
164. See A. A. Press, 'O neobkhodimosti srochnoi podgotovki kadra sotsial'nikh inzhenerov', *Gigiena, bezopasnost' i patologiia truda* (1930), 53–5.
165. For example, see M. Barsukov, 'O profile sovetskogo vracha v periode sotsialisticheskoi rekonstruktsii narodonogo khoziatsv', *Na fronte zdravookhraneniia* (1931), nos 5–6, 29.
166. The technical approach to public health was to endure for some time. In a panegyric to F. F. Erisman written in 1944 (!) the former Commissar of Public Health Semashko remarked, 'Unfortunately, the narrow laboratory approach has by no means been overcome among our hygienists.' N. A. Semashko, 'Friedrich Erisman: The Dawn of Russian Hygiene and Public Health', *Bulletin of the History of Medicine,* XX (1946), 5. The article was translated by Henry Sigerist.
167. Dorothy and Roy Porter, 'What was Social Medicine? An Historiographical Essay', *Journal of Historical Sociology* (1988), 90–106.

6

Public Health and the State: The United States

Elizabeth Fee

The United States was created out of the vast territories of North America by European colonialism. Beginning with the colonies of the eastern seaboard, the land initially occupied was gradually extended, through treaties, war, land sales and repeated violence, across the great plains to the west coast, incorporating along the way parts of Mexico. As the waves of westward migration occupied the lands of the indigenous peoples, the survivors of the territorial wars were confined in small, protected reservations.

The United States took on a separate national identity through its rebellion against the British in the mid eighteenth century, but even at that point, it was a nation as much characterized by regional diversity as by shared historical experience. As nascent capitalist enterprise formed and spread through the northeastern parts of the country, the slave-owning southern states remained semi-feudal, and the 'wild west' was being fought and won by settlers and entrepreneurs whose romantic legends reflect only part of the violence and hardships they both experienced and inflicted. Not until the Civil War, fought between the interests of the slave-holding south and the capitalist north, would the country begin to be integrated into a single system of manufacture and a single market; with slavery abolished, the southern states were opened to the railroads, cotton mills and industrial investments that would tie them more firmly into a network of national finance.

Much of the history of North America may be told in terms of the history of disease and death consequent upon the exploitation of a new continent by the various labour forces that built the new economy – millions of African slaves who grew tobacco, rice and cotton in the south; millions more of the Irish and Chinese labourers who built the railroads and mines; wave after wave of immigrants who came willingly or unwillingly, searching for a new and better life or fleeing an impoverished past; some in chains, some under contract as indentured servants bound to work for their freedom, and some eagerly expectant of the gold or land to be gained in the New World.

The particular history of North America as a colonial territory, peopled first by indigenous tribes and then by waves of immigrants, the different times and forms of settlement of the south, northeast, and western regions, the competition between slave-owning, small farming and manufacturing sectors of the economy, and the struggles of a people at once unified by their common interests and fragmented by their diversity – all provide the framework for understanding the development of public health within the context of 'the state'. The division and negotiation of powers between federal, state, and local governments and the fact that, until relatively recently, public health was mainly a local matter, follows from and reflects the complex political and economic formation of a new nation.

Colonial America

The very first colonists had found a healthy land of bracing air, clean water and acres of fertile soil. John Duffy has recounted both the enthusiastic reports of the first settlers and their subsequent struggles with hunger and malnutrition, endemic and epidemic diseases.[1] The newcomers often arrived suffering from scurvy; they also brought with them smallpox, cholera, measles, diphtheria, typhoid fever and influenza. The deadliest of the European imports was smallpox, a constant threat to the colonists, but a devastation to the Indian tribes with whom they came into contact. Historians who disagree about the size of New World populations at the time of the European contact, and therefore about the rate of depopulation, nonetheless agree that disease played an essential part in the European conquest.[2] The colonists arrived with some immunity to diseases such as smallpox and measles but, in epidemiological terms, native Americans were a virgin population.[3] The destruction caused by disease was in most cases inadvertent; in certain instances, however, transmission of infection was a deliberate act of war.[4] In some areas, smallpox is said to have wiped out 50 to 90 per cent of the Indian population.[5]

In the early colonial settlements, land was more abundant than labour. As the lands were occupied and cultivated, indentured servants who had won their freedom, the younger sons of farming families, and recent arrivals from Europe simply moved west in search of new territory. In the New England states, ownership of land was typically in small, individual plots; as Carl Degler notes, a broadly based property-owning class was 'the principal and ultimate shield of capitalism in America'.[6] Geography, climate and soil largely determined the forms of agricultural production. When tobacco, a labour-intensive crop, came to be the main agricultural product of the southern states, slavery became the favoured method of tying the labour force to the land. Slaves were first declared to be real estate in South Carolina in 1690 and in Virginia in 1705,[7] and slavery grew in significance throughout the eighteenth century. With the growth of cotton production, slavery would become even more essential to the southern economy.

In the colonies, public health consisted of activities deemed necessary to protect the population from the spread of epidemic diseases: the enactment of sanitary laws and regulations governing such matters as the construction of privies, the disposal of wastes, and the disposition of dead animals. Public health was, in the main, an urban affair. Towns and cities appointed inspectors and levied fines against the sellers of putrid meat and property owners who refused or neglected to drain their swamps. By the eighteenth century, quarantine laws had been passed in all the major towns along the eastern seaboard, although these tended to be enforced only during the immediate threat of epidemic diseases. Pest-houses were built for the immigrants arriving on infected ships and in Boston, Cotton Mather and Zabdiel Boyleston introduced the practice of inoculation for smallpox. Smallpox inoculation, while controversial, was perhaps the most successful specific preventive against disease and, when Jenner's vaccine was later announced, it was almost immediately accepted.[8] Public health, when organized at all, was a strictly local matter.

The American Revolution

At the outbreak of the Revolutionary War, America consisted of colonies with very different forms of social and economic organization, whose populations of small farmers, wealthy merchants, landholders, artisans, indentured servants and slaves had very different interests. The men who organized the Revolution, largely members of the colonial élite, owned the largest share of the country's land and wealth; George Washington was reputed to be the richest man in America. These men benefited by throwing off British controls, eliminating British trade monopolies and abolishing arbitrary taxation, but they cherished an ideal of government by a virtuous and disinterested élite – and they discouraged more radical and egalitarian ideas. Town mechanics, labourers, seamen and small farmers were, however, swept into the rebellion by revolutionary rhetoric and their hopes for the redistribution of land and wealth.[9]

The men who signed the Constitution in 1787 had become wealthy through land, manufacturing or shipping; many were slave-holders. Those unrepresented at the Constitutional Convention were slaves, indentured servants, men without property and all women.[10] The new central government would raise money through taxation to pay off government bonds, give protective tariffs to manufacturers and provide defence against Indians, unruly farmers, and any other rebellious groups in the population. All other powers, including authority over matters of public health, were left to the individual states as 'states' rights' – considered an inviolable principle by many, and especially by those in power in the southern states. According to the Tenth Amendment to the Constitution, any powers not specifically given to the national government remained with the states; each state thus had the right to endorse or outlaw slavery. Although uniting the 13 states into a single market, governed by federal laws for interstate commerce, the Constitution imposed few other restrictions. The Revolution had been 'a thoroughly upper-middle-class affair in leadership and aim', which left the existing class structure and distribution of property largely untouched.[11] The Bill of Rights, guaranteeing basic liberties of speech, assembly, a free press and a fair trial, did, however, provide real benefits – short of the redistribution of land or wealth – to those who had fought and suffered for independence.

The disruptions of the Revolutionary War and the movements of troops had brought new outbreaks of epidemic disease: the smallpox, malaria, dysentery, typhoid fever and other intestinal disorders that plagued the troops were easily carried from one part of the country to another. With the nation preoccupied by war and independence, little was accomplished in terms of building any public health infrastructure until the yellow fever epidemic of 1793 to 1806. Ravaging many of the eastern seaboard cities, the epidemic enforced a new consciousness of public health, encouraged the imposition of strict quarantine regulations, and led to the appointment of health committees, health commissioners and boards of health in the cities affected.[12]

The Early Organization of Public Health

The first organized expressions of concern for public health came not from the federal government, or even the states, but from the rapidly growing eastern cities. Each city responded in its own specific ways to the perceived threat of yellow fever and other epidemics that might be imported by boat. Quarantine regulations were either enforced and relaxed depending on the perceived threat of epidemic disease and the changing balance of power among individuals serving on city councils. Although the debates over quarantine regulations were framed in terms of contending theories of disease causation – contagionist and anti-contagionist – the laws actually passed and implemented depended more on political and economic alignments than on the inherent plausibility of one or another aetiologic theory.[13] From the first, public health interests were balanced against the interests of those engaged in international trade – the merchants, ship-builders, and craftsmen whose livelihoods depended on the ships carrying people, raw materials and manufactured goods between Europe, Africa, the Caribbean and the Americas. Local authorities tried to protect the health of the population – and the long-term economic health of the cities – while being sensitive to the immediate economic interests of, and pressures from, local merchants and investors.

Opponents of quarantine argued that diseases were internally generated and that the 'putrefactive fermentation' of rotting organic materials created the miasmatic clouds responsible for the spread of disease. City health departments attempted to regulate the filthy conditions of the docks, streets and alleys; to inspect the grave-yards, tallow chandleries, tanneries, sugar boilers, skin dressers, dyers, glue boilers and slaughter-houses and to remove dead animals and decaying vegetable matter from the streets and public spaces.[14] When reports of an impending epidemic truly alarmed city authorities, they might play it safe by taking both contagionist and anti-contagionist positions at once: enforcing strict quarantine regulations and, at the same time, instituting major clean-up campaigns to deal with offending 'nuisances'.

Although the dread of yellow fever, plague, and cholera galvanized city authorities into action, the more common endemic diseases with less spectacular lethal capacities – typhoid fever, typhus, measles, diphtheria, influenza, tuberculosis and malaria – were usually met with medical indifference or a sense of helplessness. For these diseases, little could be done beyond attempts to maintain general cleanliness, backed up by prayer and exhortations to virtue.[15] Days of prayer and fasting instituted during epidemics generated controversies about the proper separation of church and state; in 1832, President Andrew Jackson provoked a minor crisis in the midst of a cholera epidemic when he refused, on constitutional grounds, to recommend a national day of fasting and humiliation.[16]

For the most part, both poverty and disease were perceived in the late eighteenth and early nineteenth century as the consequences of moral failure at the individual and social level.[17] Disease attacked the dirty, the improvident, the intemperate, the ignorant; the clean, the pious and the virtuous tended to escape. By the same token, improvements in morality and sanitation went hand-in-hand; the moral were more likely to be clean, and the clean found it easier to be moral. The pious had a God-given responsibility to seek environmental improvements where they could; evangelicals were thus to be found in the forefront of the public health movement.[18] As John H. Griscom, a leading public health reformer in antebellum New York explained, 'Cleanliness is said to be "next to godliness", and if, after admitting this, we reflect that cleanliness cannot exist without ventilation, we must look upon the latter as not only a moral but religious duty.'[19]

If evangelicals active in public health reforms justified their work with reference to God's designs, white slave-owners in the southern states had a direct economic interest in the health of their slaves. They regulated – or more often failed to regulate – health conditions on the plantations through direct control of working conditions, housing, food, clothing, 'discipline', sanitation, maternal and infant care, and general medical care.[20] The seasons brought a familiar cycle of communicable diseases; respiratory infections in winter, and in summer, intestinal infections and fevers. Musculoskeletal deformities due to flogging were, however, testimony to the fact that the imperative of social control often overruled the slave-owners' economic interest in slave health.

The Western Expansion and the Civil War

The United States expanded dramatically in the nineteenth century. Reaching no further than the Mississippi River in 1800, its size increased by 300 per cent between 1800 and 1860. Thomas Jefferson had doubled the size of the nation by the Louisiana purchase in 1803, extending the western boundaries to the Rockies; Texas broke off from Mexico and joined the Union in 1845. The United States discovered its 'Manifest Destiny' for western expansion and found a pretext for attacking Mexico in 1846; successful in war, it then took half of Mexico in the treaty of 1848, including the lands that were to become the states of New Mexico and California. The extension of the United States to the western seaboard included what was euphemistically known as the 'Indian Removal'.[21] Removal of Indian tribes from their traditional lands cleared millions of acres to grow cotton in the south and grain in the north, to build roads, canals, railroads, and new cities and settlements, and allowed the development of a trans-continental empire reaching to the Pacific.[22]

The western expansion is obviously important to public health history but has been little discussed by public health historians who have tended to focus on the more developed east coast regions.[23] Ackerknecht's study of malaria in the Upper Mississippi Valley is one of few specialized monographs on this area; the social and demographic histories of the frontier contain many references to disease, death and violence – a frontier world not yet fully integrated into the standard histories of public health in America.[24]

The process of nation-building entered a major internal crisis with the national debate over the abolition of slavery and the outbreak of the Civil War in 1861–5. In 1790, there had been 500,000 slaves in the south; in 1860, the number had grown to four million because of the boom in cotton production, which had increased in the same period from one thousand to one million tons per year.[25] The northern élite wanted economic expansion – free land, free labour, free markets, protective tariffs for manufacturers and a national bank. When these interests conflicted with the interests of the slave-holding south, the Confederacy secede from the Union, and war was declared.

The Civil War enforced a national consciousness of epidemic disease: two-thirds of the 360,000 Union soldiers who died were killed by infectious diseases rather than by enemy bullets.[26] Joseph Jones, a surgeon in the medical department of the Confederate Army, estimated that three-quarters, or 150,000, of the Confederate soldiers' deaths were due to disease; others believed he had underestimated these losses.[27] In either case, contemporary accounts report the main causes of death on both sides as 'typho-malaria' (perhaps a combination of typhoid fever and malaria), camp diarrhoea and 'camp measles'.[28] Scurvy, acute respiratory diseases, venereal diseases, rheumatism and epidemic jaundice were widespread, and the ravages of dysentery, spread by inadequate or non-existent sanitary facilities in army encampments, were appalling. Some order was brought to the midst of this chaos by the United States Sanitary Commission, a voluntary organization inspired by Florence Nightingale's work in the Crimean War. The women of the Sanitary Commission provided nursing care to the sick and the wounded, and improved the sanitary conditions of the Union army camps; they also distributed fresh fruits and vegetables, blankets and other supplies desperately needed by the soldiers. The women tried to save their husbands, fathers and brothers from dying of typhus if they managed to survive the gunfire; the partial success of their efforts impressed a large segment of the American population with the importance of simple health and sanitary measures and thus laid a basis for public health reforms in the post-war period.[29]

Industrialization and the Expansion of Public Health

In the period after the Civil War, northern industrialists began to transform the country into a single national market. Agricultural and industrial mechanization irrevocably altered the traditional patterns of production and consumption; railroad companies competed to cross the country with railroad lines; small companies merged and collapsed into large corporations. Between 1860 and 1894, the value of manufactured goods multiplied by five. The United States was moving into first place as the most powerful industrial country in the world, bypassing England, Germany and France.

Public health lagged behind economic development. By 1860 only a few tentative moves had been made towards establishing formal public health activities beyond the confines of local city politics.[30] Local interests still shaped public health; each city made its own rules and decided its own form of organization. Indeed, this type of localism was generally characteristic of civic affairs and was supported by constitutional restraints on federal power. At the state level, state government actions tended to reflect the preferences of local property owners whose prerogatives might be challenged by any extensive concern with the public's health. The focus of public health on urban areas also reflected the widespread conviction that rural life was basically healthy. Disease was believed to derive from overcrowded, cramped, urban spaces and from foreign influences.

Until the mid nineteenth century, local élites had regarded public health matters with a certain complacency; the American environment was considered much healthier than that of Europe, and the social order more egalitarian. Poverty and disease were largely attributed to individual weakness, wickedness or laziness. The belief that epidemic diseases posed only occasional threats to an otherwise healthy social order was, however, shaken by the industrial transformation of the late nineteenth century. The burgeoning social problems of the industrial cities could not then be ignored: the overwhelming influx of immigrants crowded into narrow alleys and tenement housing, the terrifying death and disease rates of working-class slums, the total inadequacy of water supplies and sewage systems for the rapidly growing population, the spread of endemic and epidemic diseases from the slums to the homes of the wealthy, the escalating squalor and violence of the streets – all impressed members of the social élite that urban problems required concerted attention. Poverty and disease could no longer be treated simply as individual failings; they were becoming social and political problems of massive proportions.

As cities grew in size, as the flow of immigrants continued, and as public health problems became ever more obvious, city health departments mounted rearguard actions against the filth and congestion generated by anarchic urban development.[31] New York, the largest city, with some of the worst health conditions, produced energetic and progressive public health leaders; a dedicated band of reformers had passed the Metropolitan Health Bill of 1866, then the most comprehensive health legislation in the United States.[32] Boston and Providence were also noted for their active public health programmes, while Baltimore and Philadelphia trailed far behind.[33]

The Civil War, by creating massive social disruption and also generating public consciousness of the importance of communicable disease control, was a critical turning-point in public health organization. The first state board of health, created in Louisiana in 1855, was a paper organization; it was really only concerned with public health in the port city of New Orleans.[34] In the aftermath of the Civil War, however, most states created boards of health. The first working state health board was formed in Massachusetts in 1869, followed by California (1870), the District of Columbia (1871), Virginia and Minnesota (1872), Maryland (1874) and Alabama (1875).[35] The impact of these state boards of health should not be overemphasized; by 1900, only three states (Massachusetts, Rhode Island and Florida) spent more than two cents per capita for public health services.[36]

There was, however, still no organization of public health reaching beyond the level of individual cities and states. In 1872 Stephen Smith in New York City had called together a few friends and ambitiously announced the formation of a national voluntary organization, the American Public Health Association (APHA). The APHA grew rapidly, starting with ten members in 1872 and expanding to 400 members by 1880.[37] The leaders of the association immediately began to explore the need and possibilities for public health activity throughout the country. They sent questionnaires to every town with over 5,000 inhabitants and the discouraging results further persuaded them of the need for national reform. In reporting the survey results, John M. Toner noted 'how grudgingly legislatures invest Boards of Health with sufficient power to properly perform their important trust' and how reluctant the courts were to support health laws 'less they seem to abridge the rights of property and individual freedom'.[38] Deploring the lack of vital statistics, he argued that every part of the nation needed paid public health officers.

Health reformers now urged the creation of a national health board, despite the fact that the states and their political representatives in the US Congress were reluctant to give the federal government any power over local health matters. In 1879, however, a disastrous yellow fever epidemic, sweeping up the Mississippi Valley from New Orleans, finally prompted a resistant US Congress to create a National Board of Health, consisting of seven physicians and one representative each from the Army, the Navy, the Marine Hospital Service and the Department of Justice. Responsible for formulating quarantine regulations between the states, the National Board of Health soon became embroiled in fierce battles over states' rights. When it lost the struggle and was disbanded in 1883, its quarantine powers reverted to the Marine Hospital Service, originally created in 1798 to provide hospital care for sick or disabled seamen.[39] Gradually, the Marine Hospital Service extended its public health activities, assuming responsibility for the pollution of lakes and rivers as well as internal quarantine regulations. In 1887, it set aside a single room as a 'hygienic laboratory'. This initial interest in scientific investigation would later be expanded into an important centre for research on infectious diseases.[40]

Public Health as Social Reform

With the industrialization of America, the old concerns with quarantines and the threat of disease from without soon paled in comparison with the perceived threats from within. America no longer fit its own self-image as a republic of independent farmers and craftsmen; like the European countries, it now displayed extremes of wealth and privilege, social misery and deprivation. Labour agitation and social unrest forced awareness of social inequalities and widespread distress. The great railroad strike of 1877, the assassination of President Garfield in 1881, the Haymarket bombing of 1886, the Homestead strike of 1892 and the Pullman strike of 1894 were just a few of the reminders that all was not well with the republic.[41] The Noble Order of the Knights of Labor – dedicated to such measures as an income tax, an eight hour day, social insurance, labour exchanges for the unemployed, the abolition of child labour, workmen's compensation and public ownership of railroads and utilities – grew from a membership of 11 to over 700,000 within a few years. As massive strikes revealed deep class divisions, the development of democratic machine politics challenged the dominance of the traditional political and social élite, permitting some immigrant leaders to establish local bases of influence and power. The perceived social anarchy of the large industrial cities seemed to mock the pretensions to social control of the established forces of church and state, and highlighted the need for more activist responses to the multiplicity of problems.

An increasing number of reform groups devoted themselves to social issues and improvements of every variety. At the levels of both city and state, health reformers, physicians and engineers urged sanitary improvements. Medical men were prominent in reform organizations, but they were not alone.[42] Barbara Rosenkrantz has contrasted public health in the late nineteenth century with the internecine battles within general medicine: 'the field of public hygiene exemplified a happy marriage of engineers, physicians and public-spirited citizens providing a model of complementary comportment under the banner of sanitary science.'[43] The most formally organized and professional body, the American Public Health Association, thus included scientists, municipal officials, physicians, engineers and the occasional architect and lawyer.[44]

Middle- and upper-class women, seizing an opportunity to escape from the narrow bounds of domestic responsibilities, joined in campaigns for improved housing, for the abolition of child labour, for maternal and child health, and for temperance; they were active in the settlement house movement, trade union organizing, the suffrage movement and municipal sanitary reform. They declared 'municipal housekeeping' a natural extension of women's training and experience as 'the housekeepers of the world'.[45] Beginning by cleaning up their homes, neighbourhoods and cities, reforming women announced themselves ready to take on the nation as a whole. Across the country, women volunteers and public health nurses established infant feeding centres, well baby clinics and school health services.[46] In the early twentieth century, national voluntary health organizations – largely organized and staffed by women – supplied much of the impulse and energy behind public health.[47]

Progressive groups in the public health movement advocated reform on political, economic, humanitarian and scientific grounds. Although sharing the revolutionaries' perception of the plight of the poor and the injustices of the system, they usually counselled less radical solutions.[48] Politically, public health reform seemed to offer a middle ground between the cut-throat principles of entrepreneurial capitalism and the revolutionary ideas of the socialists, anarchists and utopian visionaries.[49]

As William H. Welch told the Charity Organization Society, sanitary improvement offered the best way of improving the lot of the poor, short of the radical restructuring of society.[50]

Economically, progressive reformers argued that public health should be viewed as a paying investment, giving higher returns than the stock market. In Germany, Max von Pettenkofer had first calculated the financial returns on public health 'investments' to prove the value of sanitary improvements in reducing deaths from typhoid, and his argument would be repeated many times by American public health leaders.[51] As Welch declared: '... merely from a mercenary and commercial point of view it is for the interest of the community to take care of the health of the poor. Philanthropy assumes a totally different aspect in the eyes of the world when it is able to demonstrate that it pays to keep people healthy.'[52]

Many public health leaders argued that the demand for centralized planning and business efficiency required scientific knowledge rather than the undisciplined enthusiasms of voluntary groups.[53] Public health decisions should be made by an analysis of costs and benefits 'as an up-to-date manufacturer would count the cost of a new process'. The health officer, like the merchant, should learn 'which line of work yields the most for the sum expended'.[54]

Existing health departments were, admittedly, dominated more by patronage and political considerations than by economic or administrative efficiency. Progressives regretted 'the evil of politics' and thought that by increasing the pay and minimum qualifications for health officers, they would be able to attract personnel on the basis of skill rather than influence. They argued that public health as a specialized profession must be better paid:

> We hope that every local unit of government will have its health officer and that the iceman and the undertaker will not be considered suitable candidates, but that every health officer will be trained for his work. We hope that he will receive a reasonable reward for his services, and that the pay for saving a child's life with antitoxin will at least equal that received by a plumber for mending a leaky pipe; and that for managing a yellow fever outbreak a man may receive as much per week as a catcher on a baseball nine.[55]

The attempt to insulate boards of health from local political control was part of a broader movement to make public administration more rational and efficient by training a new professional élite able to conduct social reform on scientific principles.[56]

Bacteriology and Alternative Views of Health and Disease

According to the first 'modern' public health professionals, public health was defined in terms of its aims and goals – to reduce disease and maintain the health of the population – rather than by any traditional body of knowledge. The enterprise needed many different professional skills: physicians diagnosed contagious diseases; sanitary engineers built water and sewage systems; epidemiologists traced the sources of disease outbreaks; vital statisticians counted births, deaths and reportable diseases; lawyers wrote sanitary codes; public health nurses spread popular health advice; sanitary inspectors visited markets to enforce compliance with health ordinances; and administrators tried to organize everyone within the limits of their budgets. Public health thus involved economics, sociology, psychology, politics, law, statistics and engineering, as well as the biological and clinical sciences. However, in the period immediately following the brilliant experimental work of Louis Pasteur and Robert Koch, the bacteriological laboratory became the first and primary symbol of a new, scientific public health.

The clarity and simplicity of bacteriological discoveries gave them tremendous cultural importance: the agents of particular diseases were made visible under the microscope. The identification of specific bacteria seemed to have cut through the misty miasmas of disease to define the enemy in unmistakable terms. Bacteriology thus became an ideological marker, sharply differentiating the 'old' public health, the province of politicians, physicians and reformers, from the 'new' public health, which would belong to scientifically trained professionals.

Young Americans who had studied in Germany brought back the new knowledge of laboratory methods in bacteriology and started to teach others: William Henry Welch and T. Mitchell Prudden in New York, George Sternberg in Washington and Alexander C. Abbott in Philadelphia were among the first to introduce the new bacteriology to the United States.[57] These young scientists were convinced that physicians should stop squabbling over medical ethics and politics, and commit themselves to the purer values of laboratory research.

The laboratory ideal rapidly influenced leading progressives in public health. By the 1880s, Charles Chapin had established a public health laboratory in Providence, Rhode Island; Victor C. Vaughan had created a state hygienic laboratory in Michigan; and William Sedgwick had used bacteriology to study water supplies and sewage disposal at the Lawrence Experiment Station in Massachusetts.[58] Sedgwick demonstrated the transmission of typhoid fever by polluted water supplies and developed quantitative methods for measuring the presence of bacteria in the air, water and milk. Describing the impact of bacteriological discoveries, he said: 'Before 1880 we knew nothing; after 1890 we knew it all; it was a glorious ten years.'[59]

The powerful new methods of identifying the causes of diseases through the microscope drew attention away from the larger and more diffuse problems of water supplies, street cleaning, housing reform and the living conditions of the poor. The approach of locating, identifying, and isolating bacteria and their human hosts seemed a much more efficient way of dealing with disease than environmental improvements. By focusing on the diagnosis of infectious diseases, the public health laboratory demonstrated the scientific and diagnostic power of the new public health, and began to cast doubt on the objectivity and credibility of those public health professionals who continued to insist on the necessity of social reform.

Like the new bacteriology, epidemiology now became firmly oriented to the control of specific diseases. Charles Chapin, for example, was Superintendent of Health of Providence, Rhode Island, and a leading proponent of the new epidemiology. Having published a comprehensive text on municipal sanitation in 1901,[60] he soon concluded that much effort devoted to cleaning up the cities was wasted; instead, public health officers should concentrate on controlling specific routes of infection. His new text of 1910, *The Sources and Modes of Infection,* soon became the gospel of infectious disease control.[61] Hibbert Winslow Hill, director of the division of epidemiology of the Minnesota Board of Health, popularized Chapin's work in a lively series of articles first printed in 1,100 newspapers across the United States, and later published as a book, *The New Public Health.*[62] Hill explained why modern scientific methods in public health were more efficient than old-fashioned social reforms. To control tuberculosis, for example, it was hardly necessary to improve the living conditions of the one hundred million people in the United States – only to supervise the 200,000 active tuberculosis cases *'merely to the extent of confining their infective discharges....* Need any more be said to indicate the superiority of the new principles, as practical business propositions, over the old?'[63] The vital statistician, said Hill, should become the 'cost-of-production scientific manager' of public health expenditures, 'a man who knows costs in each department in proportion to production, and where to cut costs, increase production, save time, unnecessary work and waste in general'.[64]

The dominance of this disease-oriented approach to public health was likewise evident in the first handbook for practising public health officers, *Manual for Health Officers*, published in 1915 by J. Scott MacNutt.[65] Echoing the views of Chapin and Hill, MacNutt devoted approximately half of his 600-page handbook to the contagious diseases, four pages to industrial hygiene, and gave only passing notice to housing, water supplies, public education and environmental health.

But while the narrow bacteriological view was dominant, several competing models for public health research and practice were also available. Compare, for example, Hill's narrow focus with the more expansive gaze (if wordy prose) of Charles-Edward A. Winslow of Yale University:

> Public health is the science and art of preventing disease, prolonging life, and promoting physical health and efficiency through organized community efforts for the sanitation of the environment, the control of community infections, the education of the individual in principles of personal hygiene, the organization of medical and nursing service for the early diagnosis and preventive treatment of disease, and the development of the social machinery which will ensure to every individual in the community a standard of living adequate for the maintenance of health.[66]

Winslow's was not the only alternative view. In the same year that Hill published his book on the new public health, Alice Hamilton's survey of industrial lead poisoning established the fact that thousands of American workers in pottery glazing, bath tub enamelling, cut glass polishing, cigar wrapping, can sealing and dozens of other industrial processes were being slowly killed by white lead.[67] Unaided by legislation, Hamilton argued, persuaded, shamed and flattered individual employers into improving working conditions. Almost single-handedly, she created the foundations of industrial hygiene in America.

Joseph Goldberger's epidemiological studies of pellagra for the Public Health Service offer yet another approach to public health. In 1914, Goldberger announced that pellagra was due to dietary deficiencies and not to some unknown micro-organism; he and his colleagues had cured endemic pellagra in a Mississippi orphanage by feeding the children milk, eggs, beans and meat. He then teamed up with the economist, Edgar Sydenstricker, to survey the diets of southern wage-workers' families. They showed how the sharecropping system had impoverished tenant farmers, led to dietary deficiencies and produced endemic pellagra.[68] The economic system of cotton production in the south was thus directly responsible for the high prevalence of pellagra.

Alice Hamilton, Joseph Goldberger, and Edgar Sydenstricker were minority voices amid the growing majority focusing exclusively on bacteria. As most bacteriologists and epidemiologists concentrated on specific disease-causing organisms and the individuals who harboured them, only a few tried to relate the problems of ill health and disease to the larger social environment.[69] Most public health professionals enjoyed the visibility and credibility they derived from association with the laboratory, the power of new diagnostic techniques, and the glamorous aura of scientific medicine. Given the apparent promise of scientific method, they were more than willing to dissociate themselves from local politics, street cleaning campaigns, and the agitations of 'petticoat reformers'. They were ready to demonstrate the power of their science on a larger stage.

National and International Health

By the turn of the twentieth century, public health was becoming a national and even international issue. Although the United States Congress was still reluctant to enact federal health legislation, there were mounting pressures for United States' attention to public health abroad. As American businessmen were seeking enlarged foreign markets and new sources of raw materials, a vocal group of intellectuals and politicians argued for an assertive foreign policy. The United States began to challenge European dominance in the Far East and Latin America, seeking trade and political influence more than territory, but taking territory where it could. National defence goals included broadening control of trade routes, building a Central American canal and establishing strategic bases in the Caribbean and Western Pacific.

In 1898, the United States entered the Spanish–American War, for which it sent troops to Cuba, Puerto Rico, and the Philippines, and expanded the army from 25,000 to 250,000 men. The casualties incurred showed that the United States could not afford military adventures overseas unless more attention were paid to sanitation and public health: 968 men died in battle, but 5,438 died of infectious diseases.[70] Nonetheless, the United States defeated Spain and installed an army of occupation in Cuba. When yellow fever endangered these troops in 1900, the response was efficient and effective. An Army commission under Walter Reed was sent to Cuba to study the disease and, in a dramatic series of human experiments, confirmed the hypothesis of a Cuban physician, Carlos Finlay, that it was spread by mosquitoes and showed that the mosquito itself bred in close proximity to human habitats. This was quickly followed by a quasi-military operation to destroy mosquito-breeding sites, undertaken by Surgeon-Major William Gorgas as the Sanitary Officer, which did indeed eliminate yellow fever from Havana.[71]

The United States Army in the Philippines faced even greater problems: a climate that sapped the strength of the soldiers while exposing them to disease-bearing insects, parasites and bacteria-laden water supplies.[72] The Tropical Disease Board worked on the new diseases found in the Philippines as well as on more familiar afflictions; success in the war and against the Philippine Insurrection was dependent on gaining some degree of control over malaria, dysentery, dengue fever and beriberi.[73] In Puerto Rico, the new American administration found public health measures equally important to the establishment of political control over the island and the development of American economic interests in sugar and coffee production.

These experiences confirmed the significance of public health for successful United States' efforts overseas. Earlier attempts to dig the Panama Canal had been attended by enormous mortality rates from disease.[74] But, in 1904, Gorgas, now promoted to General, took control of a campaign against the malaria and yellow fever threatening canal operations. He was finally able to persuade the Canal Commission to institute an intensive campaign against mosquitoes; in one of the triumphs of practical public health, yellow fever and malaria were brought under control and the canal was successfully completed in 1914.

US industrialists brought some of the lessons of Cuba, the Philippines, Puerto Rico and the Panama Canal home to the southern United States. The south at that time resembled an underdeveloped country within the US, with much of the population living under miserable economic and social conditions. Northern industrialists were investing heavily in southern education as well as in cotton mills and railroads; John D. Rockefeller created the General Education Board to support 'the general organization of rural communities for economic, social and educational purposes'.[75] Charles Wardell Stiles managed to convince the Secretary of the General Education Board that the real cause of misery and lack of productivity in the south was hookworm, the 'germ of laziness'. In 1909, Rockefeller agreed to provide $1 million to create the Rockefeller Sanitary Commission for the Eradication of Hookworm Disease, with Wickliffe Rose as Director.[76] This was to be the first instalment in Rockefeller's massive national and international investment in public health.

Rose went beyond the task of attempting to control a single disease and worked to establish an effective and permanent public health organization in the southern states.[77] At the end of five years of intensive effort, the campaign had failed to eradicate hookworm, but had greatly expanded the role of public health agencies. Between 1910 and 1914, county appropriations for public health work increased from a total of $240 to $110,000.[78] In 1914, the organizational experience gained in the southern states enabled the Rockefeller Foundation to extend its hookworm control programme to the Caribbean, Central America and Latin America.

Meanwhile, in Washington, the Committee of One Hundred on National Health, composed of such notables as Jane Addams, Andrew Carnegie, William H. Welch and Booker T. Washington, campaigned for the federal regulation of public health.[79] Its president, Irving Fisher, a Yale economist and a prime mover in the American Eugenics Society, argued that public health was good science and good economics, and would help conserve 'national vitality'.[80] The push for public health on a national level was thus tacitly allied to concerns about the deterioration of the national 'stock' and the idea that biologically inferior immigrants were responsible for the growing statistics of disease, alcoholism, mental illness, urban violence and criminality. Although most public health workers saw their concern for the social conditions of the poor as contradictory to the biological determinism of Social Darwinists and eugenicists, the eugenics movement no doubt spurred interest in, and analysis of, the health problems of immigrant communities.[81]

In 1912 the federal government made its first real commitment to public health by turning the Marine Hospital Service into the United States Public Health Service and authorizing it to investigate the causes and spread of diseases, study the problems of sewage, sanitation and water pollution, and publish health information for the general public.[82] The following year, the federal government made specific appropriations for field investigations of epidemic diseases, pellagra and trachoma. Among the responsibilities of the Public Health Service was the medical inspection of all immigrants arriving at Ellis Island, New York, and the attempted exclusion of those with contagious diseases or obvious physical or mental defects. By 1915, the Public Health Service, the US Army and the Rockefeller Foundation were thus the major agencies involved in public health activities, supplemented on a local level by a network of city and state health departments.

By the early decades of the twentieth century, there was an increasing demand for people trained in the new public health to direct the programmes being developed on local, state and national levels. Public health reformers agreed that full-time public health workers, not part-time physicians who would easily be distracted by the demands of private practice, were needed to staff public health departments. As William Sedgwick argued: 'Scientists and technicians alike ... must be employed and paid by the people, to rule over them as well as to guide and to guard them, to constitute a kind of official class, a kind of bureaucracy constituted for themselves by the people themselves'.[83] In 1916, the Rockefeller Foundation funded the School of Hygiene and Public Health at Johns Hopkins, the first of a series of schools of public health it was to finance in the United States and around the world. In rapid succession, schools and departments of public health were created at the universities of Harvard, Yale, Columbia, Toronto, Michigan, North Carolina and Minnesota.[84] The schools displayed a marked preference for physicians although members of other professional groups and non-physicians studying the biomedical sciences were also admitted.[85] The curricula of the schools, which for the most part emphasized the biological and laboratory sciences, helped further institutionalize the biomedical orientation of the new public health.[86]

America's entry into the First World War reinforced the new lessons being learned about the importance of public health. When selective service examinations revealed that a substantial proportion of young men were either physically or mentally unfit for combat, the sudden realization of the nation's ill health boosted political support for public health expenditures. The war years brought attention to the problems of infectious diseases and especially the sexually transmitted diseases that had hitherto been blanketed in an embarrassed silence.[87] The influenza epidemic that devastated families and communities in 1916–18 also dramatically underlined the continuing threat of infectious disease epidemics and brought public health to the centre of the nation's consciousness.

The Relationship Between Public Health and Medicine

The growing state and federal interest in public health meant new full-time public health positions in health departments, federal and private agencies, and a new demand for educational facilities to provide men and women with specialized training. These increased levels of interest and support also generated professional competition and provoked the question whether public health was a new profession or simply a specialty within one of the existing professions. Medicine, engineering, law, economics, nursing and other professional fields were clearly relevant to public health but medicine had perhaps the strongest claim to preeminence. By 1912, 15 states required that all members of their boards of health be physicians and 23 states required at least one physician member; the remaining ten states had no professional requirement for eligibility.[88]

Physicians in the mid to late nineteenth century and the early twentieth century had displayed a lively interest in public health.[89] The more élite members of the profession found urban social reform and municipal leadership positions socially and intellectually compatible as a 'natural' extension of their class standing in the community. Less well-established physicians found the income from part-time public health positions a very welcome supplement to their often meagre incomes from private practice. The overcrowding of the profession before the Flexnerian reforms meant that many physicians were happy to accept paid part-time work in dispensaries, public health departments, or medical schools, and public health work could be essential to a young physician struggling to establish a clinical practice within a highly competitive urban environment.[90]

By the second decade of the twentieth century, non-medical public health officers were beginning to protest the dominance of public health by medical men. By this time, however, the sanitary engineers were the only professional group strong enough to challenge the physicians' assumption that the future of public health should be theirs. Civil and sanitary engineers had created clean city water supplies and more adequate sewerage systems, major factors in the declining death rates from infant diarrhoea and other infectious diseases.[91] With the benefit of hindsight, we can say that they deserve much of the credit for the decline of infectious disease mortality in the late nineteenth century.[92] By the early years of the twentieth century, however, they were vociferously complaining about the 'medical monopoly' of public health. Physicians were willing to concede to the sanitary engineers responsibility for public sanitation and water supplies, but little else.

As public health activities expanded, moreover, private practitioners began to worry about the potential conflict between the public provision of services and their own economic interests. This concern was heightened as health departments abandoned urban and sanitary reform, became increasingly active in the identification and control of infectious diseases, and challenged the boundaries of medical autonomy. The claim of bacteriologists that they, and not clinicians, best knew how to diagnose diseases such as diphtheria and tuberculosis could be especially galling.[93] How could a laboratory man know more about a patient's disease than that patient's own doctor? As John Duffy has argued, the medical profession moved from a position of strong support for public health activities to a cautious, and sometimes suspicious ambivalence.[94] At times, that ambivalence turned into outright hostility.

Public health officers understood that although their interests might sometimes be opposed to those of private practitioners, it was nonetheless important to cultivate cooperative relationships with the medical profession. Indeed, Duffy has argued that this attitude had the effect of making public health officers 'cautious to the point of timidity' between 1906 and the 1930s, so reluctant were they to undertake programmes that might disturb the interests of their clinical colleagues.[95]

From the 1920s, private clinical practice gained an enormous advantage over public health in its relative status and economic rewards. Whereas incomes from private practice rose dramatically, public health salaries increased slowly, if at all. Medical knowledge and practice were transformed in the early twentieth century as medicine became more scientific, more technology-based, and more dependent on institutional settings such as the hospital.[96] Physicians were eager to join the glamorous new specialties and correspondingly less interested in community health and preventive activities. As medical practice became an ever more challenging and lucrative field, public health was increasingly perceived as an unattractive specialty, marked by low incomes and lack of autonomy.

State health departments were so keen to attract physicians that they rarely required them to have specialized public health training. As a result, the incentives for physicians to take degrees in public health were further reduced, and schools of public health began to admit ever larger numbers of nurses, engineers, statisticians and biologists. This structural problem in the relationship between medicine and public health, already clear by 1920, was never resolved. Public health in the United States would continue to be open to many professional groups and disciplines, while it maintained a special, privileged status for those with medical qualifications.

From Bacteriology to Health Education

In the 1920s state and municipal governments, in recognition of the growing practical importance of public health, offered support to health departments to develop new organizational units and increase their hiring of public health personnel, especially public health nurses. Although bacteriological laboratories continued to be important, divisions of tuberculosis, child and maternal health, venereal diseases, public health administration, and health education, along with divisions of sanitation and vital statistics, became central units of state and city health departments. After the first flush of enthusiasm for the achievements of bacteriology, public health officials had come to realize that although bacteriologists could help to diagnose diseases more accurately, they could, in most cases, neither cure nor prevent them.

Given the conservative orientation of the post-war years, public health officials now tended to focus on individual behaviour as a determinant of health and to emphasize the need for popular health education. The new professionalization of public health meant that health department divisions staffed by teams of public health nurses took the place of the older voluntary reform organizations. Broader social approaches to health and poverty were replaced by educational campaigns; rather than provide free milk for babies, public health nurses educated mothers on the proper methods of child care. Rather than attack the working conditions in sweatshops, tuberculosis nurses visited tubercular patients and cautioned against spitting.

In part, public health departments turned to health education to avoid unpleasant and unproductive controversy. The medical profession, as already mentioned, was antagonistic to the provision of medical care by public health departments; even school health clinics were regarded with suspicion, lest they interfere with the prerogatives of private practice. Efforts to deal with tenement reform or occupational health could arouse the even more determined opposition of landlords and employers. Popular health education provoked no such resistance from the powerful. In 1923, Charles-Edward A. Winslow went so far as to announce the ending of the bacteriological age and to describe popular health education as the keynote of the 'new public health':

> The dominant motive in the present-day public health campaign is the education of the individual in the practices of personal hygiene. The discovery of popular education as an instrument in preventive medicine, made by the pioneers in the tuberculosis movement, has proved almost as far-reaching as the discovery of the germ theory of disease thirty years before.[97]

Despite much agreement on principles, public health practice varied greatly throughout the states and cities across the country. A 1923 report of the Committee on Municipal Health Department Practice of the American Public Health Association displays the wide variation in public health organization across 83 United States cities in the period.[98] Some cities and states had well organized and energetic health departments, while others had half-hearted programmes and somnolent organizations.

The Growing Federal Role in Public Health

The most important federal organization in public health was the United States Public Health Service. The Public Health Service now aided the development of state health departments by giving grants-in-aid, loaning expert personnel, and providing advice and consultation on specific problems.[99] If, for example, a state was facing an unexplained outbreak of typhoid fever or other epidemic disease, the Public Health Service would send epidemiologists to trace the source of the disease and suggest means of preventing its spread. Such assistance had first to be formally requested by the state so as not to threaten closely guarded states' rights.

Other public health functions were scattered throughout the federal bureaucracy. About 40 agencies participated to some degree in public health activities, including the Department of Agriculture (home economics, entomology, plant quarantine, etc.), Department of Commerce (Bureau of the Census), Department of the Interior (Office of Indian Affairs in sanitation and medical care, Bureau of Mines in industrial hygiene), Pure Food and Drug Administration, and the Department of Labor (Children's Bureau, Bureau of Labor Statistics). The Sheppard–Towner Act of 1921 provided funds to support maternal and child health clinics but was killed in 1928 by the determined opposition of the medical profession.

A major stimulus to the development of public health practice came in response to the depression, with the New Deal and the Social Security Act of 1935. The Social Security Act expanded financing of the Public Health Service and provided federal grants to states to assist them in developing their public health services. Federal and state expenditures for public health actually doubled in the decade of the depression, fuelling the expansion of local health units. In most parts of the country, efficient provision of public health services to local communities depended on county health organizations, smaller and simpler units than the larger state health departments. In 1934, only 541 counties out of the 3,070 counties in the United States had any form of local public health service, but by June 1942, 1,828 counties could boast of health units directed by a full-time public health officer.[100] (Much of this gain would be lost during the war; by the end of the war only 1,322 counties had an organized health service.[101])

In 1935, for the first time, the federal government provided funds, administered through the states, for specialized public health education. Federal regulations required states to establish minimum qualifications for new public health personnel employed with federal grants. Faced with a growing demand for public health training, several state universities began public health programmes and existing schools of public health expanded their enrolments. By 1936, ten schools offered public health degrees or certificates requiring at least one year of attendance.[102] Between 1935 and 1938, more than four thousand individuals, including about one thousand doctors, received public health training with the new federal funds. The economic difficulties of maintaining a private practice during the depression had pushed many physicians into public health; others were attracted by the new availability of fellowships, by increased social awareness of the plight of the poor, or simply by the availability of salaried jobs. In 1939, the federal government allocated over $8 million for maternal and child health programmes, over $9 million for general public health work and over $4 million for venereal disease control.

Several important trends were stimulated by these federal funds: first, the development of programmes to control specific diseases and for services targeted at specific population groups, or what is known as the 'categorical' approach to public health. Second, the expansion in the number of local health departments; third, the increased training of personnel; and fourth, the assumption of responsibility for some phases of medical care on the part of health departments.[103] The categorical approach to public health proved politically popular; Members of Congress were willing to vote funds for specific diseases or for particular groups – health and welfare services for children were especially appealing – but they showed less interest in general public health or administrative expenditures.

Although state health officers often felt constrained by targeted programmes, they rarely refused federal grants-in-aid and thus adapted their programmes to the available pattern of funds. Federal grants came in turn for maternal and child health services and crippled children (1935), venereal disease control (1938), tuberculosis (1944), mental health (1947), industrial hygiene (1947), and dental health (1947). The pattern of funding started in the 1930s would thus shape the organization of public health departments through the post-war period. As institutionalized in the National Institutes of Health, it would also shape the future pattern of biomedical research.

Public Health and the Second World War

Mobilization for war acted as another major force in the expansion of public health in the United States. The First World War had also increased consciousness of public health, but this time, the military could build on the acceptance of social and health expenditures created by the New Deal. Public health was now declared a national priority for the armed forces and the civilian population engaged in military production. As James Stevens Simmons, Brigadier General and Director of the Preventive Medicine Division of the US Army, announced: 'A civil population that is not healthy cannot be prosperous and will lag behind in the economic competition between nations. This is even more true of a military population, for any army that has its strength sapped by disease is in no condition to withstand the attack of a virile force that has conserved its strength and is enjoying the vigour and exhilaration of health.'[104]

Politicians were now willing to vote appropriations for public health as essential to national defence.[105] As the federal government began planning and organizing new health programmes, state and local governments were urged to orient their activities to the war effort.[106] Joseph W. Mountin, Assistant Surgeon General, underlined the sense of urgency: 'If a machine is idle because the worker who should tend it is sick, that machine is doing a job for Hitler.'[107] Health departments again suffered from a critical shortage of personnel as physicians, nurses, engineers and other trained and experienced professionals left to join the armed services.[108]

The US Public Health Service in 1940 expanded its programme of grants to states and local communities, sending personnel to particularly needy areas.[109] The Community Facilities Act provided $300 million in funds for construction of public works, including health and sanitation facilities, in communities with rapidly expanding populations because of military camps and war industries. The Office of Defense Health and Welfare Services, created as part of the Office for Emergency Management, coordinated efforts to protect the health of the nation at war, while the Office of Scientific Research and Development organized the national research effort.[110]

The shock of the discovery – once again – that so many of the young men being called into the Army were unfit for military service provided a powerful impetus for increased political attention to public health.[111] In what amounted to the largest health survey ever undertaken, the Selective Service Board examined over 16 million young men and found fully 40 per cent of them physically or mentally unfit. The leading causes of rejection were defective teeth, vision problems, orthopaedic impairments (e.g. from polio), diseases of the cardiovascular system, nervous and mental diseases, hernia, tuberculosis and venereal diseases. As George St J. Perrott of the US Public Health Service noted, mortality rates from infectious diseases had declined since the First World War, but morbidity rates had changed little, if at all: in both cases, the draft had demonstrated an enormous amount of ill health in the American population.[112] One health officer noted that war forced politicians and the public to pay attention to the nation's health: 'The public is more health-minded at the present time than ever before in our generation. Publicity of the results of Selective Service examinations ... the national nutrition program ... mass health surveys ... have made health a news item.'[113]

With the movements of troops to army camps and of workers to defence industry plants, peaceful villages turned into boom towns and many cities doubled their population within a couple of years.[114] The existing infrastructure of water supplies and sewage systems were often hopelessly inadequate to cope with the increased demand.[115] Army training camps were often placed in hot southern areas where the Anopheles mosquito bred in profusion and malaria was endemic. In an effort to eradicate malaria, the Public Health Service established the Center for Controlling Malaria in the War Areas. After the war, this organization was transformed into the Centers for Disease Control which would play a major national role in addressing both infectious and chronic diseases.[116]

Post-War Feuding Between Public Health and Medicine

In the immediate post-war period, considerable optimism and energy were devoted to the possible reorganization of public health and medical care. Public health functions within state governments were now scattered among a multitude of agencies, state boards and commissions, with as many as 18 different agencies being involved in a single state.[117] In 1942, the American Public Health Association reported that only two-thirds of the people of the United States were covered by local public health units, and estimated that communities over 50,000 could provide basic health services at a cost of one dollar per capita and a superior public health service for two dollars per capita.[118] The money actually spent for public health work varied widely, from $0.13 per capita in Ohio to $1.68 in Delaware. In most cases, however, the states spending the largest sums were spending most of their money on hospital services rather than prevention.

The need for reorganization of public health was underscored by recognition of the national change in disease patterns often referred to as the 'epidemiological transition'. In 1900 the leading causes of death had been tuberculosis, pneumonia, diarrhoeal diseases and enteritis; by 1946, the leading causes of death were heart disease, cancer and accidents. Although many public health professionals in the 1930s perceived the importance of chronic diseases, the urgent wartime demands of infectious disease control had temporarily eclipsed concern with these slow killers of middle and old age. With the return to peace, however, public health officials realized they must come to terms with the problems and prevalence of chronic illness. Communicable disease control no longer provided a sufficient *raison d'être;* the major infectious disease problems of the early twentieth century, tuberculosis, syphilis, typhoid and diphtheria, were now effectively controlled.

The problem was that nobody knew how to prevent cancer or heart disease. There was little agreement or clarity about the relevance of nutritional, occupational or environmental health – or about any other aetiological factors. The only approach to prevention upon which everyone could agree was the need for screening and early diagnosis. The chronic diseases – cancer, hypertension, diabetes and others – could neither be prevented nor cured on the older public health and medical models; at best, they could be controlled through screening, education and medical supervision. Many public health leaders thought the new relevance and specific problems of chronic disease control provided a compelling argument for the long-overdue unification of preventive and curative medicine – which they hoped would take place under the leadership of public health departments. Many imagined this unification as part of a new national health programme for the post-war period, one that would provide a full range of health services to the entire population. In their enthusiasm, these reformers forgot or discounted the more than 25 years of energetic resistance by the organized medical profession to any federal or state intervention in medical care.[119]

In the late 1940s and early 1950s, some American public health professionals welcomed the concept of social medicine as seeming to offer a fresh perspective on the problems of chronic illness.[120] John E. Gordon, professor of preventive medicine and epidemiology at the Harvard School of Public Health and a prominent exponent of the 'newer epidemiology', explained how the triumvirate of 'environment, host, and disease' could be applied to non-communicable organic diseases like pellagra, cancer, psychosomatic conditions, traumatic injuries and accidents.[121] Epidemiologists increasingly rejected the notion of a single cause of disease (the agent) in favour of multiple causation.[122]

Social medicine encouraged optimism about the possibilities for new approaches to the chronic diseases, for the integration of preventive and curative medicine, and for the extension of comprehensive health programmes to the whole population.[123] But Eli Ginzberg and others introduced a note of pessimism and caution, warning more optimistic thinkers about an 'anti-government attitude' in the United States and the prevalent assumption that health depended on medical care, driving an ever-increasing demand for more doctors and hospital beds.[124]

A new specialty of preventive medicine emerged to occupy what some perceived as the middle ground between public health and the hospital-oriented clinical specialties. Its advocates were private practitioners of clinical prevention, who conducted screening tests and gave advice on an individual level; they therefore insisted that public health departments stay away from the chronic diseases: '... disturbances of the climacteric, cancer, metabolic disorders, such as diabetes, cardiovascular disease, and the like are utterly beyond the influence of public health measures ... prevention, early detection, and control of these disorders are and will continue to be individualistic and not en masse'.[125] As clinicians, they wanted to keep the state out of the doctor's office.

Public health officers were not themselves unified. Some advocated the direct administration of tax-supported medical care by health departments. Those with more traditional loyalties opposed such proposals, and felt that if public health and medical care administration were combined, preventive and educational efforts could be submerged by the demand for costly therapeutic services.[126] In 1945 Harry Mustard warned that if medical care became the responsibility of public health departments, 'Many comfortably established routines would be rudely shaken and it is possible that a hypertrophied medical-care tail would soon wag the none too robust public health dog.'[127]

While public health officials were debating whether they really wanted responsibility for medical care services, the American Hospital Association and the American Medical Association were strongly pushing a bill for the construction of hospitals. The Hospital Survey and Construction Act, more popularly known as the Hill–Burton Act, after Senators Lister Hill of Alabama and Harold H. Burton of Ohio, was passed in 1946. Hospital construction, especially in rural areas, promised to bring the benefits of medical science to all the people – without in any way disturbing the well-defended freedoms of the medical profession or the patterns of paying for their services. One third of the costs of building hospitals would be paid by the federal government, with $75 million set aside for each of the first five years.

No health programme in the US had ever been so generous or so popular. Hill–Burton answered the national demand for access to medical care in a way that posed no challenge to the private organization of medical practice and paid no more than token attention to preventive services.[128] The United States could have been completely covered by local health departments for a fraction of the cost of Hill–Burton, but public health lacked a strong political constituency to promote its cause. Curative medicine and hospital care thus gained the lion's share of public resources.

Losing Clout: The Conservative Fifties

The more pessimistic prognoses proved correct in the political climate of the 1950s. The theoretical innovations of social medicine were not translated into effective health programmes; health officer positions stood vacant because the salaries offered were so low.[129] Public health departments struggled to maintain basic services on inadequate budgets and with little political support. Post-war reconstruction meant massive expenditures for biomedical research and hospital construction, the partial payment for medical care by expanding private insurance coverage, the relative neglect of public health services, and a complete failure to implement the more radical ideas of social medicine though focused attention on the social determinants of health and disease.

There are many reasons why the United States moved towards ever more sophisticated biomedical research and high technology medicine in the post-war era. Stephen Strickland, among others, has examined the politics of research funding and shown how the priorities of research were set by the basic sciences and clinical medicine.[130] Even more to the point is the political context of the Cold War, marked by passionate anti-communism, suppression of dissent, and suspicion of any public or social services as examples of creeping socialism. In this political environment, the idealistic visions of social medicine, of integrating the social and biomedical sciences, and of combining preventive and curative services in a reorganized health system, seemed not only unrealistic but threatening. Some of the blame for the neglect of public health must also be shared by the public health profession for failing to communicate more effectively to the general public, build the political support it needed, and promote a strong and persuasive case for adequate funding of public health services.

Harry Mustard argued that the problems of public health were largely political. State health officers were of relatively low-grade rank in the hierarchy of state officials, and were limited in their freedom to introduce new proposals: 'Strained relations are inevitable if the state health officer does not hold the furthering of his health program within the bounds of the governor's interest, which is not necessarily great.'[131] Too often, state health officers accepted political constraints and bureaucratic barriers as natural and inevitable. Too seldom were they willing to risk their positions by appealing to a larger constituency. In retrospect, it also seems clear that public health failed to claim sufficient credit for controlling infectious diseases – often through the enactment of broad social and environmental reforms. In popular perception, however, scientific medicine took credit not only for specific wartime discoveries – such as DDT and penicillin – but also the longer history of controlling epidemic disease; in public relations terms, medicine and biomedical research seized the public glory, the political interest, and the financial support given for further anticipated health improvements in the post-war world.

Public health departments needed to claim their share of the credit for declining infectious diseases and to move quickly to develop programmes for the chronic diseases. But although commentators agreed public health departments should be more active in the newer areas of public health – the chronic diseases, rehabilitation, mental health, industrial health, accident prevention, environmental issues and medical care – few had any clear idea of how to begin. Most health departments simply continued running the same programmes and clinics within already established bureaucratic structures. The exceptions were notable: under Herman E. Hilleboe as State Commissioner of Health, the New York State Health Department started a screening programme to detect early cases of cardiac disease and, at the Roswell Park Memorial Institute in Buffalo, built research laboratories, a hospital and an animal farm for research on the causes and treatment of cancer.[132] Virginia started a multiple screening programme for chronic diseases and Minnesota conducted pioneering studies of atherosclerosis and nutrition.[133] For the most part, public health programmes tended to focus on screening and early detection of disease rather than on truly preventive measures; public health, in losing its social orientation, seemed to be merging with clinical preventive medicine.

The political atmosphere of the 1950s did not support aggressive new programmes and health department budgets were stagnant without the funding needed to develop fresh approaches to existing problems and the emerging new issues of the day. Health departments did implement, or try to implement, one important, new and very cost-effective public health measure; the fluoridation of water supplies to protect children's teeth. But despite virtually unanimous support from scientific authorities and professional organizations, fluoridation, denounced by the right wing as a communist plot, was effectively halted in many cities and towns through vocal local opposition.[134] Since such a simple and obviously effective measure could be so energetically opposed, health departments must have perceived the difficulty of instituting more adventurous or expensive interventions.

The one great triumph of the 1950s was the successful development of the polio vaccine and its implementation on a mass scale. The success of the polio campaign was in large part due to private funding and a massive public relations campaign by the Foundation for Infantile Paralysis which developed popular support, interest and enthusiasm. The appeal for crippled children engaged the country's attention and the polio vaccination campaign, despite some major setbacks, was a real accomplishment.[135]

Despite such public success, in the 1950s the real expenditures of public health departments failed to keep pace with the increase in population.[136] Federal grants-in-aid to the states for public health programmes steadily declined, the total dollar amounts falling from 45 million in 1950 to 33 million in 1959. Given inflation, the decline in purchasing power of these dollars had been even more dramatic.[137] At a time when public health officials were facing a whole series of new health problems, poorly understood, they were also underbudgeted and understaffed. Jesse Aronson, director of local health services in New Jersey, offered an honest if rather devastating account of the state of small public health departments:

> The full-time health officer is frequently, because of inadequate budget and staff, limited in his activities to a series of routine clinical responsibilities in a child health station, a tuberculosis clinic, a venereal disease clinic, an immunization session, and communicable disease diagnosis and treatment. He has little or no time for community health education, the study of health problems

> and trends, the initiation of newer programs in diabetes control, cancer control, rheumatic fever prophylaxis, nutrition education, and radiation control. In a great many areas the health officer position has been vacant year after year with little real hope of filling it. In these situations, even the pretense of public health leadership is left behind and local medical practitioners provide these services on an hourly basis.[138]

Many state legislatures were setting up new agencies to build nursing homes, abate water pollution, or promote mental health, and simply bypassed health departments as not active or not interested in these issues. Public health officials were expressing 'frustrations, disappointments, dissatisfactions, and discontentments' said John W. Knutson, in his Presidential Address to the American Public Health Association.[139] Public health officials, he argued, must develop more imagination, political skills and knowledge of human motivation and behaviour. 'Our graduate students', he declared, 'need a better understanding of the social and political forces swirling about them as they work professionally. In place of rapidly outdated factual information, I would have them gain from graduate education in public health a fundamental knowledge of four broad fields: cultural anthropology, human ecology, epidemiology, and biostatistics.'[140]

In 1956, the Senate Committee on Labor and Public Welfare of the United States Congress noted a 'startling and shocking drop' in the annual number of public health trainees between 1947 and 1955.[141] The Health Amendment Act then authorized a programme of traineeships in public health for physicians, nurses, sanitary engineers, nutritionists, medical social workers, dentists, health educators, veterinarians and sanitarians. In 1958, however, the official public health agencies still reported well over 2,500 vacancies in professional categories, with many vacancies being filled with inadequately trained people.[142] Over 20,000 'professionals' employed by governmental and voluntary health agencies had no specialized training in public health. Few had any idea how to cope with new health hazards such as radiation: 'The public health agencies are not staffed as they should be now. Much less are they prepared for even the known hazards that lie ahead.'[143] The First National Conference on Public Health Training held in Washington in 1958 concluded with a stirring appeal to consider public health education an important aspect of national defence:

> The great crises of the future may not come from a foreign enemy ... 'D' day for disease and death is everyday. The battle line is already in our own community. To hold that battle line we must daily depend on specially trained physicians, nurses, biochemists, public health

> engineers ... properly organized for the normal protection of the homes, the schools, and the work places of some unidentified city somewhere in America. That city has, today, neither the personnel nor the resources of knowledge necessary to protect it.[144]

The American Public Health Association at its annual meeting in 1955 asked: 'Where are We Going in Public Health?'. Leonard Woodcock, international vice-president of the United Auto Workers, opened the meeting with a rousing speech in which he both praised public health and damned public health departments.[145] State divisions of occupational health were hopelessly under-financed, he said, work-place inspections were rarely carried out, and occupational disease reporting was totally inadequate. Labour leaders had the impression that health departments had no leaders with the passion and commitment for which Alice Hamilton had been so admired.

Labour unions wanted public health officials to assess the quality of medical services, evaluate prepayment plans, and provide comprehensive preventive services. The unions had been successfully pushing their employers to provide medical insurance benefits while public health departments had simply stayed out of the fray. The public health departments, complained Woodcock, were letting commercial insurance companies dictate the future of medical care.[146] Subsequent discussions showed that many of those present at the APHA meetings admitted the truth of Woodcock's critique.[147]

A few years later, Milton Terris offered a forceful summary statement of the dilemma of public health. The communicable diseases were disappearing; their place had been taken by the non-infectious diseases which the public health profession was ill-prepared to prevent or control.[148] The public understood the fact that research was crucial, and federal expenditures for medical research had multiplied from $28 million in 1947 to $186 million ten years later. This money, however, was mainly being spent for clinical and laboratory research; there was little understanding of the importance of epidemiological studies in addressing these problems. Schools of public health had been slow to deal with the practical problems of the chronic diseases; perceiving the flow of funding for biomedical research, the schools had simply oriented themselves towards the research priorities of the National Institutes of Health. Those promoted for their abilities in research were not necessarily interested in the immediate problems of local health departments. Public health research was exciting and rewarding; public health practice seemed dispiriting and frustrating.

Most of the research funding had gone to the laboratory sciences.

Yet even the relatively small sums spent on epidemiological research had produced dramatic successes: the discovery of the role of fluoride in preventing dental caries, the relation of cigarette smoking to lung cancer, and the suspected relation of serum cholesterol and physical exercise to coronary artery disease.[149]

In the late 1950s, public health leaders recognized and lamented the failure of their profession to have asserted a strong political presence. The American Public Health Association devoted its annual meeting in 1958 to 'The Politics of Public Health'.[150] Raymond R. Tucker, Mayor of St Louis – the city hosting the APHA convention – insisted that, despite the vociferous opposition of a few special interest groups, the general public solidly defended public health reforms.[151] At least some sociological studies found that the majority of the public supported the expansion of public health services – more so than did the power élite in their communities.[152] George Rosen, editor of the *American Journal of Public Health*, wrote that the education of public health workers should begin with teaching them to think politically about their work: 'An understanding of the political process as it affects the handling of community health problems is as crucial an area of knowledge to health workers as the scientific underpinning of public health practice.'[153]

The 1960s and the War on Poverty

The 1960s saw the collapse of the conservative complacency of the 1950s, the growing power of the civil rights movement, riots in the urban black ghettos and federal support for the 'war on poverty'. The anti-poverty effort and other Great Society programmes soon became deeply involved with medical care. Growing concern over access to medical care and hospitalization, especially by the elderly population, culminated in Medicare and Medicaid legislation in 1965 to cover medical care costs for those on social security and for the poor.[154] Medicare and Medicaid reflected the usual priorities of the medical care system in favouring highly technical interventions and hospital care while failing to provide adequately for preventive services. Both programmes were built on a 'politics of accommodation' with private providers of medical care, thus increasing the incomes of physicians and hospitals and leading to spiralling costs for medical services.[155] Other anti-poverty programmes, such as the neighbourhood health centres that were intended to encourage community participation in providing comprehensive care to underserved populations, fared less well because they were seen as competing with the interests of private care providers.[156]

Most of the new health and social programmes of the 1960s bypassed the public health departments and set up new agencies to mediate between the federal government and local communities. As far as many in the federal government were concerned, state governments were too subject to local political controls and too conservative to address social issues in an egalitarian and progressive manner. Central organization, regulation and oversight were needed to overcome the structural inequalities within as well as among the states. Neighbourhood health centres and community-based mental health services were thus established without reference to public health agencies. When environmental issues attracted public concern and political attention in the 1960s and 1970s, separate agencies were also created to respond to these concerns. At the federal level, the Environmental Protection Agency was created to deal with such issues as solid wastes, pesticides and radiation. At the state level, environmental agencies, established separately from public health departments, were not necessarily aware of specific health concerns or public health expertise. Mental health agencies were also often distinct from public health agencies, the two operating quite independently of each other. The broader functions of public health were again fragmented in numerous different organizational units; losing a clear institutional base, public health further lost visibility and clarity of definition. For a field that depends so heavily on public understanding and support, such a loss was disastrous.

Beginning in the 1960s, new federal programmes encouraged a greatly expanded interest in family planning, international health and medical care administration.[157] The schools of public health responded by developing programmes in medical care organization, hospital administration, mental health, family planning, population control, international health and environmental health. In the 1960s enrolments climbed; between 1958 and 1973, they quadrupled.[158] About one-third of public health graduates in the 1960s went into public health agencies, one-quarter into medical care facilities, one-quarter into colleges and universities, and the remainder into international health agencies and voluntary organizations.[159] By the 1960s schools of public health were thus training officials for federal and international health agencies more than for local and state health departments. The federal grant system which had allowed the schools to expand their teaching and research programmes, also influenced their organization, function and orientation.[160] By the early 1970s more than half the schools' financial support came from the federal government and in some schools the figure was as high as 85 per cent.[161] This orientation to federal programmes meant new growth and development for the schools but also made them vulnerable to political shifts; when federal funds were cut, the schools would have difficulty maintaining their programmes.[162] The link between public health education and professional practice (still largely organized on the state level), had always been tenuous and was now weaker than ever – or, at least, fragmented in a way that reflected the fragmentation of the system as a whole.

Public Health Today

The organization of public health has continued to show huge variation among the states: in some states, public health may be combined with mental health, with environmental services, with Medicare and Medicaid agencies or with social welfare agencies. Where public health activities are combined with personal health care or with social welfare services, preventive activities may be swamped by these larger, more expensive programmes. In the 1970s, for example, public health departments became providers of last resort for uninsured patients and for Medicaid patients rejected by private practitioners. By 1988 almost three-quarters of all state and local health department expenditures went for personal health services.[163] As Harry Mustard had predicted some 40 years earlier, direct provision of medical care absorbed much of the limited resources – in personnel, money, energy, time and attention – of public health departments, leading to a slow starvation of public health and preventive activities. The problem of care for the uninsured and the indigent loomed so large that they eclipsed the need for a basic public health infrastructure in the minds of many legislators and the general public.

In the Reagan revolution of the 1980s federal funding for public health and most other social programmes was cut. Through the mechanism of the block grants, power was returned to state health agencies, but in the context of funding cuts, this was the unpopular power to cut existing programmes.[164] In the context of general budget cuts, state health departments were left the task of managing Medicaid programmes and delivering personal health services to the uninsured and indigent populations. They also had to deal with the adverse health consequences of reductions in other social welfare programmes, and with the problems of a growing poverty population, as evidenced in drug abuse, alcoholism, teenage pregnancy, family violence and homelessness, as well as the health and social needs of growing populations of illegal immigrants.

During the 1980s the public health was threatened by a new and lethal disease: AIDS. As Daniel Fox has argued, the AIDS epidemic made obvious a national crisis of authority in the health system and revealed the structural contradictions and weaknesses of national and federal health policy.[165] For state and local health agencies, the AIDS epidemic exacerbated their existing problems but also gave a new visibility and urgency to public health efforts. The public health community agreed that a major national effort was needed in education and prevention. Much of the AIDS funding, when it did come, went into research and medical care; as usual, education and prevention received much less attention. At the political level, it continues to be easier and less controversial to vote money for research than to deal directly with the burgeoning social problems of increasingly impoverished urban populations.[166] The issues raised by AIDS, most especially those of sexual behaviour and injection drug use, are among the most emotional social issues of the day – and ones that politicians prefer, when possible, to avoid.

Health and health care are especially important questions for the general public but are perceived by politicians mainly in terms of spiralling costs, the resistance of voters to new taxes, and an enduring legacy of racial antagonism and distrust. In recent years, public health departments have been perceived as social agencies oriented to the needs of poor, largely minority populations and have shared the fate of other social services in being left to face mounting problems with severely restricted funds. The current fragmented and unequal system of medical care serves the interests of medical supply and technology companies, the pharmaceutical industry, the health insurance industry and, to a lesser extent, the interests of hospitals and health professionals. All these interests have powerful political lobbies in the halls of Congress. Those whose interests would be best served by a radical reorganization of both public health and medical care have less voice in the political process.[167]

Public health professionals have not proved especially adept at influencing the diverse levels of government – federal, state and local – to overcome the fragmentation of public health initiatives. Nor have they been especially successful at mobilizing public concern. Many are better at conducting scientific studies than in organizing for change. A recent report by the Institute of Medicine on *The Future of Public Health* pointedly notes that: 'In a free society public activities ultimately rest on public understanding and support, not on the technical judgment of experts. Expertise is made effective only when it is combined with sufficient public support, a connection acted upon effectively by the early leaders of public health.'[168]

The growth in the technical knowledge of public health in the past one hundred years has been extraordinary – and insufficiently addressed in this brief account – but the ability to implement this knowledge in health and social reform has but little advanced. The task is made more difficult by the fragmentation of public health authority into a wide variety of federal, state, and local agencies, programmes, and committees over a large and diverse nation, and a proliferation of lobbyists representing financial stakes in the existing, chaotic system. The American political system with its checks and balances at multiple levels of government is resistant to change; political influence is a privilege largely reserved for the economically powerful. In this context, public health workers must fight to defend their contributions to the public interest. They need to build public support, clearly communicate their goals and programmes, attack the political and economic barriers to health reforms, and by responding more visibly and effectively to endemic health and social problems, as well as new crises, to demonstrate clearly the benefits of prevention to their constituency, the public at large.

Notes

1. John Duffy, *Epidemics in Colonial America* (Baton Rouge, La.: Louisiana State University Press, 1953); John Duffy, *The Sanitarians: A History of American Public Health* (Urbana, Ill.: University of Illinois Press, 1990), 9–34.
2. P. M. Ashburn, *The Ranks of Death: A Medical History of the Conquest of America* (New York: Coward-McCann, 1947); *idem, The Columbian Exchange: Biological and Cultural Consequences of 1492* (Westport Conn.: Greenwood Press, 1972); *idem, Ecological Imperialism: The Biological Expansion of Europe, 900–1900* (Cambridge: Cambridge University Press, 1986); *idem*, 'Virgin Soil Epidemics as a Factor in the Aboriginal Depopulation in America', *William and Mary Quarterly*, 33 (1976), 289–99. For a general discussion of the ways in which human population movements and long-distance contacts have spread disease across continents, see William McNeill, *Plagues and Peoples* (Garden City, N.Y.: Anchor Press, 1976).
3. Indian populations suffered from respiratory diseases and dysentery and, at least in areas of high population density, from tuberculosis and various parasitic infections, but they were unfamiliar with smallpox and measles. See John W. Verano and Douglas H. Ubelaker, 'Health and Disease in the Pre-Columbian World', in Herman J. Viola and Carolyn Margolis (eds), *Seeds of Change,* 209–23. (Washington, DC: Smithsonian Institution Press, 1991).

4. Thornton Russell, *American Indian Holocaust and Survival: A Population History Since 1492* (Norman: University of Oklahoma Press, 1987); Grant Forman, *Indian Removal* (Norman: University of Oklahoma Press, 1953).
5. As Duffy explains it, with a rather astonishing disregard for Indian lives: 'From an economic standpoint the destruction caused by smallpox among the Indians more than compensated for any damages done to the colonists. The elimination of certain tribes and the decimation of many others greatly facilitated colonial expansion. Indirectly, smallpox saved both lives and property which would otherwise have been expended in warfare with the Indians.' Duffy, *Epidemics in Colonial America,* 111.
6. Carl Degler, *Out of Our Past: The Forces That Shaped Modern America* (New York: Harper & Row, rev. edn 1970), 43.
7. *Ibid.,* 33.
8. Genevieve Miller, 'Smallpox Inoculation in England and America', *William and Mary Quarterly,* 13 (1956), 476–8.
9. John Shy, *A People Numerous and Armed: Reflections on the Military Struggle for American Independence* (New York: Oxford University Press, 1976).
10. The 13 states all required that their representatives be property owners and in most cases, embedded property qualifications for voters and office-holders in their constitutions. See especially Charles Beard, *An Economic Interpretation of the Constitution of the United States* (New York: Macmillan, 1935).
11. Degler, *op. cit.* (note 6), 100.
12. J. H. Powell, *Bring Out Your Dead: The Yellow Fever Epidemic in Philadelphia in 1793* (Philadelphia: University of Pennsylvania Press, 1949); Duffy, *The Sanitarians,* 35–51.
13. See, for example, William T. Howard, *Public Health Administration and the Natural History of Disease in Baltimore, Maryland, 1797–1920* (Washington, D.C.: Carnegie Institution, 1924). Policy debates provoked by epidemic diseases were often embedded in the particularities of local political and economic struggles; Martin Pernick, for example, has shown how the disputes surrounding the yellow fever epidemic in Philadelphia engaged the passions of party politics. See, Martin S. Pernick, 'Politics, Parties, and Pestilence: Epidemic Yellow Fever in Philadelphia and the Rise of the First Party System', *William and Mary Quarterly,* 29 (1972), 559–86. See also Powell, *op. cit.* (note 12). In the European context, Erwin Ackerknecht argued that contagionist/anti-contagionist debates over disease causation were tied to the different economic interests of those who supported and opposed quarantines: Erwin L. Ackerknecht, 'Anticontagionism Between 1821 and 1867', *Bulletin of the History of Medicine,* 22 (1948), 562–93. Margaret Pelling has, however, challenged this interpretation in a detailed account of theories of

disease aetiology in *Cholera, Fever and English Medicine, 1825–1865* (Oxford: Oxford University Press, 1978).

14. See, for example, Baltimore City Ordinance 11, approved 7 April, 1797 as cited in Howard, *op. cit.* (note 13), 50.
15. During epidemics, the clergy led days of fasting and prayer; in Baltimore, they claimed that prayer had saved the city from a threatened epidemic of yellow fever in 1819. See *ibid.*, 87.
16. Charles E. Rosenberg, *The Cholera Years: The United States in 1832, 1849 and 1866* (Chicago: University of Chicago Press, 1962), 47–53.
17. David Rosner, 'Health Care for the "Truly Needy": Nineteenth-Century Origins of the Concept', *Health and Society*, 60 (1982), 355–85.
18. Charles E. Rosenberg and Carroll Smith-Rosenberg, 'Pietism and the Origins of the Public Health Movement: A Note on John H. Griscom and Robert M. Hartley', *Journal of the History of Medicine and Allied Sciences*, 23 (1968), 16–35; see also Barbara G. Rosenkrantz, *Public Health and the State: Changing Views in Massachusetts, 1842–1936* (Cambridge, Mass.: Harvard University Press, 1972). For the larger context of evangelicism and social reform, see T. L. Smith, *Revivalism and Social Reform in Mid-Nineteenth Century America* (New York and Nashville: Abingdon, 1957).
19. John H. Griscom, *The Uses and Abuses of Air: Showing Its Influence in Sustaining Life, and Producing Disease...* (New York: Redfield, 1850), 137 n, 143, as cited in Rosenberg and Smith-Rosenberg, *op. cit.* (note 18).
20. Todd L. Savitt, 'Slave Health and Southern Distinctiveness', in *Disease and Distinctiveness in the American South*, Todd L. Savitt and James Harvey Young (eds), (Knoxville: University of Tennessee Press, 1988), 120–53.
21. Michael Rogin, *Fathers and Children: Andrew Jackson and the Subjugation of the American Indian* (New York: Knopf, 1975); Richard Drinnon, *Violence in the American Experience: Winning the West* (New York: New American Library, 1979).
22. Alvin M. Josephy Jr., *The Civil War in the American West* (New York: Knopf, 1991).
23. See, for example, John Blake, *Public Health in the Town of Boston, 1630–1822* (Cambridge, Mass.: Harvard University Press, 1959); Rosenkrantz, *op. cit.* (note 18); John Duffy, *A History of Public Health in New York City, 1625–1865* (New York: Russell Sage Foundation, 1968); *idem, A History of Public Health in New York City, 1866–1966* (New York: Russell Sage Foundation, 1974); Stuart Galishoff, *Safeguarding the Public Health: Newark, 1895–1918* (Westport, Conn.: Greenwood Press, 1975); Judith Walzer Leavitt, *The Healthiest City: Milwaukee and the Politics of Health Reform* (Princeton, N.J.: Princeton University Press, 1982).

24. Erwin H. Ackerknecht, *Malaria in the Upper Mississippi Valley, 1760–1900* (Baltimore: The Johns Hopkins Press, 1945). George Rosen, *A History of Public Health,* essentially ignores United States history before the sanitary movement of the mid nineteenth century in the east coast cities; John Duffy, in *The Sanitarians,* makes only passing reference to the frontier and westward expansion. Some interesting recent studies promise, however, to extend the canon. See, for example, Allan M. Winkler, 'Drinking on the American Frontier', *Journal of Studies on Alcohol,* 29 (1968), 413–45; Clyde N. Dollar, 'The High Plains Smallpox Epidemic of 1837–38', *Western Historical Quarterly,* 8 (1977), 15–38; Richard Slotkin, *The Fatal Environment: The Myth of the Frontier in the Age of Industrialization, 1800–1890* (New York: Harper & Row, 1986); Peter D. Olch, 'Medicine in the Indian-Fighting Army, 1866–1890', *Journal of the West,* 21 (July, 1982), 32–41; and David T. Courtwright, 'Disease, Death, and Disorder on the American Frontier', *Journal of the History of Medicine,* 46 (1991), 457–92.
25. There is a huge literature on slavery; for one classic account, see Eugene Genovese, *Roll, Jordan, Roll: The World the Slaves Made* (New York: Pantheon, 1974).
26. G. W. Adams, *Doctors in Blue* (New York: Henry Schuman, 1952). According to contemporary accounts, the main causes of death were 'typho-malaria' (perhaps a combination of typhoid fever and malaria), camp diarrhoea, and 'camp measles'; scurvy, acute respiratory diseases, venereal diseases, rheumatism and epidemic jaundice were also widespread in army encampments. See, J. J. Woodward, *Chief Camp Diseases of the United States Armies* (Philadelphia: J.B. Lippencott, 1863).
27. H. H. Cunningham, *Doctors in Grey: The Confederate Medical Service* (Baton Rouge: Louisiana State University Press, 1958).
28. Woodward, *op. cit.* (note 26).
29. Charles J. Stille, *History of the United States Sanitary Commission: Being the General Report of Its Work During the War of the Rebellion* (Philadelphia: J.B. Lippincott, 1866).
30. *Op. sit.,* (note 23).
31. John Blake, *Public Health in the Town of Boston, 1630–1822* (Cambridge, Mass.: Harvard University Press, 1959); Barbara Rosenkrantz, *Public Health and the State: Changing Views in Massachusetts, 1842–1936* (Cambridge, Mass.: Harvard University Press, 1972); John Duffy, *A History of Public Health in New York City, 1625–1865* (New York: Russell Sage Foundation, 1968); John Duffy, *A History of Public Health in New York City, 1866–1966* (New York: Russell Sage Foundation, 1974); Stuart Galishoff, *Safeguarding the Public Health: Newark, 1895–1918* (Westport, Conn.: Greenwood Press, 1975); Judith Walzer Leavitt, *The Healthiest City: Milwaukee and the Politics of Health Reform* (Princeton, N.J.: Princeton University Press, 1982).

32. Gert H. Brieger, 'Sanitary Reform in New York City: Stephen Smith and the Passage of the Metropolitan Health Bill', *Bulletin of the History of Medicine,* 40 (1966), 407–29.
33. Charles-E. A. Winslow, *The Life of Hermann M. Biggs: Physician and Statesman of the Public Health* (Philadelphia: Lea & Febiger, 1929); E. O. Jordan, G. C. Whipple, C.-E. A. Winslow, *A Pioneer of Public Health: William Thompson Sedgwick* (New Haven: Yale University Press, 1924); James H. Cassedy, *Charles V. Chapin and the Public Health Movement* (Cambridge, Mass.: Harvard University Press, 1962); Rosenkrantz, *op. cit.* (note 18).
34. John Duffy, *The Rudolph Matas History of Medicine in Louisiana,* 2 vols (Baton Rouge, Louisiana: Louisiana State University Press, 1958–1962).
35. R. G. Patterson, *Historical Directory of State Health Departments in the United States of America* (Ohio Public Health Association, 1939).
36. S. W. Abbott, *The Past and Present Conditions of Public Hygiene and State Medicine in the United States* (Boston: Wright & Potter, 1900).
37. On the early history of the APHA, see Harold M. Cavins, 'The National Quarantine and Sanitary Conventions of 1857–1858 and the Beginnings of the American Public Health Association', *Bulletin of the History of Medicine,* 13 (1943), 419–25; Howard D. Kramer, 'Agitation for Public Health Reform in the 1870s', *Journal of the History of Medicine and Allied Sciences,* 3 (1948), 473–88.
38. John M. Toner, 'Boards of Health in the United States', in *Selections from Public Health Reports and Papers Presented at Meetings of the American Public Health Association (1873–1883),* Public Health in America Series, (New York: Arno Press, 1977), 499–501, as cited in Duffy, *The Sanitarians,* 131.
39. Laurence F. Schmeckebier, *The Public Health Service, Its History, Activities and Organization* (Baltimore, Maryland: The Johns Hopkins Press, 1923).
40. For a comprehensive history of the founding of the National Institute of Health from its beginnings in this one-room bacteriological laboratory, see Victoria A. Harden, *Inventing the NIH: Federal Biomedical Research Policy, 1887–1937* (Baltimore: The Johns Hopkins University Press, 1986).
41. For a lively account of these and other social and labour struggles, see Howard Zinn, *A People's History of the United States* (New York: Harper & Row, 1980).
42. Charles E. and Carroll S.-Rosenberg, *op. cit.* (note 18), 16–35; Richard H. Shryock, 'The Early American Public Health Movement', *American Journal of Public Health,* 27 (1937), 965–71.
43. Barbara G. Rosenkrantz, 'Cart Before Horse: Theory, Practice and Professional Image in American Public Health, 1870–1920', *Journal of the History of Medicine and Allied Sciences,* 29 (1974), 55–73, 57.
44. Stephen Smith, 'The History of Public Health, 1871–1921', in

Mazyck P. Ravenel, (ed.), *A Half Century of Public Health* (New York: American Public Health Association, 1921), 1–12; Mazyck P. Ravenel, 'The American Public Health Association: Past, Present, Future', in *ibid.*, 13–55.

45. See Mary P. Ryan, *Womanhood in America: From Colonial Times to the Present* (New York: Franklin Watts, 1975), 225–34.
46. For a comprehensive and critical examination of the maternal and child health movement, see Richard A. Meckel, *Save the Babies: American Health Reform and the Prevention of Infant Mortality, 1850–1929* (Baltimore: The Johns Hopkins University Press, 1990).
47. The American Red Cross, for example, was formed in 1882, the National Tuberculosis Association in 1904, the American Social Hygiene Association in 1905, the National Committee for Mental Hygiene in 1909 and the American Society for the Control of Cancer in 1919. See Wilson G. Smillie, *Public Health: Its Promise for the Future* (New York: Macmillan, 1955), 450–8.
48. Robert H. Wiebe, *The Search for Order, 1877–1920* (New York: Hill & Wang, 1967); Samuel P. Hays, 'The Politics of Reform in Municipal Government in the Progressive Era', in *American Political History as Social Analysis* (Knoxville: University of Tennessee Press, 1980), 205–32; *idem.*, *Conservation and the Gospel of Efficiency: The Progressive Conservation Movement, 1890–1918* (Boston: Beacon Press, 1968); Daniel T. Rogers, 'In Search of Progressivism', *Reviews in American History*, 10 (1982), 115–32.
49. The debate about the nature of progressive reform is extensive. James Weinstein argues that much of the impetus for progressive reform came from protestors and radicals but that the actual reforms enacted had the tacit approval of corporate interests. Alan Dawley characterizes the period as struggle between 'progressive liberals' and 'managerial liberals', where the progressive liberals demanded public restraints on business, state-sponsored social welfare programmes, women's suffrage, legal access to birth control, regulation of working conditions and abolition of child labour; managerial liberals offered self-regulation and self-government by industry, industry-run occupational health programmes, and a carefully managed pro-corporate reform effort. From this perspective, most of the public health reformers are clearly 'progressive liberals'. See James Weinstein, *The Corporate Ideal in the Liberal State, 1900–1918* (Boston: Beacon Press, 1968); Alan Dawley, *Struggles for Justice: Social Responsibility and the Liberal State* (Cambridge, Mass.: Harvard University Press, 1991).
50. Welch, *op. sit.* (note 50), 598.
51. For a classic statement of this argument, see Max von Pettenkofer, *The Value of Health to a City.* Translated with an introduction by Henry E. Sigerist. (Baltimore: The Johns Hopkins University Press, 1941), 15–52.
52. Welch, *op. cit.* (note 50), 596.

53. Thomas M. Rotch, 'The Position and Work of the American Pediatric Society Toward Public Questions', *Transactions of the American Pediatric Society,* 21 (1909), 12.
54. Charles Chapin, 'How Shall We Spend the Health Appropriation?' in *Papers of Charles V. Chapin, M.D.,* compiled by F. P. Gorham and C. L. Scamman (New York: Oxford University Press, 1934), 28–35.
55. Chapin, 'Pleasures and Hopes of the Health Officer', *ibid.,* 11.
56. Martin J. Schiesl, *The Politics of Efficiency: Municipal Administration and Reform In America, 1880–1920* (Berkeley and London: University of California Press, 1980).
57. For the development of bacteriology in the United States, see especially Patricia P. Gossel, 'The Emergence of American Bacteriology, 1875–1900', (Ph.D. Dissertation, The Johns Hopkins University, 1988).
58. For Sedgwick's rather lyrical view of bacteriology, see William T. Sedgwick, 'The Origin, Scope and Significance of Bacteriology', *Science,* 13 (1901), 121–8.
59. As cited in Jordan, Whipple, & Winslow, *op. cit.* (note 33), 57.
60. Charles V. Chapin, *Municipal Sanitation in the United States* (Providence, R.I.: Snow & Farnham, 1901).
61. Charles V. Chapin, *The Sources and Modes of Infection* (New York: John Wiley & Sons, 1910).
62. Hibbert Winslow Hill, *The New Public Health* (New York: Macmillan, 1916).
63. *Ibid.*, 19–20.
64. *Ibid.*, 134–5.
65. J. Scott MacNutt, *A Manual for Health Officers* (New York: John Wiley & Sons, 1915), 85.
66. Charles-Edward A. Winslow, 'The Untilled Fields of Public Health', *Science,* 51 (1920), 23; see also, C.-E.A. Winslow, *The Evolution and Significance of the Modern Public Health Campaign* (New Haven: Yale University Press, 1923).
67. See Barbara Sicherman, *Alice Hamilton: A Life in Letters* (Cambridge and London: Harvard University Press, 1984), 153–83.
68. Milton Terris, (ed.), *Goldberger on Pellagra* (Baton Rouge: Louisiana State University Press, 1964). See especially, Joseph Goldberger and Edgar Sydenstricker, 'Pellagra in the Mississippi Flood Area', 271–91.
69. For a detailed examination of this point in the case of tuberculosis, see Bonnie Kantor, 'The New Scientific Public Health Movement: A Case Study of Tuberculosis in Baltimore, Maryland, 1900–1910', (Sc.D. Dissertation, School of Hygiene and Public Health, The Johns Hopkins University, 1985).
70. George M. Sternberg, 'Sanitary Lessons of the War', in *Sanitary Lessons of the War and Other Papers* (Washington, D.C.: Byron S. Adams, 1912), 2; see also, Graham A. Cosmas, *An Army for Empire: The United States Army in the Spanish–American War* (Columbia,

Mo.: University of Missouri Press, 1971).

71. One classic older account is Howard A. Kelley, *Walter Reed and Yellow Fever* (Baltimore: Medical Standard Book Company, 1906). See, however, the fascinating rewriting of this history by François Delaporte, *The History of Yellow Fever: An Essay on the Birth of Tropical Medicine* (Cambridge: Mass.: MIT Press, 1991).
72. Mary C. Gillett, 'Medical Care and Evacuation During the Philippine Insurrection, 1899–1901', *Journal of the History of Medicine and Allied Sciences,* 42 (1987), 169–85; see also Rodney Sullivan, 'Cholera and Colonialism in the Philippines, 1899–1903', in *Disease, Medicine, and Empire: Perspectives on Western Medicine and the Experience of European Expansion,* Roy MacLeod and Milton Lewis (eds), (London: Routledge, 1988), 284–300.
73. J. M. Gates, *Schoolbooks and Krags: The United States Army in the Philippines, 1898–1902* (Westport, Conn.: Greenwood Press, 1973).
74. Sternberg, 'Sanitary Problems Connected with the Construction of the Isthmian Canal', *op. cit.* (note 70), 39–40.
75. Raymond B. Fosdick, *Adventure in Giving: The Story of the General Education Board* (New York and Evanston: Harper & Row, 1962), 57–8.
76. For a detailed account of the Rockefeller Sanitary Commission, see John Ettling, *The Germ of Laziness: Rockefeller Philanthropy and Public Health in the New South* (Cambridge, Mass.: Harvard University Press, 1981).
77. Wickliffe Rose, *First Annual Report of the Administrative Secretary of the Rockefeller Sanitary Commission,* (1910), 4, as cited in Raymond B. Fosdick, *The Story of the Rockefeller Foundation* (New York: Harper & Brothers, 1952), 33.
78. Ettling, *op. cit.* (note 76), 220–1.
79. George Rosen, 'The Committee of One Hundred on National Health and the Campaign for a National Health Department, 1906–1912', *American Journal of Public Health,* 62 (1972), 261–3; Alan I. Marcus, 'Disease Prevention in America: From a Local to a National Outlook, 1880–1910', *Bulletin of the History of Medicine,* 53 (1979), 184–203.
80. Irving Fisher, *A Report on National Vitality, Its Wastes and Conservation,* Bulletin 30, Committee of One Hundred on National Health (Washington, D.C.: Government Printing Office, 1909).
81. A starting point for the large and growing literature on the influence of the eugenics movement is Daniel J. Kevles, *In the Name of Eugenics: Genetics and the Uses of Human Heredity* (New York: Knopf, 1985).
82. For a detailed history of the Public Health Service, see Ralph C. Williams, *The United States Public Health Service, 1798–1950* (Washington, D.C.: Government Printing Office, 1951); for a briefer, but more engaging account, see Fitzhugh Mullan, *Plagues*

and Politics: The Story of the United States Public Health Service (New York: Basic Books, 1989).

83. William T. Sedgwick, 'Scientists and Technicians in the Public Service', as cited in Jordan, Whipple, & Winslow, *op. cit.* (note 33), 133–4. For the history of subsequent developments in professional public health education, see Elizabeth Fee and Roy M. Acheson (eds), *A History of Education in Public Health: Health That Mocks the Doctors' Rules* (Oxford and New York: Oxford University Press, 1991).
84. Fee & Acheson *ibid.*
85. Arthur J. Viseltear, 'C.-E. A. Winslow and the Early Years of Public Health at Yale, 1915–1925', *Yale Journal of Biology and Medicine*, 55 (1982), 137–51; Arthur J. Viseltear, 'The Yale Plan of Medical Education: The Early Years', *Yale Journal of Biology and Medicine*, 59 (1986), 627–48; Elizabeth Fee, *Disease and Discovery: A History of the Johns Hopkins School of Hygiene and Public Health, 1916–1939* (Baltimore: Johns Hopkins University Press, 1987). See also Fee & Acheson, *op. cit.* (note 83).
86. See especially Fee, *op. cit.* (note 85).
87. See especially Allan M. Brandt, *No Magic Bullet: A Social History of Venereal Disease in the United States Since 1880* (New York: Oxford University Press, 1987).
88. Morris Knowles, 'Public Health Service Not a Medical Monopoly', *American Journal of Public Health*, 3 (1913), 111–22.
89. For a useful discussion of the relationship of physicians to public health, see Rosenkrantz, *op. cit.* (note 43), 55–73.
90. Charles Rosenberg, 'Making It in Urban Medicine: A Career in the Age of Scientific Medicine', *Bulletin of the History of Medicine*, 64 (1990), 163–86.
91. Joel A. Tarr, 'The Separate Vs. Combined Sewer Problem: A Case Study in Urban Technology Design Choice', *Journal of Urban History*, 5 (1979), 308–99.
92. It is difficult to be confident about mortality rates in the United States before 1900, when the death registration areas began regular reporting. The evidence seems, however, to suggest that mortality rates between 1850 and 1880 remained relatively constant, with wide annual variations depending on the presence of epidemics. In the 1880s the mortality rates began to decline, and continued this decline, with minor fluctuations, throughout the period from 1890 to 1915. The major component of the decline was in infant mortality, especially mortality rates from the infectious diseases and infant diarrhoea. This pattern is consistent with the thesis that the extension of municipal water systems and the filtration of water supplies played a major role in the decline in mortality. The pasteurization of milk was probably also an important contributing factor. On the estimation of mortality rates for the period, see Edward Meeker, 'The Improving Health of the United States,

1850–1915', *Explorations in Economic History,* 9 (1972), 353–73; Michael R. Haines, 'The Use of Model Life Tables to Estimate Mortality for the United States in the Late Nineteenth Century', *Demography,* 16 (1979), 289–312; Frederick L. Hoffman, 'The General Death Rate of Large American Cities, 1871–1904', *Publications of the American Statistical Association,* 10 (1906–1907), 1–75. For a general discussion of the social impact of infectious diseases, see John Duffy, 'Social Impact of Disease in the Late Nineteenth Century', *Bulletin of the New York Academy of Medicine,* 47 (1971), 797–811.

93. Daniel M. Fox, 'Social Policy and City Politics: Tuberculosis Reporting in New York, 1889–1900', *Bulletin of the History of Medicine,* 49 (1975); 177–80; Elizabeth Fee and Evelynn M. Hammonds, 'Science, Politics, and the Art of Persuasion: Promoting the New Scientific Medicine in New York City', in *Epidemic! Public Health Crises in New York,* David Rosner (ed.), (New Brunswick, N.J.: Rutgers University Press, forthcoming).
94. John Duffy, 'The American Medical Profession and Public Health: From Support to Ambivalence', *Bulletin of the History of Medicine,* 53 (1979), 1–22.
95. *Ibid.*, 21.
96. E. Richard Brown, *Rockefeller Medicine Men* (Berkeley: University of California Press, 1979); Paul Starr, *The Social Transformation of American Medicine* (New York: Basic Books, 1982); Charles Rosenberg, *The Care of Strangers: The Rise of America's Hospital System* (New York: Basic Books, 1987).
97. Charles-Edward A. Winslow, *The Evolution and Significance of the Modern Public Health Campaign* (New Haven: Yale University Press, 1923), 53, 55. See also, Charles-Edward A. Winslow, 'Public Health at the Crossroads', *American Journal of Public Health,* 16 (1926), 1075–85.
98. *Report of the Committee on Municipal Health Department Practice of the American Public Health Association, in Cooperation with the United States Public Health Service.* Public Health Bulletin, no. 136. (Washington, D.C.: Government Printing Office, 1923).
99. Harry S. Mustard, Director of the School of Public Health at Columbia University, stated that: 'The United States Public Health Service occupies an enviable and commendable position in its relationships with the health authorities of the several states ... through high standards of performance and through demonstration and efficiency, the Public Health Service has raised the level of work performed in every county, city, and state health department with which it has had even indirect contact.' Harry S. Mustard, *Government in Public Health* (New York: The Commonwealth Fund, 1945), 59.
100. F. K. Kratz, 'Status of Full-Time Local Health Organizations at the End of the Fiscal Year 1941–1942', *Public Health Reports,* 58 (1943), 345–51.

101. Corwin (ed.), *Ecology of Health* (New York: The Commonwealth Fund, 1949), 125. See also, Mustard, *op. cit.* (note 99), 190.
102. W. S. Leathers *et al.*, Committee on Professional Education of the American Public Health Association, 'Public Health Degrees and Certificates Granted in 1936', *American Journal of Public Health,* 27 (1937), 1267–72.
103. Corwin *op. cit.* (note 101), xii.
104. James Stevens Simmons, 'The Preventive Medicine Program of the United States Army', *American Journal of Public Health,* 33 (1943), 931–40.
105. Harry S. Mustard, Editorial, 'Yesterday's School Children are Examined for the Army', *American Journal of Public Health,* 31 (1941), 1207.
106. See, for example, Alfred L. Burgdorf, 'War and the Health Department', *American Journal of Public Health,* 33 (1943), 26–30; for the disarmingly pessimistic view of a local health officer, see Hubert O. Swartout, 'Wartime Problems of a County Health Officer', *American Journal of Public Health,* 34 (1944), 379–82.
107. Joseph W. Mountin, 'Evaluation of Health Services in a National Emergency', *American Journal of Public Health,* 32 (1942), 1128.
108. *Idem,* 'Responsibility of Local Health Authorities in the War Effort', *American Journal of Public Health,* 33 (1943), 35–40.
109. For a detailed account of the activities of the US Public Health Service during the war, see Ralph Chester Williams, *The United States Public Health Service, 1798–1950* (Washington, D.C.: Commissioned Officers Association of the United States Public Health Service, 1951), 612–768; Bess Furman, *A Profile of the Public Health Service, 1798–1948* (Bethesda, Md.: National Institutes of Health, 1973), 418–58.
110. Frances Sullivan, 'Public Health Planning for War Needs: Order or Chaos?' *American Journal of Public Health,* 32 (1942) 831–6.
111. G. St J. Perrott, 'Findings of Selective Service Examinations', *Milbank Memorial Fund Quarterly,* 22 (1944), 358–66. 'Selective Service Rejection Statistics and Some of Their Implications', *American Journal of Public Health,* 36 (1946), 336–42.
112. *Ibid.,* 341–2; Felix J. Underwood, 'The Role of Public Health in the National Emergency', *American Journal of Public Health,* 32 (1942), 530.
113. Alfred L. Burgdorf, 'War and the Health Department', *American Journal of Public Health,* 33 (1943), 28. According to Hubert O. Swartout, Health Officer of Los Angeles County, the public was more anxious about health issues than ever before: '... there is the public, more upset and more fearful about almost everything now than ever before, and more often and more insistently than ever demanding that the health department "do something about it"'. *op. cit.* (note 106), 379.

114. Kenneth F. Maxcy, 'Epidemiologic Implications of Wartime Population Shifts', *American Journal of Public Health*, 32, (1942), 1089–96.
115. For wartime concern with water supplies, see for example, R. F. Goudey, 'Wartime Protection of Water Supplies', *American Journal of Public Health*, 31 (1941), 1174–80; W. H. Weir, 'Lessons Learned from the Internal Security Program of the War Department', *American Journal of Public Health*, 35 (1945), 353–7.
116. Elizabeth W. Etheridge, *Sentinel for Health: A History of the Centers for Disease Control* (Berkeley: University of California Press, 1992).
117. Joseph W. Mountin and Evelyn Flook, 'Distribution of Health Services in the Structure of State Government: The Composite Pattern of State Health Services', *Public Health Reports*, 56 (1941), 1676; *idem*, 'Distribution of Health Services in the Structure of State Government: State Health Department Organization', *Public Health Reports*, 58 (1943), 568.
118. Haven Emerson, *Local Health Units for the Nation* (New York: The Commonwealth Fund, 1945).
119. Ronald L. Numbers, *Almost Persuaded: American Physicians and Compulsory Health Insurance, 1912–1920* (Baltimore: The Johns Hopkins University Press, 1978); *idem* (ed.), *Compulsory Health Insurance: The Continuing Debate* (Westport, Conn.: Greenwood Press, 1982); Daniel S. Hirshfield, *The Lost Reform: The Campaign for Compulsory Health Insurance in the United States from 1932 to 1943* (Cambridge, Mass.: Harvard University Press, 1970); Richard Harris, *A Sacred Trust* (New York: New American Library, 1966); Monty M. Poen, *Harry S. Truman Versus the Medical Lobby* (Columbia, Mo.: University of Missouri Press, 1979); Starr, *op. cit.* (note 96); Frank D. Campion, *The AMA and U.S. Health Policy Since 1940* (Chicago: Chicago Review Press, 1984); Daniel M. Fox, *Health Policies, Health Politics: The British and American Experience, 1911–1965* (Princeton, N.J.: Princeton University Press, 1986).
120. Iago Galdston, Secretary of the New York Academy of Medicine, organized the Institute on Social Medicine in 1947. See Galdston (ed.), *Social Medicine: Its Derivations and Objectives* (New York: The Commonwealth Fund, 1949).
121. John E. Gordon, 'The Newer Epidemiology', in *Tomorrow's Horizon in Public Health*, Transactions of the 1950 conference of the Public Health Association of New York City (New York: Public Health Association, 1950), 18–45; *idem*, 'The World, the Flesh and the Devil as Environment, Host and Agent of Disease', in *The Epidemiology of Health*, Iago Galdston (ed.), 60–73.
122. Ernest L. Stebbins, 'Epidemiology and Social Medicine', in *Social Medicine: Its Derivations and Objectives* (New York, The Commonwealth Fund, 1949).
123. Wilson G. Smillie, 'The Responsibility of the State', in *Tomorrow's*

Horizon in Public Health, 95–102.
124. Eli Ginzberg, 'Public Health and the Public', *ibid.*, 104.
125. Edward J. Stieglitz, *A Future For Preventive Medicine* (New York: The Commonwealth Fund, 1945), 32–3.
126. Bernard J. Stern, *Medical Services by Government: Local, State, and Federal* (New York: The Commonwealth Fund, 1946), 31–2.
127. Mustard, *op. cit.* (note 99), 191.
128. The act did include some funds for building public health centres, but this component of the bill was far overshadowed by the emphasis on acute care facilities.
129. In 1947, the Committee on Medicine and the Changing Order, supported by the Commonwealth Fund, the Milbank Memorial Fund and the Josiah Macy Jr. Foundation, had recommended the extension of public health services and argued that the quality of public health officers must be improved by better recruitment, training, assured tenure and adequate salaries: 'The mean salary of state health officers is now only a little over $5,000, which is certainly inadequate. Only when tenure and better salaries are provided will it be possible to attract the more competent individuals and to insist upon higher training standards.' Report of the New York Academy of Medicine, Committee on Medicine in the Changing Order, *Medicine in the Changing Order* (New York: The Commonwealth Fund, 1947), 109.
130. Stephen P. Strickland, *Politics, Science, and Dread Disease* (Cambridge, Mass.: Harvard University Press, 1972).
131. Mustard, *op. cit.* (note 99), 112.
132. Herman E. Hilleboe, 'Public Health in a Changing World', *American Journal of Public Health*, 45 (1955), 1517–24.
133. *Idem*, 'Editorial: Research in Public Health Practice', *American Journal of Public Health*, 47 (1957), 216–17.
134. Donald R. McNeil, *The Fight for Fluoridation* (New York: Oxford University Press, 1957).
135. For a triumphant account of the polio vaccine, see, for example, R. Carter, *Breakthrough: The Saga of Jonas Salk* (New York: Trident Press, 1966); Allan M. Brandt provides a more critical, although brief, analysis in 'Polio, Politics, Publicity, and Duplicity: Ethical Aspects in the Development of the Salk Vaccine', *International Journal of Health Services*, 8 (1978), 257–70.
136. B. S. Sanders, 'Local Health Departments: Growth or Illusion?' *Public Health Reports*, 74 (1959), 13–20.
137. Milton Terris, 'The Changing Face of Public Health', *American Journal of Public Health*, 49 (1959), 1119.
138. Jesse B. Aronson, 'The Politics of Public Health – Reactions and Summary', *American Journal of Public Health*, 49 (1959), 311.
139. John W. Knutson, 'Ferment in Public Health', *American Journal of Public Health*, 47 (1947), 1489.

140. *Ibid.*, 1490–1.
141. Senate Committee on Labor and Public Welfare, 29 May, 1956. As cited in *Report of the National Conference on Public Health Training to the Surgeon General of the Public Health Service, 28–30 July, 1958* (Washington, D.C.: US Department of Health, Education, and Welfare, 1958), 1.
142. Howard Ennes, 'Manpower – The Achilles' Heel in Public Health', *American Journal of Public Health,* 47 (1957), 1390.
143. Senate Committee on Labor and Public Welfare, 29 May, 1956. As cited *op. cit.* (note 141), 3.
144. *Ibid.*, 15.
145. Leonard Woodcock, 'Where Are We Going in Public Health?' *American Journal of Public Health,* 46 (1956), 278–82.
146. *Ibid.*, 280.
147. Hugh R. Leavell, 'Where Are We Going in Public Health? Association Symposium (Part II) – Resolving the Basic Issues', *American Journal of Public Health,* 46 (1956), 408.
148. Terris, *op. cit.* (note 137), 1113–19.
149. *Ibid.*, 1114.
150. APHA Symposium – 1958, 'The Politics of Public Health', *American Journal of Public Health,* 49 (1959), 300–13.
151. The Honorable Raymond R. Tucker, 'The Politics of Public Health', *American Journal of Public Health,* 49 (1959), 300–5.
152. Julius S. Prince, 'A Public Philosophy in Public Health', *American Journal of Public Health,* 48 (1958), 903–12.
153. George Rosen, 'Editorial: The Politics of Public Health', *American Journal of Public Health,* 49 (1959), 364–5.
154. Robert Stevens and Rosemary Stevens, *Welfare Medicine in America: A Case Study of Medicaid* (New York: Free Press, 1974).
155. Starr, *op. cit.* (note 96), 374–8.
156. Karen Davis and Cathy Schoen, *Health and the War on Poverty* (Washington, D.C.: Brookings Institution, 1978); Alice Sardell, *The U.S. Experiment in Social Medicine: The Community Health Center Program, 1965–1986* (Pittsburgh: University of Pittsburgh Press, 1988).
157. John C. Hume, 'The Future of Schools of Public Health: The Johns Hopkins School of Hygiene and Public Health', in *Schools of Public Health: Present and Future,* John Z. Bowers and Elizabeth F. Purcell (eds), (New York: Josiah Macy Jr. Foundation, 1974), 64.
158. By 1960 there were 13 schools of public health in the United States, the newest ones being in California at Los Angeles, Puerto Rico and Pittsburgh. Six more schools would be established between 1965 and 1972: Hawaii, Oklahoma, Texas, Washington, Illinois and Loma Linda, and seven more schools between 1973 and 1988.
159. Cecil G. Sheps, 'Trends in Schools of Public Health in the United States Since World War II', *op. cit.* (note 157), 1–10.

160. Frank C. Ramsey, 'Observations of a Recent Graduate of a School of Public Health', *ibid.*, 130–3.
161. 'Summary', *ibid.*, 172–6.
162. John R. Hogness, 'The Future of Schools of Public Health in Relation to Government', *ibid.*, 124–9.
163. Institute of Medicine, Committee for the Study of the Future of Public Health, *The Future of Public Health* (Washington, D.C.: National Academy Press, 1988), 110.
164. G. S. Omenn, 'What's Behind Those Block Grants in Health?' *New England Journal of Medicine,* 306 (1982), 1057–60.
165. Daniel M. Fox, 'AIDS and the American Health Polity: The History and Prospects of a Crisis of Authority', in *AIDS: The Burdens of History,* Elizabeth Fee and Daniel M. Fox (eds), (Berkeley; University of California Press, 1988), 316–43.
166. See Warwick Anderson, 'The New York Needle Trial: The Politics of Public Health in the Age of AIDS', *American Journal of Public Health,* 81 (1991), 1506–17.
167. For an analysis of the political context of medical care organization, see Vicente Navarro, *Medicine Under Capitalism* (New York: Prodist, 1976) and *idem, Crisis, Health, and Medicine: A Social Critique* (New York: Tavistock Publications, 1986).
168. Institute of Medicine, *op. cit.* (note 163), 130.

7

Public Health in Canada

Jay Cassel

Public health measures in Canada were only slowly organized. This state of affairs was due to a number of factors, including the political climate, social and economic conditions, and the limitations of medicine. It was also because the concept of itself only grew slowly into a coherent form. Though we now recognize that communities have for centuries responded to collective health problems, the term 'public health' is relatively recent, as is its present definition and the particular way of thinking associated with it. The key period of development in Canada is about 1880–1920. What emerged was in many senses a new way of doing things and, however obvious it may seem to us today, it was anything but a foregone conclusion at the time. Moreover, the particular concepts with which Canadians operated, and the cultural characteristics of the society, gave to health measures a distinct form, and led to emphasis being skewed away from some issues and towards others. More attention was focused on curative medicine and on assuring access to care for the individual than was devoted to factors influencing the health of individuals and communities.

Accounts of the history of public health in Canada are distinctly uneven. The concept and definition of 'public health' assumed a fixed form at the beginning of the twentieth century, a rather narrow definition – heavily influenced in the English-speaking world by the British concept. The accounts currently available are often evidently influenced by the authors' acceptance of the classic definition – most authors write from within the paradigm and offer very conventional narratives. These may reflect Canadian conditions or they may indicate the degree to which historians themselves have internalized the public health paradigm: instead of looking at the way the subject was defined, they have accepted the definition. Being a colony, and then a junior partner in a powerful empire, Canada was strongly influenced by the metropolitan society; it is not surprising that it would adopt British models. Uneven coverage of the country is also a problem. There is considerable geographic and social variation across Canada – many provinces are as large as whole countries elsewhere – but not all regions have been as thoroughly studied. Nor have all topics been the subject of diligent historical research. A marked tendency toward institutional studies has the effect of beginning the story when permanent structures are in place. One has to turn to others, chiefly urban historians, to broaden the discussion to consider, for example, the role of civil engineers.

The history of public health in Canada must be understood in the context of the intellectual paradigm that most heavily influenced Western thinking about health and disease for much of the nineteenth and twentieth centuries. The medical model considers the human body as a set of parts and functions analagous to a machine, beyond that it conceives of the body as a series of chemical reactions. Any breakdowns are due to either the failure of a part or the interference of some agent. Attention, therefore, focuses on devising a repair system aimed at rectifying individual breakages or problems. From this line of reasoning emerged the idea, or hope, that any breakdown might be treated or prevented by a specific technology. As a corollary to this, attention was focused on the individual involved, which was in keeping with the general cultural pattern of the Victorian era. The medical model spread from the profession to the public, and its acceptance was steadily increased by a succession of discoveries until by the mid-twentieth century the idea was verging on certainty. With that came an almost unshakable confidence in medical science. Preservation, restoration and improvement of health came to be seen as largely, if not exclusively, dependent on the development and employment of medical techniques. The medical paradigm became institutionalized; it shaped health care delivery and was reinforced by the way care was provided. The very success of scientific medicine, however, contributed to a determination in the public to have access to it. Some doctors and others in society began to speak of assuring everyone access to the best health care possible. People, therefore, began to turn their attention to systems of health insurance – still aimed at providing for the event of a breakdown in health.

Such reasoning became a rate-determining factor in the evolution of a collective response to health problems confronting people as a group. More attention was placed on treatment than on prevention.

However, there were problems that obviously affected the community as a whole. These usually drew attention to themselves when a disease spread, often rapidly, to many people, hence the prominence of epidemics in the early history of 'modern' public health. Such crises prompted a recognition that collective action was needed and that the activity of individuals and groups might have to be constrained for the collective good. This appealed to another feature of Victorian politics: an inclination to reason along utilitarian lines. Crises also led some observers to recognize that health was affected by more than just biological causes, notably lifestyle (though they would not have used that term), social conditions and, particularly, economic structures, which affected access to essential resources such as food, clothing and shelter. The focus on essential resources had radical implications, and Canadians trod gingerly around it for decades.

Early Action, 1800–1880

British North America comprised several colonies and territories strung along a rugged coast and spreading over a vast, often harsh interior. At the time of Confederation, the start of an independent country in 1867, there was only a limited amount of public health legislation in any of the colonies, either the four that originally joined or those which came in the following decade.[1] The colonies passed what amounted to their first substantial public health legislation in reaction to the cholera epidemic of 1832. Most created a Board of Health to supervise special measures against the disease, and authorized local governments to appoint boards of health and assume certain powers in their efforts to cope with the crisis. The boards, however, were temporary, ceasing to exist once the epidemic was over; there was no standing body of disease-control legislation. In 1849, again in response to cholera, the united colony of Canada (present-day Quebec and Ontario) created a board of health which issued regulations from time to time that served as general guidelines for local boards of health. But all the boards and their regulations only came into operation during an epidemic. Legislation in various colonies during the 1850s and 1860s provided for the appointment of a board or medical officer of health during any serious epidemic. The general terms of this legislation allowed local boards to adopt a range of measures at the discretion of local doctors and officials.

Until the 1880s, responsibility for what today falls under the purview of 'public health' was largely left to the municipalities. Towns and cities made as many by-laws and regulations as they deemed necessary. The most extensive measures were adopted by the major centres, which were also the principal ports – Halifax, Nova Scotia and St John, New Brunswick, on the Atlantic coast, Quebec and Montreal on the St Lawrence River, and the new, rapidly growing cities on the Great Lakes such as Toronto and Hamilton.

There were two broad types of legislation: regulation of the everyday activity of inhabitants, and emergency powers to fend off serious threats. These, in a limited sense, are the roots of 'modern' public health measures. The first was intended to control nuisances and assure a minimum standard in living conditions. This legislation touched on basic concerns such as water supply (not water quality for the most part but actual supply, such as the creation of waterworks in Montreal in 1801), waste disposal, animal control, traffic, building standards, the slaughter of animals, and the condition, storage and sale of food (e.g. at markets). Most of these by-laws and regulations remained on the books until superseded by later legislation, but the early measures were limited in scope and lightly enforced. Later historians have been tempted to see in these the roots of public health, but much of this legislation was not so much concerned with health *per se* as with facilitating activities in places of concentrated population, smoothing co-existence. The second type of legislation comprised emergency measures adopted in response to an epidemic, notably recurring cholera outbreaks between 1832 and 1866, and other diseases, especially smallpox, diphtheria and typhoid. The cause of most diseases was not established at the time and there were frequent debates between contagionists (those arguing that something passed from person to person), environmentalists (arguing that there was something in the immediate surroundings, particularly the atmosphere) and constitutionalists (arguing that the individual's 'constitution' or personal make-up was in some way deficient or disposed to a particular disorder). Cholera in particular was baffling, following no known pattern of contagion, so any plan to control its spread was inevitably challenged. The measures most readily adopted were those that in some way might persuade a majority comprising people of different views. Most, therefore, were aimed at cleaning up surroundings: removal of waste, washing and fumigation. Governments also relied on quarantine, the classic device for keeping diseases from entering a community or trying to contain their spread when individuals fell sick, but in such a vast territory, quarantine was inevitably a very leaky sieve. Some attempts were made to isolate the sick but this measure met with resistence and evasion. As long as the cause of diseases was disputed, many measures did not have strong support among doctors, politicians or the public. The exception to the rule was smallpox, against which authorities knew they could use Jenner's vaccine (until the early nineteenth century the earlier procedure of inoculation was used by a few). This, however was done only in a fitful way. There were a few instances of compulsory vaccination for people facing an outbreak, but the provisions were not readily complied with. People did not understand why the vaccine worked and the idea of having animal matter introduced into their bodies repelled some.

The political, economic and social life of Canadian cities during much of the nineteenth century was dominated by a growth-conscious commercial élite which did not think in terms of collective social welfare.[2] They could, when it suited them, adhere to a *laissez-faire* policy on many issues. In general there was a reluctance to raise taxation, so local governments were troubled by a shortage of money. As a rule, municipalities were preoccupied with 'essential services' (roads, rail lines, water and, later, electricity). Early regulations with a 'public health' component were an extrapolation of attention to economic activity and essential services. This fitted into the Canadian preoccupation with development. The tendency to avoid doing something explicit about health was only broken by a spectacular indication of the need for action – epidemics. Permanent health boards, if the idea was actually floated, were considered costly and unnecessary. Despite recent revisionist history in other countries, the pattern for Canada is quite obvious: action was often in response to a disaster. Unlike the United States, Pietism and philanthropic traditions do not seem to have played a significant role in the early development of Canadian public health programmes.

Native Peoples

The greatest health disaster in nineteenth-century Canada befell its native peoples.[3] Isolated from the disease pools of Europe and Asia for millenia, they had little or no resistence to diseases brought into their midst by Europeans. Pandemics spread westwards and northwards as whites penetrated the continent. Disease ran deep into the interior, carried along the fur trade routes. Smallpox was most devastating, but tremendous damage was also done by measles, influenza and tuberculosis, and probably others such as diphtheria and typhoid. Repeated devastations might have shaken peoples' faith in their healers, but an even greater challenge came from some of the newcomers who sought to change the native health care system.

The efforts of colonial authorities to Westernize the native people extended to changing economic activities, religious beliefs and medical practice.[4] Treaties signed in the 1870s and later with Indians on the

Prairies included a clause assuring Indians the provision of a 'medicine chest'. This would become the basis of Indian claims to provision of health care by the federal government. The organization of a new health care system was fitful. European Canadians wanted the Indians to be assimilated or disappear. The settlement of the interior coincided with the rise of Social Darwinism, and the principle of survival of the fittest seemed to be working out in all its various ways in the new Dominion. Rather belatedly, officials sent in their own healers. This created two problems: a system of dependence on outside help, and a position of subordination to the authority of 'experts'. Health care and public health measures were imposed from outside. It was an alien system in which the people barely participated. Slowly marginalized economically and forced out of their traditional lifestyles, the natives succumbed to diseases of poverty and the inevitable psychological complications of misery.

The health of the native population in general was very different from the European peoples of Canada, a contrast that remains up to the present. The record of public health on reserves has been one of conspicuous failure. Throughout the twentieth century, tuberculosis and other infectious diseases remained endemic in many parts of the country. Alcoholism and suicide were and are common. Only in the 1980s did native healing start to return, largely in a bid to find a better way to cope with psychological problems. Only then did attention shift to the social and economic elements of health.[5]

The Politics of Public Health, 1880–1920

The idea which emerged during the French Revolution, and reappeared in 1848, that health was a right of citizenship and health preservation was an obligation of the state was quite literally foreign to Canadians. Indeed, the British North America Act (BNA Act, 1867) which forms the basis of the Canadian constitution, made no specific provision for public health.[6] Three things taken together can broadly be said to have touched off and sustained public health reform: concern for living conditions and the level of disease in the populace; breakthroughs in medical research; and social reform concepts. At the same time, the political culture of the country and tensions between ethnic groups limited developments.

Canada experienced major changes in the final quarter of the nineteenth century.[7] Montreal, Toronto, Hamilton and other cities rapidly became industrialized. The country as a whole experienced a tremendous increase in population, largely through immigration from a growing number of countries. Between 1881 and 1901 the population of cities in central Canada nearly doubled and new cities grew out of small towns in the west. Cities such as Winnipeg and Vancouver came out of nowhere in the 1880s and 1890s. Between 1901 and 1911 the population of major centres increased at a staggering rate: Montreal went from 267,730 to 490,504; Toronto from 209,892 to 381,833; Winnipeg from 42,340 to 136,039; Vancouver from 27,010 to 100,401. With this growth emerged the classic problems of the era: pollution, crowding, inadequate housing, poor sanitation, inadequate roads and water supply, poor work conditions, increased incidence of disease. The spectacle of these problems, drawn to people's attention by periodic disasters such as fire and disease which touched more than the newly arrived and the poor, triggered a reform movement. Though preoccupied by the need to increase population to fill the 'empty spaces', Canadians emphasized immigration and economic opportunity rather than health promotion and disease treatment. Maternal and infant mortality, worker injury and death remained higher than in most Western countries.

Just as pressing in some circles, as recent historians have shown, were the interests of middle-class citizens. While there was a genuine concern among some for the health of slum dwellers, energetic action only emerged when diseases threatened the community as a whole. Once the contagiousness of diseases which flourished among the poor was clearly established, they were seen as a threat to members of the middle class and, therefore concern about slums increased. Measures were also tied into the efforts of various cities to boost development by attracting new industries and other employers. Parks and housing codes would help 'embellish' a city, preventing unsightly slums which, among other things, could affect the value of property near problem areas, and this would attract 'the better sort' of people.[8] The desire to attract new investors, however, could cut both ways. A certain resistance to stringent regulations developed if they were perceived as discouraging a new venture.

Even in the context of an age of reform, crises continued to serve as triggers for the expansion of public health activities. The national anthem proclaimed Canada to be the 'true north strong and free'. Canadians imagined that their northern climate, with its bracing winter cold, purified the environment. Certainly they did not face the miseries of the tropical world. In fact, the country enjoyed all the features that Victorians thought were conducive to good health: sunshine, space and an abundance of food. People were unprepared for the poor results of medical examinations at recruiting stations during the First World War. Doctors were shocked by the number of deformities and physical deficiencies, as well as the high rates of tuberculosis, sexually transmitted disease, and other preventable diseases. The appalling number of deaths in combat led to increased worries about population. These played on earlier concerns of the Anglo-Canadian élite about 'race suicide' – the declining birth rate among 'the better sort'. Problems encountered during the First World War increased acceptance of the need for an organized response to ill health and a greater willingness to accept government intervention.[9]

Implementation of public health measures and their acceptance by the community often hinged on what physicians could or could not do about disease. The bacteriological revolution of the 1870s and 1880s made a major difference. The timing of legislation in Canada is remarkable: as shall be seen, a great wave of new legislation began around 1884, followed by greater attention to water supplies. Scientific medicine provided a logical theoretical structure and an apparently sound empirical basis for action. With spectacular discoveries and the establishment of the germ theory, 'regular' practitioners were much better able to explain the cause of physical disability and disease, and believed they could identify more effective action against them. Still, confidence was neither overwhelming nor universal because not enough was known about some diseases, disagreements still persisted over what should be done and, for many diseases, there was still no effective treatment. By the 1920s, however, success in some areas, such as smallpox, diphtheria, and typhoid prevention, even the decline in tuberculosis, led to a rapidly increasing confidence in medicine.

As in the United States and other Western countries, there was a strong reform movement in the late nineteenth and early twentieth centuries. Public health activists' reaction to the economic, political and moral consequences of disease was influenced by broader social reform concepts.[10] To simplify a very complex phenomenon, the reform movement can be said to have comprised two different strands. The first was an attempt to reaffirm and secure old social and moral values, usually defined by Anglo-American attitudes and by ideals derived from Christian, particularly Protestant religion. As with the first strand of reform, the second had an underlying desire to restore order and a sense of community to an increasingly complex urban society, but instead of placing the greatest weight on the reassertion of moral values, the second group of reformers set out to reorder the affairs of society. During the Progressive Era, public interest in reform, influenced by American concepts, centred on 'efficiency' and 'order' which played into the case for public health reform. The argument was increasingly presented that ill health was a significant drain on national economic resources, exceeding the cost of public health measures that would prevent sickness. An increasing respect for the 'expert' also worked in favour of public health specialists. This was not limited to physicians who interested themselves in public health matters, however; different professions were entrusted with other aspects of city life – architects and civil engineers were involved in town planning and the construction of public works, for example – but judging from the historical literature, the boundaries between their responsibilities remained quite distinct. The one area of overlap was 'sanitary engineering' which dealt with matters such as water supply and sewerage, and building regulations.

Another influence on the development of public health in Canada was the gradual political organization of the medical profession and the efforts of regular practitioners to secure and promote their position in the community, both for their own benefit and for the public good, as doctors perceived it.[11] In the mid nineteenth century regular physicians formed local organizations, and in 1867 the Canadian Medical Association was established. However, the professionalization of Canadian medicine proceeded slowly. Regulars set out to increase their control over education, licensing and practice. However, there had to be a clear benefit in the eyes of the public before regulars would be accorded major control over medical business. The great successes of scientific medicine certainly accelerated the process. Even then, the last big step only came in 1902 with the passage of the Canada Medical Act (which only came into effect in 1912 because of the need for provincial approval). Public health became another vehicle for extending the profession's standing in the community.

Not surprisingly, the promoters of public health measures were first and foremost physicians and other specialists, many of whom went on to become public health officers.[12] Physicians developed a network with other reform-minded individuals among the clergy, journalists and politicians. A few lay people became prominent in health reform campaigns, notably J. S. Woodsworth, a prominent Methodist minister and socialist politician. Campaigns attracted a limited number of wealthy philanthropists, including some Americans like Rockefeller. They also appealed to a fair number of middle- and upper-class people, particularly women, willing to put a moderate amount of time and money into the cause. No lay people, however, had a major influence on the development of ideas about health reform in this period.

Reticence to support public health measures still was evident in many quarters and had several origins. Public health measures involved governments dictating certain actions defined by certain individuals to all citizens, obliging citizens to take collective action for the health of themselves and others. In both the nineteenth and twentieth centuries there was a noticeable tension between a distinctly Canadian tradition of looking to government to resolve certain problems (particularly in the area of economic development), and a dislike of government involvement in people's lives. Much discussion was coloured by the liberal concept of separate 'public' and 'private' spheres. To many, public health regulation implied government intervention in 'private' activities. Physical well-being was considered a personal matter, and illness was often seen as a personal failing. Many observers noted that morbidity and mortality were associated with certain kinds of environment, especially poor hygiene, overcrowding and poverty, and these were likewise often considered to be in some way signs of personal failing. For the most part, the middle classes became concerned only when there was a danger of disease reaching them. Opposite such views was a sense that the way one person lived affected others. Because of the social nature of so many activities, people felt a need to influence the way individuals thought and acted with regard to many things – eating, waste disposal, sex. This was expressed in the system of taboos, moral imperatives and behavioural norms instilled in children as they grew up. Around the turn of the century there was a growing belief that there had to be an overriding authority to cope with serious problems; one instance of this was a begrudging recognition that individual physicians could not cope with health problems effectively enough on their own. The hesitant nature of public health action in Canada and the halting progression towards state medicine had much to do with tensions between these two positions.

Acceptance of public health measures by physicians was also qualified. Though useful at first to establish the profession's position, doctors were wary of the state. They were suspicious of the creation of a medical bureaucracy with the potential for growing outside-supervision and a corresponding diminution of their autonomy. They were also concerned that collective health measures could affect their economic interests in terms of the work they might get. Medicine preserved its own version of free-enterprise, enshrined in the direct doctor–patient relationship and the freedom of the doctor to practise as he and his peers saw fit. In Canada, the government was often called on to help launch an enterprise, such as canals or railways, or to protect a commercial operation from outside competition; but once things were up and running, Canadians preferred the state to stand back and leave them to run their own affairs. So it was with medicine. Doctors relied heavily on the state to secure a monopoly, the crowning achievement being the Canada Medical Act, but then resented anything that looked like state intervention in their practice. The profession, then, was often torn between doctors who favoured public health initiatives, and those who were suspicious of the effect on medical practice.[13]

The reform process was given a further boost when the Canadian Public Health Association was formed in 1910 by a group of doctors and dentists.[14] It was modelled on the American association, founded in 1872, and there remained close links between the two (Canadians were often members of both). The *Public Health Journal* was also begun in 1910, before its American counterpart, though the CPHA only took it over in 1929. This was not, however, the first attempt to establish an association; several efforts, also by physicians, had been made between 1874 and 1895. French Canadians were more successful, creating the Société d'hygiène de la province de Québec in 1884. The faltering early efforts in English Canada and the limited effect of the Quebecois organization on public health reform in that province indicate that support was not exactly intense. By the time the national organization was in place, commitment was much stronger and legislation far more extensive. The CPHA then became concerned with pressing reform forward and attending to the detailed working out of plans, and extension of professional and public education. Formal organizations such as the CPHA and CMA had the effect of taming the impulses of radicals and modified the extremism of conservatives. The CPHA was generally a mainstream organization which aimed at achieving its broad goals by engineering a consensus. But that meant courting middle-class opinion and the Anglo-Protestant élite. Its proposals were often couched in terms that reinforced their views, and since the Association, in the early years, was largely comprised of English professionals, it was in effect their agent.

In much of Canada, men of English and Scottish descent largely dominated the political and economic world, shaping things as they saw fit. Politicians, doctors, bureaucrats, all largely drawn from British or German stock set out to deal with the problems of immigrants and native-born labourers who, after 1890, often came from different cultures. Perceptions of problems were coloured by the view of one ethnic group by another and one class by another. Generally, infectious diseases were concentrated most heavily in the working classes, often recent immigrants or French Canadians. Tuberculosis was thought to be especially common among immigrants, which touched off nativist prejudices and defensive reactions from immigrants. Deep suspicion born of the way they were treated by the majority could lead people in some communities to resist or simply ignore public health programmes. There were many different points of conflict, ranging from housing inspection to food regulations, to measures against infectious diseases. (This problem persisted right up to the stand-offs between officials and the gay community during the AIDS crisis of the 1980s.) The most abiding Canadian problem, however, was that of 'the two solitudes'. Almost everywhere in medical and public health activities, in associations, journals, planning and regulation, there was some evidence of an English–French split. In Montreal there was a clear division between the large English minority and the French majority, further complicated by a host of immigrants of different nationalities, and the traditional animosity between the English and the Irish. This led to complex politics that jammed action, even frustrating lobbies which often remained rooted in one community with only token representatives from elsewhere. In particular, the French Catholic populace was suspicious and wary of the Protestant Anglophone élite who were most often behind public health initiatives.[15]

Government and Public Health, 1880–1920

The Canada which emerged in the second half of the nineteenth century was more like sandstone than granite, an artificial creation of empire fashioned from disparate colonies, each of which retained important powers in the new federation. The central government, despite the desires of the first Prime Minister, was not that strong, and criss-crossing or overlapping powers led to epic disputes between the federal and provincial governments. The subject of health care was only very vaguely covered in two now-famous sections which set out the powers and responsibilities of the federal and provincial governments. In 1894 the BNA Act was interpreted as giving the majority of the various responsibilities for citizens' health to the provinces.[16]

Beginning with Ontario in 1882–4, each province passed wide-ranging Public Health Acts, setting out the basic administrative framework and gathering the different regulatory functions of the past together with new spheres of authority covering sanitation, inspection and disease control.[17] Ontario was spurred to action by developments in Britain, notably the passing of the Consolidated Public Health Act of 1875 which was the basis for its own legislation. The matter became pressing in 1877 with a serious outbreak of yellow fever in the US. The government was also lobbied by physicians led by William Oldright, a professor of hygiene at the University of Toronto. One after another the provinces established permanent boards of health between 1882 (Ontario) and 1908 (Prince Edward Island). The then independent Dominion of Newfoundland was something of an exception, creating its board in 1929 and passing its first comprehensive Public Health Act in 1931. Provincial boards initially had a modest role, overseeing operations, passing general regulations and accumulating vital statistics, but in the next 25 years they gradually evolved more elaborate bureaucracies with more ambitious programmes (discussed later). Heading operations at each level were officers of health, invariably physicians, often with further training in public health. The Chief Officer of Health presided over the provincial board; most provinces were divided into large districts each with an officer, and then into towns or counties with a local Medical Officer of Health. Below the Chief Officer of Health in the central board was an increasing number of division heads. By 1920 boards usually had divisions responsible for: administration, communicable diseases, laboratories, public health nurses, child welfare, VD, TB, Sanitation (or Sanitary Engineering), statistics/epidemiology and health education. The rising political status of health was reflected by the recasting of the provincial board as a full ministry, beginning with New Brunswick in 1918. Having assumed the bulk of responsibility, the provinces, in turn, continued to lay a large measure of the responsibility for routine operations on local governments until the explosion of centralized bureaucracy in the 1960s and 1970s.[18]

Municipal, county or district health boards (some later renamed health departments) were begun in many places during the 1880s and 1890s.[19] These were often based on British models, particularly London's board, occasionally revised with a glance at arrangements in the United States and elsewhere. Toronto established its first permanent health officer in 1883. From this evolved the present Health Department. The success of health departments was often determined by municipal politics. For example, in Ontario until provincial legislation was changed in 1909, local health officers had to persuade aldermen to provide funding for operations or increases of staff. Divisions grew in number according to the areas of concern. By 1920 larger city boards included statistics, communicable disease control and quarrantine, sanitation, food, laboratories, water, public health nursing, TB, VD, pest control and sanitation. The core of the office was its full-time staff: the MOH, usually with a deputy, both of whom were doctors. Then there were division heads, with qualifications suited to their position. Below them were the largest occupational groups: health inspectors and nurses. In addition some boards employed doctors, dentists and lay people part-time for specific activities. Public health measures relied heavily on teams of public health inspectors to ensure compliance and to identify problems. The positions were occupied by laymen who, until 1935 generally received their training on the job, though many were encouraged to complete British-based certificates. Not before 1950 were inspectors encouraged to pursue university education, a very different state of affairs from the doctors and nurses with whom they worked. Low salaries and limited benefits usually ensured that boards were unable to attract as many as they really needed. Public health nursing began with volunteer organizations active against TB (1905 in Toronto, 1909 in Nova Scotia). Between 1911 (Toronto) and 1929, local boards began to employ public health nurses themselves for a variety of functions and illnesses. Nurses visited homes and schools identifying new cases, trying to ensure that patients complied with treatment, looking for signs of trouble among others, and educating people. The influenza epidemics of 1918/19 revealed the need for better training, prompting special courses in several universities across the country. Public health work was not that attractive and only a small fraction of all nurses chose it. Working conditions, the difficulties of the work itself, lack of interest in many cities and the low esteem in which people working with the poor were held, all discouraged individuals.

In the nineteenth century, the federal government's role in health was restricted to the two responsibilities assigned to it in the BNA Act: screening and quarantine of people arriving from abroad and regulating the production and marketing of food and drugs.[20] Regulation of the preparation, content and sale of food, liquor and drugs began with provisions in the omnibus Inland Revenue Act (revised 1874), supplemented by the Adulteration Acts (1884, 1885), and the Proprietary or Patent Medicines Act (1909), the latter prompted largely by recent controversy over patent medicine in the US. A new systematic approach to regulation is evident in the Food and Drugs Act of 1920 which was substantially influenced by the

American Act of 1906. With time, Canada developed what are now some of the most stringent regulations in the world. The federal government also maintained strict control on narcotics with the passage of the Opium Act in 1908, which was extended to include cocaine and heroin in 1911. It was superseded by the Opium and Narcotic Drug Act of 1920.

A Federal Department of Health was not created until 1919. The idea was that the central government would serve as a coordinating authority. Its measures generally amounted to a standardization of programmes across the country through the device of conditional grants to the provinces. These grants-in-aid, with their string of conditions, went a considerable distance towards dictating the broad form of certain health programmes. No provincial government was likely to turn down a sizeable amount of money, so the federal conditions helped shape local programmes. Health grants also helped establish the Canadian tradition of linking the amount contributed by the federal government to the amount spent by the province on particular programmes, though subsequently adjustments were made to redistribute some wealth in favour of poorer provinces. Constitutionally, this was quite significant, marking the beginning of the federal 'spending invasion' of provincial responsibilities. Not surprisingly, one or more of the provinces often viewed the coordinating efforts of the federal government with suspicion bordering on hostility. Federal activities became an issue at almost every conference touching on constitutional reform. Ottawa remained determined to provide a central planning role, using its larger tax resources to encourage recalcitrant provinces to accept the general plan worked out in inter-governmental meetings. The federal role remained a peculiar one: indirect and largely at one remove from most public health activity. This was reflected in the department's small staff and in its divisions: food and drugs, narcotic drugs, proprietary and patent medicines, quarantine and immigration, child welfare, venereal disease, scientific research and publications. In addition, Ottawa maintained a central epidemiological office to monitor conditions across the country and correlate the data with those from other countries.[21]

The Evolution of Public Health Measures I: 1880s–1920s

Despite the creation of an institutional framework, action varied considerably between cities and between provinces in the later nineteenth and early twentieth centuries. Toronto produced the most extensive public health programme, and it would retain its preeminent status throughout the twentieth century.[22] Generally, however, action remained quite limited. Canadians were particularly concerned to assure that treatment facilities were in place should they fall ill. The argument that it was better to spend hundreds on prevention than thousands on cure had only a limited impact. In many areas, action was still often prompted by crises, such as improvement of water supply after the 1911–12 typhoid epidemics in Ottawa.[23] Political forces and economic resources affected measures. But while some poor regions predictably had to make do with less, others like New Brunswick, and later Saskatchewan, attempted to compensate by organizing thoroughgoing, even radical, programmes to assure the best health measures possible given their limited resources.[24] Wealth, however, was not necessarily a decisive factor. Montreal was for a long time the most important city economically, and yet it had a poor health record, underlined by one of the worst levels of infant mortality in the developed world.[25]

General patterns appear in the history of public health problems from the 1880s to the 1920s, persisting in some ways up to the present. Canadian measures followed the classic British public health model with attention to sanitation, food inspection, water supply, waste disposal, epidemiology and communicable disease control. Action most often began as a local response, followed by provincial measures, though provincial governments might then have to press tardy local governments. Rarely did the federal government initiate action, though it attempted to coordinate measures and bring along stragglers through financial incentives. Many Public Health Acts were at first quite loose in defining what was covered and what local health officers could do. During the first two decades of the twentieth century, therefore, there was a second wave of legislation and regulation, tightening up wording, elaborating measures, and filling in holes. The flood of legislation, the political commitment and eventually the money, diminished around the mid-1920s.[26]

A great amount of local authorities' attention, was directed at sanitation and living and working conditions.[27] The earliest measures generally related to waste disposal, nuisances and pest control. From the 1890s onward there were increasingly extensive provisions for building inspection. Housing Acts aimed at eliminating unsafe, ill-lit, poorly ventilated, and overcrowded buildings but they did not address the problem of an inadequate supply of inexpensive housing. The one could be clearly seen as a health problem while the other could be separated off as an economic matter best left to the working of the market. In fact, building regulations exacerbated the housing problem by discouraging tenement construction and boarding house conversion. To the surprise of some, they could also breed resentment of inspectors who intruded in people's homes. Attention to the work-place came a little later; Factory Acts and other legislation regarding occupational health and safety were brought in around the turn of the century in eastern provinces but most were limited in scope. Divisions of Industrial Hygiene appeared in the inter-war years, starting with Ontario (1919).

The food supply was the other major preoccupation of all levels of government. Standards were often set with reference to those elsewhere, particularly in England but also in the United States.[28] Local boards undertook inspection of premises, supervision of production, and testing of samples in everything from abbatoirs and bakeries to restaurants. Similar attention was paid to the milk supply. In the 1890s regulations sought to eliminate contaminants and adulteration. After 1912, in reaction to British research on bovine tuberculosis, pasteurization was made compulsory, first in parts of Ontario and gradually everywhere during the 1920s.

Assuring adequate amounts of good water was another longstanding concern periodically intensified by water-borne epidemics.[29] New regulations from the 1880s onwards touched on plumbing, drainage and sewerage. Filtration was adopted by individual cities and towns in the 1890s and gradually extended across the country. Massive growth helped prompt major construction projects for both water mains and sewerage systems. Not surprisingly, the first divisions of sanitary engineering appeared in provincial boards soon after (Quebec 1908, Ontario 1911). Chlorination was begun as an emergency measure against typhoid in Toronto in 1910, and then Ottawa after its epidemic in 1912. In the light of such experience, and with a nudge from provincial boards of health, many places adopted chlorination between 1915 and 1925. Not all citizens took this in their stride. Some objected to tampering with their water and complained about the taste, prompting more testing and a diligent education campaign in the 1920s.

The rapid expansion of cities and the reform mentality of the turn of the century contributed to a greater attention to town planning.[30] This was influenced by the City Beautiful and Garden City movements of Britain, Europe and the United States, popular since the Chicago Exhibition of 1893. In this field, public health activists added their voices to those leading the plans, both laymen and engineers, influencing planning in part by directing attention to features they thought were conducive to health – parks, adequate space for housing and transportation, and water and sewerage facilities.

The legacy of epidemics ensured a continuing preoccupation with infectious diseases.[31] This, of course also influenced the measures already noted. Strategies to limit the spread of infection initially relied on prompt reporting, isolation of the sick, quarantine and fumigation. These all met with resistence, particularly in the first decade of the new regime, 1885–95. Reporting was opposed both by members of the profession and the public. It was only considered generally satisfactory in the 1910s. This was said to be partly a generational phenomenon: there was better acceptance among the young who grew up in the presence of the measures. Isolation, quarantine and fumigation were all invasive and had a stormier time, especially with distraught family members. Opposition, however, was tempered by a fear of the disease and acceptance increased in face of bacteriological discoveries. Enforcing regulations, given small staff and large distances, remained difficult. With the development of effective treatment, vaccines and toxoids, more attention was focused on treatment or prevention by vaccination. Epidemiology as a basis for public health action was limited before the 1890s and only developed gradually. The rise of bacteriology made the laboratory a central institution, and from the 1900s to the 1920s the provinces embarked on a flurry of laboratory construction. With them came increased reliance on testing, sometimes compulsory, to identify cases early on. Research laboratories working in microbiology and immunology followed soon after with the foundation of what became the Connaught Medical Research Laboratories of the University of Toronto in 1913.

Development of effective treatment and prevention did not automatically produce action. Immunization campaigns were considerable but so were the devastations of diseases such as diphtheria, and smallpox remained a problem for a century after Jenner's vaccine was introduced. The major smallpox epidemic of 1885 helped trigger reforms, but there was another in 1892, and again from 1900–2. This led to piecemeal adoption of compulsory vaccination. In the 1880s and 1890s provincial governments gave local boards authority to order compulsory vaccination in the face of an outbreak and to appropriate land for isolation hospitals. Part of the reason for the gradual approach was cost, but it was also due to opposition which was considerable in some localities. In 1888 the Toronto Anti-Compulsory Vaccination League was established – by a physician. Two decades later, in 1919 there was an alarming spread of the smallpox in Alberta, Ontario and Quebec. Compulsory vaccination touched off strong protests from members of the public, and health officials' arrogant dismissal of objections did nothing to improve their standing with opponents. In the inter-war years, growing respect for medical science reduced resistence, and vaccination programmes were ultimately successful in eliminating the disease from the country.

Diphtheria antitoxin was discovered 1893, and soon after provincial boards began making arrangements to supply it at little or no charge, first to the poor, and then to everyone. Prevention with a toxoid was discovered in 1907. In the 1910s Ontario assisted in providing this to the public as well, an example followed by the other provinces in the 1920s. Mass immunization of children was attempted by cities like Edmonton, Alberta in the 1920s, following the example of New York. Others, like Toronto, continued to rely on antitoxin to control the disease. During and after the First World War municipal and provincial governments, particularly Ontario, provided sera, vaccines and toxoid at cost, or little or no charge to individuals, in a bid to to ensure that everyone received them. On occasion such arrangements prompted opposition from the medical profession which viewed such activities as infringing on their practice. Large-scale immunization of schoolchildren in Ontario cities began in 1927 but was cancelled in 1929 because doctors objected. It only went ahead two years later in the face of further outbreaks. The result was a plunge in incidence; Toronto was one of the only cities in the world to record no deaths from diphtheria in some years during the 1930s.

Tuberculosis and sexually transmitted diseases were the focus of still more ambitious programmes. These were prompted to a considerable extent by statistics indicating that there was a high prevalence of both. TB campaigns were begun at the start of the century by private volunteer organizations such as the Montreal Anti-Tuberculosis Association and the Canadian Tuberculosis Association. In 1911 Ontario gave in to a decade of pressure and made reporting compulsory, a move that immediately prompted protests, but the regulation remained and was soon adopted by other governments. The campaign only got up to speed when government stepped in at the end of the 1910s, and it remained a public–private venture. Sanitoria had begun to appear at the turn of the century, and government-funded institutions appeared in the 1910s and 1920s. With a glance at European and American examples, Canadians devised case-finding and case-supervision proceedures. Many health departments offered free examinations and tuberculin tests, and operated travelling X-ray clinics in the 1920s. Eliminating the disease by treating those found to be infected and controlling contact between the infected and the general populace were expected to lead to a rapid reduction of the prevalence of these infections. This is evident in the statistics which showed a steep decline in incidence during the inter-war period.[32]

The other major preoccupation of the inter-war period was venereal disease.[33] Major programmes were established at the local, provincial and federal levels. The first VD Act was devised by Ontario (1918), closely modelled on the legislation in Western Australia (1915). This, in turn, influenced the legislation in other provinces. Governments established special VD clinics offering diagnosis and treatment free of charge, and embarked on ambitious education campaigns. The results, however, were not as gratifying as they were with TB: the incidence of infection did not show any substantial change. This had much to do with the social response to these diseases and the limitations in diagnosis, treatment and actual medical facilities.

Substance abuse also attracted attention because of its effect on the health of the individual and his or her dependents, as well as on public order.[34] When health reformers turned their attention to alcohol and narcotics they gained the support of temperance and prohibition groups and, in particular women. Federal restrictions on opiates, hashish and related drugs remained stringent; indeed sale and use was either forbidden or closely controlled. Toleration of alcohol varied. Beginning in the mid nineteenth century, the federal, and some provincial governments, passed temperance laws aimed at limiting consumption. Total prohibition came during the First World War but was abandoned by one province after another beginning in 1923. Thereafter provincial governments tried to limit consumption of alcohol by regulating sales.

In the early twentieth century, efforts also began to focus on mothers and young children.[35] Biological determinism influenced theories of social development and, by extension, public policy. From the later nineteenth century well into the twentieth century there was an almost obsessive concern among people of British descent over the declining birth rate and the perception that it was 'the better sort' whose numbers were dropping. This prompted a rising concern with maternal and infant mortality. Child Welfare or Child Hygiene divisions were created by provincial and some local boards and departments of health between 1914 and 1929. Well-Baby Clinics, inspired in part by the example of New Zealand, emerged in English Canada during the 1920s. Such clinics, however, met with resistance from doctors. They did not object to being relieved caring for the poor but they resented losing paying patients. The programmes were further complicated by ethnic, linguistic and religious differences. The fixation with 'the quality of the race' also led some provinces to embark on the sterilization of the 'mentally deficient'. In another direction, medical inspection of schoolchildren began in Hamilton and Montreal in 1907, and Toronto in 1910, some ten years after American cities adopted the measure. Again, the measure was opposed by some doctors who resented the lost work and what they thought was easy pay for those who worked in schools. Still, medical examination of schoolchildren became a major operation in many places during the inter-war years. When this revealed that a substantial number of children were malnourished, nutrition classes and school milk programmes were begun.

Attention extended beyond regulation and treatment to health education.[36] Most of the key subjects – motherhood, sex, sexually transmitted disease, even some aspects of personal hygiene – were fraught with controversy since they were loaded with personal and moral considerations. With the exception of personal hygiene, initiatives were therefore limited until after the First World War, when more attention was paid to motherhood, tuberculosis and STD. Pamphlets were produced by various governments from the 1920s onwards, but a significant amount of the material was American or British in origin. Some training in motherhood was attempted, mostly by nurses, who also attended to children in nurseries and schools. At the same time, paediatricians and child psychologists were gaining public recognition and their ideas were extended by increasing coverage in the press.

Concern about madness during the nineteenth century was guaranteed to prompt attention to mental health in the years following.[37] Attention concentrated on treatment or care of the insane and mentally ill until after the Great War. Then in 1918 the National Committee for Mental Hygiene was established (later renamed the Canadian Mental Health Association). It was followed soon after by Divisions of Mental Hygiene in the federal department and in the Alberta board of health. Efforts remained concentrated on children until after the Second World War. The objective was to prevent various conditions leading to mental retardation, but with limited understanding of the causes and limited capacity to prevent or treat conditions, it was not possible to make much headway. Beyond that, efforts were made to identify cases early on and to provide special education for the retarded. Aside from simple observation, the chief instrument was the intelligence test, first employed in Toronto in 1917.

The Evolution of Public Health Measures II: 1930s–1960s

The evolution of public health in Canada between the 1930s and the 1960s was affected by both economic conditions and medical knowledge and technology. The Depression of 1929–39 did not prompt new measures in most areas of public health. The country experienced the severe distress that befell resource-based exporting economies at the time. Provinces generally cut back to bare essentials.[38] Concerns that poverty would lead to inadequate care for people with TB or STD prompted governments to maintain funding of diagnosis and treatment, and even expand their role in TB care. The next burst of activity was touched off during the Second World War, particularly with the introduction of penicillin which seemed to promise the eradication of many diseases including syphilis, gonorrhoea and tuberculosis. Curative medicine took centre stage in the later 1940s and 1950s – that was where striking progress was being made. 'Damage control' and 'repair' rather than prevention continued to be the principal concern of Canadians in general. There was a much greater acceptance of the need to pour resources into facilities to treat the ill and the injured than there was support for preventive measures, many of which were perceived as restricting freedom of the individual or commerce. Given this outlook, it is not surprising that attention focused on government assistance in the construction of hospitals and other institutions.[39] The federal government made many planning and construction grants to the provinces between 1947 and 1970. Canada built up an elaborate, often excellent system of care for the sick. Institutions like the Toronto Hospital for Sick Children, Toronto General Hospital and Montreal Neurological Institute developed international reputations. Every city and many towns wanted their own facilities. Tremendous political pressure developed around the institutions. This further skewed health policy, including commitment to other public health measures.

Much of the public health work from the 1940s through the 1960s was an elaboration of the arrangements made earlier.[40] Provincial and local health departments developed larger and increasingly complex bureaucratic structures. Regulations and inspection proceedures were elaborated. Prevention of disease continued along well-established lines. Education campaigns encouraged periodic check-ups by both doctors and dentists. Other programmes were organized for groups such as food handlers. Immunization programmes persisted, reaching extensive proportions in the 1950s and 1960s.[41] This was facilitated by increased public acceptance and by technical improvements such as the production of combined vaccines. Canadian doctors remained wary of 'state medicine' and campaigns relied alternately on government staff and general practitioners. BCG was used to prevent tuberculosis in some juridsictions in the 1940s and 1950s but only limitedly. Polio was undoubtedly the most alarming 'new' epidemic. There were outbreaks in parts of Canada in 1930, 1934 and most notably in 1937 and 1953/4. Canadians were involved in the initial testing of the Salk vaccine, and then in the first immunization drive between 1955 and 1957. Fluoridation of water to prevent tooth decay prompted considerable debate. Again, tampering with the water supply and the use of poisonous compounds or 'mass medication', was seen by some as an infringement of individual freedoms. Despite support from the CPHA and many dental associations in the 1950s, the programme was only slowly adopted in the 1960s in many, though not all, parts of the country.[42]

Attention to STD wavered.[43] A tremendous amount of money and effort was expended on STD in the 1940s and early 1950s in reaction to increased infection in the armed forces and then in response to the promise of penicillin. Once incidence dropped to relatively low levels in the mid-1950s, budgets were cut back. In the later 1960s incidence began to rise, veering sharply upward in the 1970s and triggering a new STD campaign. Education regarding both sex and sexually transmitted disease was inadequate until the 1970s and remained insufficient until the mid-1980s when the AIDS crisis very slowly persuaded the circumspect Canadian public to accept candid discussion among young people.

Mothers and young children remained a priority.[44] Canadians prided themselves on the decline in both maternal and infant mortality in many parts of the country during the 1940s, although there had been a marked decline ever since 1918. Prenatal classes, pioneered in the 1930s, were extended in later decades. Providing advice about birth control and selling contraceptives, however, were illegal until 1969. The economic distress of the 1930s gave birth control a certain respectability but did not prevent activists from facing controversial trials. A few clinics and mail-order advice companies were operated by private citizens, while health departments coyly relied on nurses visiting the poor at home. The process of change really began with the formation of organizations like Planned Parenthood Association of Toronto in 1961 and the feminist challenge to the patriarchal legal system in the 1960s. Family planning clinics and other services were begun by local health departments or private groups from 1969 onwards, though departments continued to rely heavily on family physicians. Pre-school clinics remained controversial with physicians through the 1930s and 1940s. Child Health Centres reached their peak during the baby boom in 1950s then declined – the effect of the 'baby bust', changing attitudes, and changing work patterns of women. Medical inspections of schoolchildren were extensively undertaken. In addition, dental programmes for schoolchildren began in some jurisdictions in the 1930s and were extended after the Second World War. Unlike doctors before them, dentists generally did not object to school programmes. The Great Depression had raised concerns about nutrition and led to relief efforts in schools. Emphasis, however, generally remained on education, telling children what they should be eating, rather than grappling with the enormous challenge of the socio-economic order that created nutritional problems.

Growing public awareness of other problems led to expansion in new directions after the Second World War. Concern about air pollution was triggered by famous 'fogs' in London and elsewhere in the 1940s. New by-laws in Toronto (1949) and Hamilton (1950) stiffened regulations against smoke.[45] During the 1960s and 1970s many cities paid increasing attention to pollution of air, water and soil, slowly increase the stringency of their regulations and testing programmes. The persistent problem of alcoholism prompted the foundation of the Addiction Research Foundation in Toronto in 1948. The spectacular outburst of 'youth culture' in the 1960s and increasing awareness of problems with alcohol and drug abuse led to an intensification of law enforcement and the development of education and addiction programmes in the later 1960s and 1970s.[46]

Attention to mental health increased markedly after the Second World War, coinciding with the increased acceptance of psychiatry in Canadian society.[47] During the 1930s the provincial departments of health in Saskatchewan, Manitoba and Quebec had joined Alberta in establishing Mental Health divisions, and the other provinces followed suit in the 1940s. More attention was finally devoted to adults. Initially attention concentrated on severe disorders and emergency cases unable to afford medical care, but slowly more efforts were made to improve psychiatric clinics which remained in short supply. Consultation and testing were expanded in the 1940s and 1950s, followed in the next decade by counselling, supportive therapy and the employment of mental health nurses. In the 1960s efforts were also made to get people out of institutions, which led to a rise in suicides. This highlighted the need for continued counselling and attention to problems such as retraining and housing. Concerns about mental retardation persisted. In the 1960s and 1970s the development of a better understanding of causes, and tests for some of the associated disorders, led to a redoubling of efforts to identify possible cases very early with the hope of preventing damage leading to retardation.

Canada also extended its concern about health to the international forum. George Brock Chisholm, a psychiatrist who came into public health during military service in the 1940s, became heavily involved in the establishment of the World Health Organization. He went on to serve as its first Director General from 1948 to 1953. The constitution of WHO, though devised by a committee, bears his stamp, particularly in the definition of health as 'a state of complete physical, mental and social well-being, and not merely the absence of disease or infirmity'. Canada has continued to play a significant role in WHO from then to the present with the aim of extending to other parts of the world the prospect of health which had gradually become a significant feature of its own policy.[48]

The Cost of Health, and Medical Insurance

Eliminating disease and ill health from the community became intimately bound up with the economics of health care. While the two are not synonymous, public health and health insurance became inseparable as policy issues.[49] Yet the paradigm of the medical model continued to dominate thought, prompting people to concentrate on disease and injury rather than contend with social and economic conditions. Much less was spent on preventive medicine and health promotion than was spent on curative facilities. Moreover, Canadians were most willing to support preventive measures if they were in the form of medical technology – vaccines, sanitizing proceedures, water treatment. They were reluctant to countenance extensive regulation, they were not particularly interested in education, especially if it broached sensitive topics, and they were not prepared to look very closely at their lifestyle or such politically-loaded issues as access to essential resources (food, clothing, shelter). Assuring everyone roughly equal access to medical care appeared to be the most effective way of dealing with a wide range of problems, and so attention turned to health insurance.

Early insurance arrangements in Canada operated on a 'private' basis; shifting this to the public sphere was fraught with controversy. Private insurance grew in the later nineteenth century among the urban middle class. It worked well for those it served, but it did not cover a significant part of the population. Companies generally did not cover the poor, or high risk cases, nor, in practice, many ethnic minorities. Ideas about larger state programmes were influenced by German and British reforms, but the system introduced under Bismarck was rejected in the 1900s by Canadian physicians as too extreme, even before it was brought to the attention of politicians. Government health insurance was first discussed publicly during the First World War but the proposal was again abandoned. The Depression reactivated the issue but new measures encountered intense opposition from physicians. Efforts to provide a system of relief in Manitoba led to Canada's first doctors' strike in which physicians withdrew many services from July 1933 to February 1934. British Columbia attempted to implement government health insurance in 1936 but backed down after the legislation was passed. The same thing occurred in neighbouring Alberta. During the Second World War, the British *Beveridge Report* (1942) inspired a similar Canadian document, the *Marsh Report* (1943). The federal government then drafted a national health insurance plan, which gained further impetus at the end of the war when Britain introduced its National Health Service. But the scheme was frustrated by objections from provincial governments and medical associations. Although it had favoured an insurance scheme during the Depression, the Canadian Medical Association was much less interested when prosperity returned and from 1949 onwards it was explicitly opposed to universal coverage by the state. So instead Canadians relied on the private system, which was expanded in the 1930s and 1940s by companies formed by doctors themselves.

In this atmosphere, governments turned their attention instead to assisting in assuring effective treatment for the sick. They set out to improve health care by contributing to the construction of the most expensive element: hospitals. They also moved to help cover the most expensive part of treatent: hospitalization. State insurance was adopted by the province of Saskatchewan in 1947 and it was soon followed by three others. The federal government passed the National Hospital and Diagnostic Services Act in 1957, providing 50 per cent federal cost-sharing for hospital services. This prompted the remaining provinces to introduce hospital insurance by 1961.

Government health insurance came into being during the 1960s. In 1962 Saskatchewan became the first province to establish full health insurance and the next year it was followed by British Columbia and Alberta. The federal government appointed a royal commission to study the matter, and from this came the *Hall Report* (1964), which favoured universal health insurance. The government then passed the Medical Care Act establishing the Medicare system, which was supposed to begin in 1967, a symbolic move in the year of Canada's centennial (in fact, it only slowly became operational across the country). From this point on, anyone needing almost any kind of care would have access to it (in theory at least), including routine check-ups, medical tests and preventive procedures. Medicare would operate on the basis of cost-sharing grants; the federal government would assist provinces, on condition that they meet certain stipulations, but implementation of the programmes would take place at the provincial level.

These moves met with resistence from the medical profession. In 1962 government insurance prompted a doctors' strike in Saskatchewan. The reorganization of the health care system and introduction of state insurance touched off a doctors' strike in Quebec in 1971. In both, the majority of the public perceived the medical profession as being concerned above all with status and income, and since this was one of the wealthiest groups on a per capita basis in the country, sympathy was low. In addition, the public was determined to have a system that assured them access to the best possible health care. Scientific medicine succeeded almost too well, convincing people that what it offered was indispensable. Not surprisingly, each strike failed.

During the 1970s Canadians were faced with the nightmare of rapidly escalating costs. Expenditure rose from 6 per cent of gross national product at the time state health insurance was introduced, to 7.4 per cent in 1977, and almost 9 per cent in 1990. This was not a uniquely Canadian problem. In the United States, with its 'free enterprise' system, which covered the population much less thoroughly, the figure stood at 11.5 per cent in 1990. Some alleged that the new system was too bureaucratic but in Canada administrative costs are 2.5 per cent of the total while in the US they are 10 per cent.[50] Still, in Canada, health care became one of the largest items in federal and provincial budgets. We now know that the demand for health care is infinite, and that this is as likely to be led by producers as by consumers. Developments in medicine during the second half of the twentieth century have been both dramatic and expensive: new medicines, new technology, more tests, combined with a willingness to use them, led to spiralling costs. Yesterday's high technology became today's routine procedure. Added to this was a period of rapid inflation and escalating pay raises for hospital staff. At the same time, increased demand, rising expectations, and the needs of an ageing population propelled expenditure upwards. The hope had been that universal coverage would make it easier to eliminate disease, and by degrees expenditure on health care would fall. Such was not the case.

As costs continued to mount and the state's fiscal capacity was endangered, public authorities inevitably began to question the effectiveness of treatment strategies.[51] State intervention expanded beyond bureaucratic rationalization of health care – as doctors had feared. Cost overruns also became a source of disputes between the federal and provincial governments, particularly as the federal government grew more reluctant to commit further amounts to an expensive operation, ducking behind the BNA Act which made health largely a provincial responsibility. Between 1977 and 1991 the federal government several times altered the cost-sharing formula, effectively reducing its portion of the total expenditure. Some provinces allowed physicians to 'opt out' of Medicare. Patients would receive payment from the government plan, then pay the doctor, who might charge more than the plan's rate. This was seen as jeopardizing the principle of universal access, and extra-billing was banned, beginning with British Columbia in 1981. Federal legislation in 1984 tried to force all provinces to conform. When Ontario reluctantly passed legislation in 1986 it was faced with a strike which, like earlier ones, failed. Nonetheless, curative medicine was cripplingly expensive.

Revising Public Health, 1970s–1990s

Mounting problems with the conventional medical system drove Canadians to look seriously at the broader problems affecting the health of the population and from this, more wide-ranging initiatives emerged. As earlier activists had predicted, public health would become a paying proposition. Officials began to stress the need to reduce use of the facilities by preventing illness, and they were dissatisfied by programmes that sought to prevent further illness largely by treating those who were ill. In 1974 Marc Lalonde, then federal Minister of Health and Welfare, brought out *A New Perspective on Health for Canadians.* This marked a significant shift in government priorities away from treatment facilities and towards prevention and the reduction of illness associated with lifestyle and environmental factors.[52] More attention turned to risk factors, including the physical and social environment, food, drink, smoking, work and psychological problems.

New health promotion campaigns were begun in the later 1970s and 1980s.[53] Campaigns were launched to encourage more attention to fitness and nutrition. Efforts to reduce smoking were begun by CPHA in 1960 and the federal government in 1964 but they produced limited results in the era of 'sex 'n drugs 'n rock 'n roll'. A second campaign was begun in the late 1970s. This was more coercive, employing aggressive anti-smoking notices, bans on advertising and prohibition of smoking in many public spaces. Measures were implemented to reduce traffic accidents and alcohol abuse. More attention was paid to occupational safety and health. Rising concern among the public about ecological damage, which found its most radical expression in the Greenpeace organization, slowly persuaded governments to be more stringent in pollution control. In the 1980s accidents at Three Mile Island near the US–Canada border, and at Chernobyl in the USSR made many Canadians increasingly wary of the use of nuclear energy. There was also greater criticism of the widespread use of additives in food and drink. Yet only after an alarming rise in STD and a protracted debate did Canadians embark on programmes to encourage safer sexual practices. The initial response to AIDS, from 1981 to 1988 was excessively guarded and as a result education campaigns remained weak until the problem clearly required bold action.[54]

These initiatives met with a guarded reaction. Many, particularly those relating to lifestyle, required behavioural modification which people were not very willing to countenance. Others, particularly environmental regulations, impinged on business and required companies to spend money on what appeared to be non-revenue-generating activities. Closer economic ties with the United States, where resistance to such action is often higher, will probably limit change in this direction. Budgets for public health programmes remained generally small compared to funds devoted to care for the ill. Much has been left to local officials. The combined effect was evident in the oddly uncoordinated beginning of campaigns against smoking, and the poor beginning to the AIDS campaign. AIDS exposed a number of problems in public health – tensions between different levels of government, between strategies for prevention and treatment, the problems of cost and moral expectations.

The shift to a new approach to health care has been most dramatic in the province of Quebec which embarked on a reorganization of its entire health care system during the late 1960s and early 1970s.[55] The Catholic Church had played a major role in medical care since the time of New France (1608–1760). In a breathtaking arrangement typical of the Quiet Revolution (a period of extensive social and political change in the 1960s), the Castonguay–Nepveu Commission gained nearly complete control over health reform. Elsewhere in Canada an élite group never received such legitimacy or such control over governmental activity in a particular sector. The commission's reforms were more radical than anything attempted elsewhere in Canada. It favoured 'social medicine': an open social model in place of the traditional closed medical model. To achieve this, the commission proposed to decentralize services and decision-making, open up participation in the decision process, and equalize the rights and privileges of health workers. In response to its report a *ministère des affaires sociales* (department of social affairs) was created, grouping the old departments of health, family affairs and social welfare. *Départements de santé communautaire* (departments of community health) in 32 Quebec hospitals replaced the public health units a nd municipal health services. Their aim was not just to maintain traditional public health operations but to instil in hospitals, the strongholds of specialized curative medicine, a new community orientation emphasizing prevention. Alongside this were 70 (now 140) centres locaux de services communautaires (local community service centres, or local health centres). Although more democratic in principle, in practice the reforms led to greater centralization; the different levels facilitated handing down commandments from on high regarding everything from physician reimbursement to placement of facilities. This was in part the legacy of top–down reform. The CLSCs were troubled by everything from the location of the buildings to pressures from local politicians and the shuffling of details between departments. Everywhere, officials came up against the stubborn opposition of physicians. Multi-disciplinary programmes proved to be unwieldy and touched off disputes that destroyed all hope of refashioning medical thinking to take into consideration the multi-causal nature of illness. Private practice and the more traditional polyclinics continued to attract most physicians and patients.

The experience in Quebec is illustrative of the larger problems in health care delivery and public health in Canada at present. While recognition of the nature of health and disease is changing and new systems are being devised, it is difficult to get health care workers and the public in general to take in these concepts and respond effectively to them. This, paradoxically, is in part the consequence of the dazzling success of scientific medicine in the twentieth century. There is a tendency to say 'why mess with success?' So it is at the points where current systems are in difficulty that change is pressed for – in the cost of care, and in the elimination of disease – rather than in the way we promote and maintain health. Public health continues to serve several different objectives: reducing the cost of illness to society, assuring the health of individuals, and sustaining or reinforcing the standards of conduct set by the prevailing culture.

Notes

1. R. D. Defries (ed.), *The Development of Public Health in Canada* (Toronto: Canadian Public Health Assiociation, 1940); *idem, The Federal and Provincial Health Services in Canada* (Toronto: CPHA, 1959); J. J. Heagerty, *Four Centuries of Medical History in Canada* (Toronto Macmillan, 1928) Parts 1 and 4; Jacques Bernier, *La médicine au Québec, naissance et évolution d'une profession* (Quebec: Presses de l'université Laval, 1989); Melvin Baker, 'The Development of the Office of a Permanent Medical Health Officer for St John's Newfoundland 1826–1905', *History of Science and Technology of Canada, Bulletin,* 7 (1983); Geoffrey Bilson, *A Darkened House: Cholera in Nineteenth Century Canada* (Toronto: University of Toronto Press, 1980); Kenneth Pryke, 'Poor Relief and Health Care in Halifax, 1827–1849', in W. Mitchinson and J. P. Dickin McGinnis (eds), *Essays in the History of Canadian Medicine* (Toronto: McClelland & Stewart, 1988), 39–61; Barbara Tunis, 'Inoculation for Smallpox in the Province of Quebec, a Reappraisal', in Charles Roland (ed.), *Health Disease and Medicine: Essays in Canadian History* (Toronto: Hannah Institute, 1984), 171–93; D. Baldwin, 'Smallpox Management on PEI, 1820–1940: From Neglect to Fulfilment', *Canadian Bulletin of the History of Medicine,* 2 (1985), 147–82; Barbara Craig, 'Smallpox in Ontario: Public and Professional Perceptions of Disease, 1884–5', *ibid.,* 215–49; *idem,* 'State Medicine in Transition: Battling Smallpox in Ontario 1882–1885', *Ontario History,* 75 (1983), 319–47; Michael Bliss, *Plague: A Story of Smallpox in Montreal* (Toronto: Harper-Collins, 1990).
2. G. A. Stelter and A. F. J. Artibise (eds), *The Canadian City: Essays in Urban History* (Ottawa: Carleton, 1977); Christopher Armstrong and H. V. Nelles, *Monopoly's Moment: The Organization and Regulation of Canadian Utilities, 1830–1930* (Philadelphia: Temple University Press, 1986).
3. *Handbook of North American Indians* (Washington DC: Smithsonian Institute), 6 vols, (1981), 15 (1987); Robert Fortuine 'The Health of the Eskimos, as Portrayed in the Earliest Written Accounts', in S. E. D. Shortt (ed.), *Medicine in Canadian Society. Historical Perspectives* (Montreal: McGill-Queen's University Press, 1980),

19–43; A. J. Ray, 'Diffusion of Diseases in the Western Interior of Canada, 1830–1850', *ibid.*, 45–73.

4. George Graham Cummings, 'Health of the Original Canadians, 1867–1967', *Medical Services Journal*, 23 (1967), 115–66; J. R. Miller, *Skyscrapers Hide the Heavens, A History of Indian-White Relations in Canada* (Toronto: University of Toronto Press, 1989); *Handbook of North American Indians*, 6 vols, 15; Corinne Hodgson, 'The Social and Political Implications of Tuberculosis among Native Canadians', *Canadian Review of Sociology and Anthropology*, 19 (1982), 502–12; T. K. Young, 'The Health of Indians in Northwestern Ontario, a Historical Perspective', in David Coburn *et al.* (eds), *Health and Canadian Society. Sociological Perspectives* (Markham: Fitzhenry & Whiteside, 2nd edn 1987), 109–26; Paul Grescoe, 'A Nation's Disgrace', *ibid.*, 127–40; John O'Neil 'Health Care in a Central Canadian Arctic Community: Continuities and Change', *ibid.*, 141–58; special issue on Native Health, *Canadian Journal of Public Health*, 77 No. 4 (1986).
5. See note 4.
6. Great Britain, *An Act for the Union of Canada, Nova Scotia, and New Brunswick, and the Government Thereof*, 30 & 31 Vict. 1867 C3, s. 91 ss. 6, 11 and 25, and s. 92 ss. 7.
7. Leroy Stone, *Urban Development in Canada* (Ottawa: Dominion Bureau of Statistics, 1968).
8. Paul Bator, 'The Struggle to Raise the Lower Classes: Public Health Reform and the Problem of Poverty in Toronto, 1910–1921', *Journal of Canadian Studies*, 14 (1979); John Weaver, '"Tomorrow's Metropolis" Revisited: A Critical Assessment of Urban Reform in Canada, 1890–1920', in Stelter & Artibise (eds), *op. cit.* (note 2), 393–418.
9. Jay Cassel, *The Secret Plague: Venereal Disease in Canada, 1838–1939* (Toronto: University of Toronto Press, 1987); Paul Bator, 'Saving Lives on the Wholesale Plan: Public Health Reform in the City of Toronto, 1900–1930' (Ph.D Dissertation, University of Toronto, 1979); Janice Dickin-McGinnis, 'From Health to Welfare: Federal Government Policies regarding Standards of Public Health for Canadians, 1919–1945' (Ph.D Dissertation, University of Alberta, 1980); Carl Berger, 'The True North Strong and Free', in J. M. Bumsted (ed.), *Interpreting Canada's Past*, Vol. 2 (Toronto: Oxford University Press Canada, 1986), 157–74.
10. Bator *op. cit.* (note 9), Cassel, *op. cit.* (note 9), chs 5 & 7.
11. Heagerty, *Four Centuries*, ch. XIV; Ronald Hamowy, *Canadian Medicine: A Study in Restricted Entry* (Vancouver: Fraser Institute, 1984); Bernier, *op. cit.* (note 1); Elizabeth McNab, *A Legal History of the Health Professions in Ontario* (Toronto: 1970); R. D. Gidney and W. P. J. Millar, 'The Origins of Organized Medicine in Ontario, 1850–1869', in Roland *op. cit.* (note 1), 65–95; David Naylor, 'The

CMA's First Code of Ethics: Medical Morality or Borrowed Ideology?' *Journal of Canadian Studies,* 17 (1982), 20–32; and 'Rural Protest and Medical Professionalism in Turn-of-the-Century Ontario', *Journal of Canadian Studies,* 21 (1986), 5–20; Colin Howell, 'Reform and the Monopolistic Impulse: The Professionalization of Medicine in the Maritimes', *Acadiensis* (1981), 3–22, and 'Elite Doctors and the Development of Scientific Medicine: The Halifax Medical Establishment and 19th Century Medical Professionalism', in Roland *op. cit.* (note 1), 105–22.

12. George Wherrett, *The Miracle of the Empty Beds: A History of Tuberculosis in Canada* (Toronto: University of Toronto Press, 1977); Gina Feldberg, 'An Antitoxin of Self-Respect: North American Debates over Vaccination against Tuberculosis, 1882–1960' (Ph.D Dissertation, Harvard University, 1989); Katherine McCuaig, '"From Social Reform to Social Service" The Changing Role of Volunteers: The Anti-Tuberculosis Campaign, 1900–1930', *Canadian Historical Review,* 61 (1980), 480–501; Claudine Pierre-Deschênes, Claudine, 'Santé publique et organisation de la profession médicale au Québec 1870–1918', *Revue d'histoire de l'Amérique française,* 35 (1981); Cassel, *op. cit.* (note 9).
13. Heather MacDougall, *Activists and Advocates: Toronto's Health Department, 1883–1983* (Toronto: Dundurn, 1990); Cassel, *op. cit.* (note 9), Pierre-Deschênes, *op. cit.* (note 12).
14. Defries, *Health Services in Canada,* iv–v; CPHA, *Proceedings of Annual Meetings.*
15. Terry Copp, *The Anatomy of Poverty: The Condition of the Working Class in Montreal, 1897–1929* (Toronto: McClelland & Stewart, 1974); Bliss, *op. cit.* (note 1). MacDougall, *op. cit.* (note 13).
16. A. H. Birch, *Federalism, Finance, and Social Legislation in Canada, Australia and the United States* (Oxford: Oxford University Press, 1955), 72–3.
17. Defries, *Public Health In Canada* and *Health Services in Canada; Provincial Statutes and boards of health, Annual Reports*
18. *Provincial Health Reports;* Defries, *Public Health in Canada* and *Health Services in Canada*; Pierre-Deschênes, *op. cit.* (note 12).
19. In addition to note 18, see: A. Groulx, *Le Service de Santé de la Ville de Montréal: Evolution et Organization actuelle* (Montreal: 1954); Michael Farley, Othmar Keel, and Camille Limoges, 'Les commencements de l'administration montréalaise de la santé publique 1865–1885', *HSTC Bulletin,* 6 (1982); MacDougall, *op. cit.* (note 13). Maureen Riddell, *Edmonton Local Board of Health, 1871–1980* (Edmonton: 1980); Monica Green, *Through the Years with Public Health Nursing* (Ottawa: CPHA, 1984).
20. Tom Nesmith, 'The Early Years of Public Health: The Department of Agriculture 1867–1918', *The Archivist,* 12 (1985); L. I. Pugsley, 'The Administration and Development of Federal Statutes on Food and

Drugs in Canada', *Medical Services Journal* (1967), 387–449; G. D. W. Cameron, 'The Department of National Health and Welfare', in Defries (ed.), *Health Services in Canada*, 1–2; R. E. Wodehouse and J. J. Heagerty, 'The Health Section of the Department of Pensions and National Health', in Defries (ed.), *Public Health in Canada*, 143–78; Janice Dickin McGinnis, '"Unclean, Unclean" Canadian Reaction to Lepers and Leprosy', in Roland *op. cit.* (note 1), 250–75.

21. Canada, Department of Health/ Pensions and National Health, *Annual Reports 1919–1939*; Wodehouse and Heagerty, 'National Health Section'; Dickin-McGinnis, *op. cit.* (note 9).
22. MacDougall, *op. cit.* (note 13), especially 29.
23. Sheila Lloyd, 'The Ottawa Typhoid Epidemics of 1911 and 1912', *Urban History Review*, 8 (1979); Chris Warfe, 'The Search for Pure Water in Ottawa 1910–1915', *Urban History Review*, 7 (1979), 90–112.
24. New Brunswick and Saskatchewan, Departments of Health, *Annual Reports*; J. A. Melanson, 'New Brunswick Department of Health and Social Services', in Defries (ed.). *Health Services*, 57–68, F. B. Roth and R. D. Defries, 'Saskatchewan Department of Public Health', *ibid.*, 105–15.
25. Copp, *op. cit.* (note 15), 88–105; Bernier, *op. cit.* (note 1).
26. *Provincial Statutes*; Defries (ed.), *Public Health in Canada*; MacDougall, *op. cit.* (note 13), Riddell, *op. cit.* (note 19), Mary Powell, 'Public Health Litigation in Ontario, 1884–1920', in Roland, *op. cit.* (note 1), 412–35.
27. Eric Tucker, *Administering Danger in the Workplace: The Law and Politics of Occupational Health and Safety Regulation in Ontario, 1850–1914* (Toronto: University of Toronto Press, 1990); Michael Piva, *The Condition of the Working Class in Toronto 1900–1921* (Ottawa: University of Ottawa Press, 1979), ch. 3; Copp, *op. cit.* (note 15); Bernier, *op. cit.* (note 1); MacDougall, *op. cit.* (note 13), 70–85; Riddell, *op. cit.* (note 19); Weaver, *op. cit.* (note 8); Janice Sandormirsky, 'Toronto's Public Health Photography', *Archivaria*, 10 (1980), 145–55.
28. MacDougall, *op. cit.* (note 13), ch. 5; Riddell, *op. cit.* (note 19); Defries, *Public Health in Canada* and *Health Services in Canada*.
29. See note 28.
30. A. F. J. Artibise and G. A. Stelter (eds), *Shaping the Urban Landscape: Aspects of the Canadian City-Building Process* (Ottawa: Carleton, 1982), and *The Canadian City: Essays in Urban and Social History* (Ottawa: Carleton, 1977) and *The Useable Urban Past: Planning and Politics in the Modern Canadian City* (Toronto: Macmillan, 1979); Geoffrey Wall and John Marsh (eds), *Recreational Land Use: Perspectives on Its Evolution in Canada* (Ottawa: Carleton, 1982); Robert McDonald, '"Holy Retreat" or "Practical Breathing Spot?"

Class Perceptions of Vancouver's Stanley Park, 1910–1913', *Canadian Historical Review,* 65 (1984), 127–53.

31. Margaret Andrews, 'Epidemic and Public Health: Influenza in Vancouver, 1918–1919', *BC Studies,* 34 (1977) 21–44; Janice P. Dickin McGinnis, 'The Impact of Epidemic Influenza: Canada, 1918–1919', in Shortt *op. cit.* (note 3), 447–77; Paul Bator, 'The Health Reformers versus the Common Canadian: The Controversy over Compulsory Vaccination against Smallpox in Toronto and Ontario 1910–1921', *Ontario History,* 75 (1983), 348–73; Baldwin, *op. cit.* (note 1); Jane Lewis, 'The Prevention of Diphtheria in Canada and in Britain, 1914–45', *Journal of Social History,* 20 (1986), 163–76; MacDougall, *op. cit.* (note 13), chs 6 & 7; Riddell, *op. cit.* (note 19); David Gagan, 'For "Patients of Moderate Means": The Transformation of Ontario's Public General Hospitals, 1880–1950', *Canadian Historical Review,* 70 (1989), 151–79; R. D. Defries, *The First Forty Years, 1914–1955; Connaught Medical Research Laboratories, University of Toronto* (Toronto: University of Toronto Press, 1968); Paul Bator and Andrew Rhodes, *Within Reach of Everyone: A History of the University of Toronto School of Hygiene and the Connaught Laboratories* (Toronto: CPHA, 1990).
32. Wherrett, *op. cit.* (note 12); Feldberg, *op. cit.* (note 12); Katherine McCuaig, 'From Social Reform to Social Service', and 'Tuberculosis: the Changing Concepts of the Disease in Canada, 1900–1950', in Roland *op. cit.* (note 1), 296–307.
33. Cassel, *op. cit.* (note 9).
34. Puglsey, *op. cit.* (note 20); Gerald Hallowell, *Prohibition in Ontario, 1919–1923*; James H. Gray, *Booze: the Impact of Whiskey on the Prairie West* (Toronto: Macmillan, 1972); Robert Campbell, 'Liquor and Liberals: Patronage and Government Control in British Columbia, 1920–1928', *BC Studies,* (1988), 30–53.
35. Neil Sutherland, *Children in English Canadian Society: Framing the Twentieth Century Consensus* (Toronto: UTP, 1976); Angus McLaren, *Masters of Our Own Race: Eugenics in Canada 1885–1940* (Toronto: McClelland & Stewart, 1990); MacDougall, *op. cit.* (note 13), ch. 8; Jo Oppenheimer, 'Childbirth in Ontario: the Transition from Home to Hospital in the Early Twentieth Century', *Ontario History,* 75 (1983), 36–60; Veronica Strong-Boag, 'Intruders in the Nursery: Childcare Professionals Reshape Years One to Five, 1920–1940', in Joy Parr (ed.), *Childhood and Family in Canadian History* (Toronto: 1982); V. Strong-Boag and Kathryn McPherson, 'The Confinement of Women: Childbirth and Hospitalization in Vancouver, 1919–1939', *BC Studies,* 69 (1986), 142–75; Nora Lewis, 'Physical Perfection for Spiritual Welfare: Health Care for the Urban Child, 1900–1939', in P. T. Rooke and R. L. Schnell (eds), *Studies in Childhood History, a Canadian Perspective,* 135–66; Andrée Levesque, 'Mères ou malades? Québecoises de l'entre-deux-guerres

vues par les médecins', *Revue d'histoire de l'Amérique française*, 38 (1984), 23–37.

36. *Provincial Health Reports 1920–1939*; Cassel, *op. cit.* (note 9), chs 6, 7 & 9; MacDougall, *op. cit.* (note 13), Chs 3, 5, 8, 9 & 10.
37. MacDougall, *op. cit.* (note 13), 194–8.
38. *Provincial Health Reports 1930–1940.* See numerous articles in *Canadian Public Health Journal* (1929–42). Cassel, *op. cit.* (note 9); Wherrett, *op. cit.* (note 12).
39. *Provincial Health Reports*; Harvey Agnew, *Canadian Hospitals 1920–1970, a Dramatic Half-Century* (Toronto: 1974); Gagan, *op. cit.* (note 31); George Torrance, 'Hospitals as Health Factories', in Coburn, *op. cit.* (note 4), 479–500.
40. Defries (ed.), *Health Services in Canada; Provincial Health Reports.* See numerous articles in *Canadian Journal of Public Health* (1943–1969).
41. *Provincial Health Reports*; MacDougall *op. cit.* (note 13), 147–58; Riddell, *op. cit.* (note 19); Defries (ed.), *Health Services in Canada*; Wherrett, *op. cit.* (note 12); Feldberg, *op. cit.* (note 12); Bator & Rhodes, *op. cit.* (note 31).
42. MacDougall, *op. cit.* (note 13), 201–3, 265–70
43. Jay Cassel, 'Making Canada Safe For Sex: Government Measures To Control Sexually Transmitted Diseases in the Twentieth Century', in David Naylor (ed.), *Canadian Medicine and the State: A Century of Evolution* (Kingston & Montreal: McGill-Queen's University Press, 1992).
44. Angus McLaren, *The Bedroom and the State: the Changing Practices and Politics of Contraception and Abortion in Canada, 1880–1980* (Toronto: McClelland & Stewart, 1986); MacDougall, *op. cit.* (note 13), 170–84, 204–9, 224–30.
45. MacDougall, *op. cit.* (note 13), 270–3
46. Canada, *Report of the Commission of Inquiry into the Non-Medical Use of Drugs* (Ottawa: the commission, 1972); MacDougall, *op. cit.* (note 13), 244–8; Terry Chapman, 'Drug Use in Western Canada', *Alberta History*, 24 (1976), 3–26.
47. Harvey Simmons, *Unbalanced: Mental Health Policy in Ontario, 1930–1989* (Toronto: 1990); MacDougall, *op. cit.* (note 13), 233–42; Defries (ed.), *Health Services in Canada.*
48. Jay Cassel, 'George Brock Chisholm', in Warren Kuehl (ed.), *Biographical Dictionary of Internationalists* (Westport Cn: Greenwood, 1983); Canada, External Affairs, *Canada and the World Health Organization* (Ottawa: External Affairs, 1975).
49. David Naylor, *Private Practice, Public Payment: Canadian Medicine and the Politics of Health Insurance, 1911–1966* (Montreal: McGill-Queen's University Press, 1986), and 'Canada's First Doctors' Strike: Medical Relief in Winnipeg, 1932–4', *Canadian Historical Review*, 67 (1986), 151–80; Malcolm Taylor, *Health Insurance and Canadian*

Public Policy: The Seven Decisions that Created the Canadian Health Insurance System (Montreal: McGill-Queen's University Press, 1978); Robert Bothwell and John English, 'Pragmatic Physicians: Canadian Medicine and Health Care Insurance, 1910–1945', in Shortt *op. cit.* (note 3), 479–93; Michael Stevenson and Paul Williams, 'Physicians and Medicare: Professional Ideology and Canadian Health Care Policy', *Canadian Public Policy,* 11 (1985), 504–21; Gwendolyn Gray, *Federalism and Health Policy: the Development of Health Systems in Canada and Australia* (Toronto: University of Toronto Press, 1991).

50. Malcolm Brown, 'Health Care Financing and the Canada Health Act', *Journal of Canadian Studies,* 21 (1986), 111–32; Michael Rachlis and Carol Kushner, *Second Opinion: What's Wrong with Canada's Health Care System and How To Fix It* (Toronto: 1989); Anne Crichton, David Hsu and Stella Tang, *Canada's Health Care System: Its Funding and Organization* (Ottawa: Canadian Hospital Assn., 1990).
51. Gray, *op. cit.* (note 49); Brown, *op. cit.* (note 49); S. Heibert and R. Deber, 'Banning Extra Billing in Canada: Just What the Doctor Didn't Order', *Canadian Public Policy,* 13 (1987), 62–74; Howard Palley, 'Canadian Federalism and the Canadian Health Care Program: A Comparison of Ontario and Quebec', *International Journal of Health Services,* 17 (1987), 595–616.
52. Marc Lalonde, *A New Perspective on the Health of Canadians* (Ottawa: National Health and Welfare, 1974); D. D. Gelman, R. Lachaine and M. M. Law, 'The Canadian Approach to Health Policies and Programmes', *Preventive Medicine,* 6 (1977), 265–75; Barry Edginton, *Health, Disease and Medicine in Canada, A Sociological Perspective* (Toronto and Vancouver: Butterworths, 1989).
53. *Public Health in the 1980s: Report of the Health Planning Steering Committee* (Toronto: the committee, 1978); MacDougall, *op. cit.* (note 13), ch. 12; Edginton, *op. cit.* (note 52).
54. Cassel, *op. cit.* (note 43).
55. Marc Renaud, 'Reform or Illusion? An Analysis of the Quebec State Intervention in Health', in Coburn *op. cit.* (note 4), 590–614.

8

A New World? Two Hundred Years of Public Health in Australia and New Zealand

Linda Bryder

British colonization of Australia began with the transportation of the first British convicts in 1788 and that of New Zealand in 1840 when the Maori chiefs signed the Treaty of Waitangi, seceding the land to the British Crown. Most of the early white settlers in both countries came from Britain, and these settlers brought with them local customs and traditions (their 'cultural baggage') including their own medicine and approaches to health and disease. The British background is important in understanding the development of public health in Australia and New Zealand. While the two countries increasingly gained independence from Britain, they maintained close links with the 'Mother Country' through immigration and identification well into the twentieth century. Of equal importance, however, was the fact that in the New World they were confronted with a different physical environment and set of problems from the Old World as well as a different social and political environment which influenced the direction of public health policies.

The British influence on 'Antipodean' medicine was strong. Medical education followed British models, and doctors frequently pursued post-graduate study in Britain.[1] Dr J. H. L. Cumpston, involved in the Australian public health service from 1908 to 1945, and described by the historian Milton Lewis as 'undoubtedly the most important figure in public health in Australia this century', had gained the London Diploma in Public Health (DPH) in 1906 and worked briefly at the Lister Institute of Preventive Medicine in London.[2] Dr J. S. C. Elkington, another leading figure in Australian public health, also held the London DPH. Dr J. A. Thompson, the head of the Department of Public Health of New South Wales in its formative years from 1896 to 1914, had a DPH from the University of Cambridge. Dr W. C. Armstrong, Sydney's medical officer from 1898 to 1913 and recognized as the founder of the infant welfare movement in Australia,[3] also held a DPH from Cambridge. The founder of the infant welfare movement in New Zealand, Dr (later Sir) Truby King, gained the new B.Sc. in public health at Edinburgh University in 1887. Dr J. M. Mason, appointed the first Chief Health Officer under New Zealand's Public Health Act of 1900, had also been awarded a Cambridge DPH, as had Dr R. H. Makgill who framed the 1920 Health Act in New Zealand.[4]

The close contact with the 'Mother Country' continued well into the twentieth century. Almost every member of a committee set up by the medical profession to look at reform of the health services in New Zealand in 1935, had some experience of the British system.[5] The governments of Australia and New Zealand invited British 'experts' to advise them when they came to propose reform of the health services around that time.[6] Until 1962 in Australia, and 1967 in New Zealand, the medical profession was organized locally as branches of the BMA. The annual subscription gave members access to the *British Medical Journal*, keeping them in touch with British developments.[7]

Much public health legislation is said to have followed British models. The historian D. H. Coward asserted that the sanitary reforms which took place in Sydney in the second half of the nineteenth century were based on the ideas and practices developed in Britain. Indeed, he wrote that the Sydney sanitary reformers enjoyed an advantage over their counterparts in Britain – i.e. that in Australia British-derived ideas possessed an intrinsic authority.[8] Nineteenth-century sanitary reforms in Australia and New Zealand followed the English Acts of 1848 and 1875.[9] The infant welfare movement in Australia after 1918 was greatly influenced by the Maternity and Infant Welfare Act passed in England and Wales that year.[10] Measures against tuberculosis in both countries appeared to have precedents in Britain.[11] According to the historian G. W. Rice, the establishment of the Ministry of Health in Britain in1919 'seems very likely to have been the model for New Zealand's 1920 Health Department'.[12]

However, it does not follow that the colonies merely copied Britain, for there were important differences – in timing, in priorities, and in allocations of powers and responsibilities between central and local authorities as well as between public and private, medical and non-medical, authorities. While Britain may have provided the models, these were transformed in the colonial context. Only by examining local environments, political structures, and the ideological and social beliefs of dominant groups in society, can the differences be explained. British world beliefs and structures could not, and would not, be transplanted intact to the New World.

The history of public health in Australia and New Zealand can be conveniently divided into four phases. The first encompasses the colonial period of the nineteenth century. 1901 was to be an important date in public health reform in both countries – it was the year the six Australian colonies federated (Northern Territory, Victoria, New South Wales, South Australia, Western Australia and Tasmania), and New Zealand set up its first Department of Public Health. The second phase covers the first two decades of the twentieth century when preoccupations with the future of the population led to a greater concern for infant health in particular. The third phase is the inter-war period, the two decades following the establishment of new or restructured Departments of Health intended to rationalize and improve health services. The final phase starts about the time of the Second World War when both became involved in attempts to establish a national health service integrating preventive and curative medicine. The public health provision for the indigenous populations, the Aborigines of Australia and the Maori of New Zealand, does not fit neatly into this chronology and therefore must be considered separately, as indeed it was by the governments of the day for much of this period.

Australia and New Zealand were slow to adopt effective public health legislation in the nineteenth century. Public health at this time did not extend far beyond quarantine and vaccination measures. The first comprehensive Public Health Act in Australia was passed by the state of Victoria (modelled on the English Act of 1848) in 1854. Yet, the functions of the central board established under the Act were merely 'advisory and admonitory'. According to Coward, the board's main activity was 'pontificating in bulky, impressive-looking annual reports'.[13] Another historian, Stephen Garton, has written that when legislation comparable to that in Britain was passed in Australia in the 1880s it was 'limited, poorly enforced and ineffectual'.[14] New Zealand's Public Health Acts of 1872 and 1876 were also largely ineffective. The Central Board of Health, set up under the latter Act, 'failed to initiate any public health policy' and local authorities 'displayed a complete indifference to the cause of public health', according to the public health historian, F. S. Maclean.[15] The largest Australian colony, New South

Wales, did not even go through the motions; it did not adopt a comprehensive Public Health Act until 1896.

This lack of commitment to public health reform in the nineteenth century despite a population increasing rapidly through immigration, was explained at the time and subsequently quite simply in terms of the absence of the health problems of the Old World in the colonies. Coward pointed out that the objective urban living conditions in England and in New South Wales offered considerable contrasts: 'Sydney, with its sea breezes, equable temperatures, ample sunshine ... [and] its hilly, well-drained land' provided a healthy environment.[16] Melbourne was said in the nineteenth-century to be 'naturally healthy', possessing a 'salubrious climate'.[17] The belief that Queensland possessed a healthy and health-giving environment, with its unlimited space, fresh air, pure water, warmth and sunshine, persisted throughout the colonial period and to the present.[18]

There are many examples of the supposedly healthy conditions of the colonies. In 1859, a visiting doctor, A. S. Thomson, wrote of the salubrious climate of New Zealand. This, he claimed, provided ideal conditions for those suffering from consumption (tuberculosis).[19] Dr Samuel Dougan Bird published a book in 1863, *On Australian Climates, and their Influence in the Prevention and Arrest of Pulmonary Tuberculosis.* Dr Bird asserted that the Australian climate had saved him from dying of consumption and recommended the colonies for consumptives. Many of the latter did indeed go to the colonies in search of health.[20]

Not only was the climate supposedly healthy, but the New World, as a 'workingman's paradise', offered opportunities for a healthy lifestyle. Poverty, it was claimed, was non-existent. This view has persisted in, for example, the argument of the economic historian R. V. Jackson: 'Australians were well fed, well clothed and well housed ... Australian cities were spacious, healthy, and free of large areas of extreme poverty'.[21] From the 1870s, the average workingman's consumption of meat in Australia was 'almost legendary'.[22]

These conditions appeared to suggest that minimal government intervention was necessary since people were able to maintain their own health standards. Yet other sources reveal a less than rosy picture of this 'southern Arcadia'. Infant death rates were indeed low by world standards, but it was the rural rates which kept them low.[23] The infant death rates in large Australian cities were much the same as those in English cities.[24] Until about 1890, infant mortality in Sydney was as high as, and sometimes higher than, that in London.[25] Sydney's Health Officer, Dr Henry Graham, reported to a Select Committee as early as 1859–60 that the conditions of the working classes in some areas of the city were 'worse than in any part of the world'.[26] Epidemics of typhoid, sometimes known as the 'colonial or pauperising fever',[27] were frequent. In New Zealand the typhoid rates in the cities in the 1890s were greater than in British cities. Typhoid fever was more prevalent in Melbourne than in comparable British cities.[28] It reached epidemic proportions of 357 per 100,000 population in Western Australia during the gold rushes of the 1890s.[29] Mortality from gastro-intestinal diseases in Sydney, Melbourne and Brisbane was twice the rate of London and Birmingham.[30] In 1901 Dr W. C. Armstrong, Medical Officer of Health for Sydney, recorded that in a year's public health work in Whitechapel, London, he had not seen dwellings as bad as some he knew of in Sydney.[31]

It is clear then that the tardiness of public health reform cannot be explained in terms of an absence of public health deficiences. Rather, it is to be explained in terms of the failure to acknowledge mounting health problems. The colonists were intent on attracting immigrants and investment for the further development of the colonies. This desire led them to turn a blind eye to anything which would tarnish the proclaimed attractiveness of the colonies. For this reason, as the historian Miles Fairburn has written of nineteenth-century New Zealanders, they were intolerant of social criticism and tended to discourage objective social analysis.[32] When poor living conditions were discussed, the focus tended to be on the habits and morals of the poor. This was especially so in the 1870s when epidemic diseases and mortality rates had reached new heights in Australia.[33] Not only was there a reluctance to acknowledge social and health problems which would affect the image of the 'working-man's paradise', but there was also a strong belief in individualism and the virtues of self-reliance among the nineteenth- century colonists which kept social intervention to a minimum.[34] Attempts at sanitary reform were thus hindered by the social beliefs and perhaps financial priorities of local ratepayers.

The 'shock diseases' of the nineteenth century are generally given the credit for stimulating such reform in public health as occurred, galvanizing local communities into action during, for example, the smallpox epidemics of the 1880s and bubonic plague in 1900. Yet, as noted above, the implementation was often half-hearted, and the shock effect did not last long beyond the crisis itself – leaving impressive legislation but little commitment to it. The 1900 plague scare in particular was thought to have shocked the public out of its complacency. In Sydney it dramatically highlighted poor conditions. However, as soon as the threat of plague subsided the push for municipal reform lost momentum.[35] The plague scare was also said to have inspired the enactment of the 1900 Public Health Act in New Zealand, establishing the first public health department under Ministerial control in the British Commonwealth. Yet it appears that the Government was already considering the establishment of such a department before the plague scare.[36] Moreover, in practice little use was made over the next two decades of the draconian powers bestowed upon health officers under the Act.[37] The preventive side of the new department lost any impetus it might have had when the Department of Public Health was amalgamated with the Department of Hospitals and Charitable Institutions in 1909 and the offices of Chief Health Officer and Inspector General of Hospitals were combined. The incumbent, Dr T. H. A. Valintine, it appears, was more interested in the latter role.[38]

The early twentieth century did, however, see new initiatives in public health in both countries, partly voluntary and partly government supported, which cannot be attributed to the 'shock epidemics', but to a new political climate and new national concerns.

The governments in office at this time – the Progressives in Australia and the Liberals in New Zealand – were highly nationalistic. Their nationalism included an 'imperial strategy'. Loyalty to Mother Britain was not incompatible with local nationalism – indeed it was believed that in this new environment transplanted Britons could be made healthier and fitter. Environmentalism and eugenics both found their place in this new climate.[39] Concern for 'national efficiency', or the future of the Anglo-Saxon race, was shared with Britain but had its own local component, which was the 'Yellow Peril', the fear that Asian 'hordes' would descend upon these southern lands if the Anglo-Saxon population were not maintained. Japanese expansionism was especially feared. The 1903/4 New South Wales Royal Commission on the Decline of the Birth-rate and on Infant Mortality warned of the dangers of Australia's small population. The President of the Commission, Sir Charles K. Mackellar, a pronatalist, admonished Australia to 'populate or perish'.[40] The empty spaces of the Australian continent had to be filled to keep it in white hands. The Commission claimed that the 'newborn child is our best immigrant', a frequently repeated slogan.[41] Dr J. H. L. Cumpston, at that time working for the Western Australian public health service, also spoke in 1910 of the urgent need to raise the birthrate and populate the continent.[42]

This pronatalist concern was shared by New Zealand. The Prime Minister, Richard Seddon, published a pamphlet in 1904 on the 'Preservation of Infant Life' and two Acts on Infant Life Protection were passed in 1894 and 1907. However, it was not the Department of Public Health that took the initiative with regard to infant health in New Zealand but rather a voluntary organization, the Society for the Promotion of the Health of Women and Children (known in short as the Plunket Society), founded by Dr Frederick Truby King in 1907. King, who acquired international fame for his child-rearing doctrines, was a pronatalist and eugenist.[43] The Society, under King, was concerned only with the population of European descent.

As in Britain, the solution to improving infant health for the sake of national efficiency was sought in the education of mothers in child-rearing. The bulk of the 1903/4 New South Wales Royal Commission's report was devoted to infant mortality, and it found 'very strong' medical evidence that infant mortality was primarily the result of improper feeding, related to women's laziness or fondness for pleasure.[44] Similar views were expressed by Truby King in New Zealand.[45]

The infant welfare movement in Australia is said to have originated in Sydney in 1904 when Dr W. G. Armstrong appointed a 'lady sanitary inspector' for home visiting.[46] In 1912 the Australian Federal Labor Government gave a tremendous boost to the movement when it introduced a 'baby bonus' of £5 for every new-born live white baby, regardless of the mother's 'character'.[47] This encouraged parents to register babies so that they could claim the allowance, which in turn enabled nurses to visit homes soon after a birth. Aboriginal and Asiatic women living in Australia, and indigenous women in Australia's colony, Papua, were not eligible, indicating its eugenist aims. As Milton Lewis has asserted, 'Infant health and "white Australia" went hand in hand'.[48]

In New Zealand, non-Maori mothers were to be educated by the Plunket nurses and district health nurses (who were to reach rural mothers under the Backblock District Health Service established in 1909). The 1907 Infant Life Protection Act reduced the period for the notification of births from two months to three days, in order to allow the nurse to visit as soon as possible. In 1904 the Midwives Registration Act had been passed to improve the quality of midwifery, and St Helens Hospitals were set up from 1905 to provide state-subsidized maternity care for wives of working men. Medical care for other sectors of the community was organized privately at that time, or on a charitable basis through the Hospitals and Charitable Institutions Acts of 1885 and 1909.

Schoolchildren also became a target for early twentieth-century health reformers, as in Britain. In Tasmania, Dr J. S. C. Elkington, the local Commissioner of Public Health and later an influential member of the Federal Health Department, succeeded in establishing medical inspection and health education in government schools by 1908.[49] He also campaigned for child health at the national level. School medical services were initiated in Victoria in 1909 and South Australia in 1913. Children were to be inspected and teachers were to be taught health education. However, school medical officers and nurses were not to encroach upon private medical practice by administering treatment. The same restrictions, imposed by a medical profession opposed to state medicine, applied to the school medical service established in New Zealand in 1912.[50]

The First World War further intensified the concern for the fitness of the people and in particular the next generation. During the war it was claimed that 'the hope of Australia lies in healthy living babies, fewer dead babies, stronger children, and a fitter race'.[51] While fewer men were rejected as unfit for overseas military service in Australia and New Zealand than in Britain (the respective rejection figures were 36 per cent for Australia, 31 per cent for New Zealand, and 51 per cent for Britain),[52] the Antipodean figures were still held to be high enough to cause concern.

Some active steps were also taken in the first decade of the twentieth century to combat tuberculosis, as in other Western countries. Tuberculosis, striking at adults in the prime of life, was considered a threat to national efficiency. In New Zealand tuberculosis was made a notifiable disease in 1901, and the first government sanatorium for the treatment of the disease was set up in 1902.[53] Tuberculosis had been made a notifiable disease in South Australia in 1898, and other states followed, although New South Wales did not make it notifiable until 1915 and then only in proclaimed districts and not in the whole State until 1929. Sanatoria and dispensaries were also set up by state governments in Australia.[54]

The influenza epidemic of 1918/19, coming close on the heels of the First World War, provided a further stimulus for health reform and the demand for greater efficiency in health administration. In New Zealand a Health Act was passed in 1920, reforming the former Department of Public Health and dividing it into Divisions of Public Hygiene, Hospitals, Nursing, School Hygiene, Dental Hygiene, Child Welfare[55] and Maori Welfare. An individualist rather than an environmental orientation of the restructured Department of

Health was indicated by the way in which three departments dealt with the child ('Dental Hygiene' meant School Dental Hygiene), one with Maori, and two with hospitals ('Nursing' was mainly concerned with hospital nursing).

In Australia the influenza epidemic severely tested the quarantine powers of the federal authority and seemed, at least to Cumpston, at that time the Director of Quarantine, to highlight the need for stronger central control. Cumpston couched his arguments in terms of national efficiency.[56] Aided by the Rockefeller Foundation which was conducting a worldwide campaign against the tropical disease, hookworm, Cumpston persuaded the Federal Government to create a Department of Health of which he became Director-General. Tropical health was central to the argument for a federal department as it transcended state boundaries and because the Federal Government (and not individual states) was responsible for public health in Australia's newly extended colony of Papua New Guinea.[57] The desire to settle northern Australia by whites, as part of the White Australia policy, was important in focusing attention on tropical health and in the decision to set up a federal department of health.[58]

One of the few institutions operated by the new Federal Department of Health was the Australian Institute of Tropical Medicine (AITM), which had been founded in Queensland in 1911. The 'tropical-frontier' emphasis of the department continued until the late 1920s. The AITM was closed down in 1930 when the School of Public Health and Tropical Medicine was set up in Sydney, under the aegis of the University of Sydney. This move south was part of a strategy by Cumpston to consolidate the new Department of Health in the federal bureaucracy, by focusing attention away from tropical questions to the problems of urban temperate Australia, where the great majority of the electorate lived.[59]

Not only did the interest in tropical diseases subside but much of the reformist zeal of the early twentieth century had also disappeared.[60] Cumpston, who was to head the Federal Department of Health for 24 years, admitted in 1945 that the Department achieved considerably less than full success.[61] The federal structure itself has been held chiefly responsible. There were interstate rivalries, which were probably largely responsible for the failure to implement the national health plan proposed by the 1925 Royal Commission on Health.[62] There was also a general reluctance on the part of states to cooperate with the Federal Government on any issue not specifically demanded by the constitution. Under the 1901 constitution of the Commonwealth of Australia, individual states retained total control over health provision and even when the Commonwealth extended its health powers by referendum in 1946, these were still limited. The medical profession in particular was in a powerful position in respect of local health reform.[63]

Infant health continued to claim attention. A Baby Clinics Service was set up in Queensland following the Maternity Act of 1922. The 1932 Notification of Births Act enabled clinic nurses to contact mothers soon after the birth of their babies and to invite them to the clinics where they would be given instruction in child-rearing.[64] Despite a pretence of universalism, Aboriginal women were discouraged from attending the baby clinics and hospitals.[65]

Truby King's work with the Plunket Society in New Zealand was endorsed by the Government in 1921 when he was appointed Director of Child Welfare in the new Department of Health. In the 1920s the Government sent a copy of King's book, *The Expectant Mother and Baby's First Month,* to every married woman under the age of 35, and a copy was to be issued to anyone applying for a marriage licence.[66] The number of Plunket nurses as well as district nurses continued to grow, although they were instructed not to encroach on private medical practice.[67]

Similarly, in the school medical service, care had to be taken not to usurp the territory of private practitioners. The most successful aspect of the school medical service in New Zealand, for which it attracted international fame, was the school dental service, run by dental nurses who were trained in dental schools from 1921. With their separate and minimal training, these nurses were not seen as a threat to the 'real' dentists.[68]

Concern for infants extended in the 1920s in Australia and New Zealand, as in Britain, to concern for the health of their mothers.[69] In Australia, the Federal Health Council, established in 1927, attempted to improve maternity services. That it did not achieve its aim has been attributed largely to a hostile medical profession.[70] The New Zealand Health Department met similar obstructions when it attempted to reform maternity services in the 1920s. Doctors mobilized themselves through the Society for Obstetrics and Gynaecology, founded in 1927, primarily in response to the challenges to their authority emanating from the Health Department's enthusiastic reformers, Dr Henry Jellett and Dr Tom Paget. By inspecting private hospitals and improving the training for midwives and for the new category of maternity nurse, the Department had forced the doctors on to the defensive. Doctors resented state interference and feared state medicine.[71]

Thus, by 1939 public health services included infant welfare clinics, antenatal clinics and school medical services. This period also saw the expansion of tuberculosis dispensaries and sanatoria, and the establishment of venereal disease clinics. In both countries at this time the medical profession resisted encroachment into their terrain; they were totally devoted to private practice and were also well-organized to stand up for themselves.[72]

In New Zealand the medical profession led by the anti-socialist Dr J. P. S. Jamieson successfully thwarted the first Labor Government's attempts (1935–49) to introduce free health care. The 1938 Social Security Act was intended to provide free medical attendance in hospitals and by general practitioners. The medical profession, however, refused to cooperate. Free maternity care was soon agreed to (1939), as this favoured doctor-controlled hospital deliveries over a midwifery service. The eventual agreement relating to general practitioner services indicated the bargaining strength of the medical profession. The state was to subsidise medical attendance charges (on a fee-for-service basis), while the patient was to pay a 'token' amount. As time passed this amount lost its token character, and general practitioner services became more and more expensive. Hospital treatment was now free, but private hospitals were allowed to remain in existence – it was assumed they would eventually disappear owing to a lack of clientele. On the contrary, private hospitals grew in popularity as public hospitals were left to run down. These two trends – in general practitioner and hospital services – encouraged the growth of private insurance from the 1960s and a growing inequality of health care services. Those most adversely affected by this trend were the Maori and the more recent immigrants from the Pacific Islands, generally located at the lower end of the socio-economic scale.

In Australia opposition from the organized medical profession led to the abandonment of the Federal Government's National Health and Pensions Insurance Act in 1939.[73] During the Second World War the Labor Government considered introducing a national health service, and in 1948–9 this was attempted. The service was to be administered by the Director-General of Health and the country was to be divided into health areas under district medical officers who would be advised by committees consisting of local medical practitioners. Preventive work was to be carried out by regional clinics staffed on a sessional basis. Remote areas would have a salaried service, but most of the country would continue to use private practitioners. The patient and the Government would each pay half the doctor's scheduled fee. The scheme was, however, rejected by the medical profession which feared nationalization.

In late 1949 the more conservative Menzies Liberal-Country Party was elected to office, and a national health service was introduced on a fee-for-service basis. It was financed by government-subsidized voluntary insurance. This was acceptable to the doctors. Thus the Government provided public funds to supplement private insurance, which continued until the 1970s when universal health insurance schemes – Medibank (1975) and later Medicare (1983) – were introduced. Those who benefited least from the 1949 scheme were the poor, who included the indigenous population, the Aborigines.

One public health problem encountered by white settlers in both countries related to the health of the indigenous populations, the Aborigines in Australia and the Maori in New Zealand, who showed little resistance to the diseases introduced by the Europeans. When concern was expressed and action taken regarding the health of these peoples in the early years of white settlement, it was largely as a result of the fear of the spread of the diseases to the contiguous white communities. Indeed, it has been argued that a 'genuine' concern for the health of the Aboriginal population of Australia was not evident before the 1960s.[74] At least until the 1930s medical efforts in Papua New Guinea were almost wholly directed towards protecting the health of ex-patriots, or native males working for Europeans.[75]

Until the turn of the century in New Zealand and much later in Australia, it was believed that the non-white indigenous populations were dying out in the face of a superior civilization (a belief arising from Social Darwinism) and that it was the duty of the white administration merely 'to smooth the pillow of the dying race'.[76] It was noted in *The Queenslander* in 1880, 'By these laws the native races were doomed on the advent of the white man, and the only thing left for us to do is to assist in carrying them out with as little cruelty as possible'.[77] It was predicted in the *Australian Handbook for 1888* that another decade would bring the 'extinction of the race within Victoria's boundaries... They were inevitable victims of that all ruling influence of the law of survival of the strongest'.[78] As late as 1937 Donald Thomson, apparently a 'very sympathetic student of Aboriginal life', noted that it was 'evident to any scientific observer who examines the evidence, that wherever the white or Asiatic races come into contact with the aboriginals the latter first become degenerate and ultimately die'.[79]

The 1901 Australian Commonwealth constitution stated that 'In reckoning the numbers of the people... Aboriginal natives shall not be counted'. Health statistics on Aborigines therefore remained inaccurate. However, the existence of poor health was indisputable. The prevalence of smallpox among the Aboriginal population was already noted in 1790 by the commander of the first convict ship to arrive in Australia, Captain Arthur Phillip. He wrote that the small-pox epidemic of 1789 had killed fully one half of the Aborigines living in the area (New South Wales).[80] A severe epidemic of smallpox also occurred in 1829–31. In the absence of statistics, the role of other infectious diseases remains unclear, but it appears that tuberculosis was a major killer as well as influenza, pneunomia and measles.

In 1788 the Aboriginal population totalled somewhere between 300,000 and 750,000. By 1901 there were about 67,000 Aborigines, most of whom lived in the north-western tropical areas of the continent.[81] The nineteenth-century approach to Aboriginal welfare, when anything was done, was paternalistic. From about 1850 a 'protection policy' was adopted; legislation was introduced under which Aborigines were to be segregated and 'protected'. The main benefactors of this policy appeared to be white employers who were ensured a cheap source of labour through the missions and reserves established.[82] The first Aborigines Protection Board was set up in 1883 by the New South Wales government, but was given no specific statutory powers until 1909 when the Aborigines Protection Act (New South Wales) was passed. Legislation enacted between the 1880s and the 1930s established reserves throughout Australia.[83]

1927 saw the establishment of the Northern Territory Medical Service, covering an area where about 46,000 or two-thirds of the Aboriginal population resided. The Service consisted of a chief protector who was also chief medical officer, an assistant chief protector, a patrol officer, a clerk, four employees on reserves in Darwin and Alice Springs and fewer than 40 police officers throughout the Territory. In addition to the police duties, protectors in remote areas were expected to supervise the employment of Aborigines, report cases of ill-treatment and illness, order and distribute rations to the aged and indigent, and diagnose, order medicines for, and treat people who fell ill.[84] In practice, the housing conditions and nutritional status of Aborigines remained poor for those on the reserves and missions as well as for those who lived in towns or on fringe camps, in the Northern Territory and elsewhere.[85]

From the late 1930s the Commonwealth authorities adopted a policy of assimilation in relation to the Aboriginal population. While full-blooded Aborigines were still to be kept on reserves, those of mixed descent were to be directed away from their own culture towards Western education, jobs and medicine.[86]

The Second World War saw some improvements in the material conditions of Aborigines (largely as a result of their involvement in the war effort),[87] but it was not until the 1960s that the actual health status of the Aboriginal population entered the wider political arena. Aborigines themselves were partly responsible for the heightened concern, inspired by the Black Rights movement in the USA. A combination of international and internal pressures led to the adoption of a new policy of integration in 1965.[88] Aborigines were included in the national census following a referendum in 1967. In 1968 E. Gough Whitlam, the leader of the Opposition, claimed, 'The health of Aboriginals is an indictment of this country.' He referred to a 1963 survey carried out under the auspices of the Australian National University and the Australian Institute of Aboriginal Studies which showed a death rate of 208 per 1,000 live births among Aborigines in central Australia, and quoted the report on the survey that this 'must be among the highest infant mortality rates in the world'. The Aboriginal infant mortality rate in general, Whitlam noted, was about ten times greater than that for other Australian infants. The incidence of leprosy among Aborigines in the Northern Territory was one of the highest in the world. In 1960 members of an American–Australian scientific expedition claimed that in four places they had visited in the Northern Territory, 'leprosy is considered endemic'.[89]

With the election of the Whitlam Labor Government in 1972, Aboriginal affairs became a prominent part of the political agenda for all parties.[90] However, despite the development from the 1970s of self-help organizations such as the Aboriginal Medical Services (the first established in the Sydney suburb of Redfern in 1971), and the Commonwealth government's National Plan for Aboriginal Health adopted in 1973,[91] vast discrepancies in health status between Aborigines and the rest of the population remained, related to the continued poverty and poor living conditions of the former.[92] As one observer has noted, 'Where Aboriginal and white health are concerned ... we are still two nations'.[93]

New Zealand is usually credited with a better record in respect to its indigenous population.[94] Steps to improve Maori health were taken in 1900 at a time when the Maori population had reached an all-time low of around 45,000 (the pre-Western-contact population was estimated to lie somewhere between 100,000 and 500,000). Maori Councils were set up to look after the health and welfare of the Maori people in 1900. However, these Councils were chronically under-funded by the Government and consequently did not achieve much. Some initiatives came from the Maori themselves around the turn of the century. The *Te Aute* College Students' Association (also known as the Young Maori Party) worked towards the improvement of Maori health and welfare. One member of the Association, Dr Maui Pomare, the first Maori to qualify in medicine, was the government's 'native' health officer from 1901 to 1911. Pomare sought to improve Maori health by assimilation or total adoption of European ways. The 1907 Tohunga Suppression Act, which Pomare campaigned for, is indicative of a reluctance to work through traditional Maori channels. (The *tohunga* was the traditional Maori medical and priestly figure.) Assimilation was also the aim of the scheme of 'native' district nurses sent into Maori communities from 1911, the year the Public Health Department became responsible for Maori health. The 1920 Health Act established a separate Division of Maori Welfare, directed by another member of the Young Maori Party, Dr Te Rangi Hiroa (also known as Peter Buck) until 1927, although lack of funds was once again an inhibiting factor. In 1930 the Maori Welfare Division of the Department of Health was abolished and it was announced that the Maori would no longer be treated as a race apart.

Few detailed studies were made of Maori health before the 1930s. In 1933 Dr H. B. Turbott carried out a study of tuberculosis in a Maori district on the East Cape, financed by the British Medical Research Council.[95] Tuberculosis was found to be ten times higher in this community than in the general population. His recommendations included total adoption of Western cultural ways. The number of district nurses was increased, but little financial aid was given to improve the housing conditions which were in all probability at the root of the high tuberculosis rates.

The health of the Maori people showed some improvement in the post-Second World War period, probably related to urbanization of the Maori.[96] Tuberculosis declined, partly owing to an active campaign of BCG vaccination and mass radiography to detect early cases, but also related to the urban drift of the Maori which improved living conditions, at least initially in the prosperous economic climate of the 1950s and 1960s. While some improvements in health occurred in the 1950s and 1960s, health differentials between Maori and non-Maori remained stark.[97] Maori, along with Pacific Islanders who had immigrated to New Zealand in the 1950s and 1960s in response to employment opportunities, were the first to suffer from the economic downturn from the late 1960s. The decline in public health services and the growth of private health insurance also adversely affected that sector of society.

Australia and New Zealand's tardy response to public health

problems lay not in the absence of such problems. The reasons can be found rather in an unwillingness to abandon the view of these southern colonies as 'naturally' healthy, allied to a firm belief in individualism prevalent in frontier societies and a reluctance of local ratepayers to devote the necessary finances. When action was taken in the early twentieth century, it was in response to concerns about national efficiency, the future of the Anglo-Saxon race and the rising belief in the powers of medical science to solve social problems. The approach was initially educational, although public health increasingly encroached on the terrain of private practice. Largely as a result of the intransigence of a well-organized medical profession devoted to private practice, a national health service was never implemented, despite the political will in both countries around the time of the Second World War.

Public health in the early twentieth century aimed to improve the quality of the white population. When attention was later focused on the non-white indigenous populations, there was no attempt to work through or show any respect for traditional channels – indeed medicine and public health, as far as the indigenous populations of both countries were concerned, could be described as yet another cultural agency, and did not serve their health needs well. More recent initiatives in both countries show some attempt to reverse this cultural insensitivity,[98] although health differentials remain stark.

Notes

1. C. Thame, 'Health and the State. The Development of Collective Responsibility for Health Care in Australia in the first half of the Twentieth Century' (Ph.D. Thesis, Australian National University (ANU), 1974), iii.
2. M. Lewis, 'Editor's Introduction', J. H. L. Cumpston, *Health and Disease in Australia. A History,* (Canberra: 1989), 1, 2.
3. P. Mein Smith, 'Reformers, Mothers and Babies. Aspects of Infant Survival. Australia 1890–1945' (Ph.D. Thesis, ANU, 1990), 73.
4. G. W. Rice, 'The Making of New Zealand's 1920 Health Act', *New Zealand Journal of History (NZJH),* 22, 1 (1988), 5.
5. D. G. Bolitho, 'Some Financial and Medico-Political Aspects of the New Zealand Medical Profession's Reaction to the Introduction of Social Security', *NZJH,* 18, 1 (1984), 34–49.
6. See E. Hanson, *The Politics of Social Security: The 1938 Act and Some Later Developments* (Auckland: 1980); R. Watts, 'The Origins of the Australian Welfare State', *Historical Studies,* 19 (1980–1), 185. 6 Thame, *op. cit.* (note 1), iii.
7. D. H. Coward, *Out of Sight, Sydney's Environmental History*

1851–1981, (Canberra: 1988), 7 & 8; P. Curson and K. McCracken, *Plague in Sydney. The Anatomy of an Epidemic,* (New South Wales: 1987, 49).

8. K. M. Reiger, *The Disenchantment of the Home. Modernising the Australian Family 1880–1940,* (Melbourne: 1985), 136–52. It was also influenced by the New Zealand infant welfare movement, Mein Smith, *op. cit.* (note 3), 148–52.
9. R. Walker, 'The Struggle against Pulmonary Tuberculosis in Australia, 1788–1950', *Historical Studies,* 20 (1982–3), 439–61; L. Bryder, '"If Preventable Why Not Prevented?" The New Zealand Response to Tuberculosis, 1901–40', in L. Bryder (ed.), *A Healthy Country. Essays on the Social History of Medicine in New Zealand,* (Wellington: 1991), 115.
10. Rice, *op. cit.* (note 4), 20. In fact it is incorrect to assume a single system for the whole of Britain. The Ministry of Health covered only England and Wales; Scotland established a separate Board of Health under the Secretary of State for Scotland in 1919.
11. Coward, *op. cit.* (note 7), 169.
12. S. Garton, *Out of Luck. Poor Australians and Social Welfare 1788–1988,* (Sydney: 1990), 41.
13. F. S. Maclean, *Challenge for Health. A History of Public Health in New Zealand,* (Wellington: 1964), 12 & 13. Maclean, unlike the other historians cited, was not a professional historian but a doctor who worked for the Department of Health from 1927 to 1957 and wrote the history following his retirement.
14. Coward, *op. cit.* (note 7), 169.
15. D. Dunstan, *Governing the Metropolis. Politics, Technology and Social Change in Victorian Melbourne. 1850–1891,* (Melbourne: 1984), 121.
16. H. R. Woolcock, '"Our Salubrious Climate": Attitudes to Health in Colonial Queensland', *Disease. Medicine and Empire. Perspectives on Western Medicine and the Experience of European Expansion,* R. MacLeod and M. Lewis (eds), (London & New York: 1988), 176, 180, 183. For a contrast with conditions in Britain, see A. Wohl, *Endangered Lives. Public Health in Victorian Britain,* (London: 1983).
17. *Ibid.*
18. *Ibid.*
19. A. S. Thomson, *The Story of New Zealand: Past and Present. Savage and Civilised. I,* (London: 1859).
20. Walker, *op. cit.* (note 9), 441; Woolcock, *op. cit.* (note 16), 184; L. Williams, 'Feminine Frontiers. Queensland's Early Medical Women', *Fevers and Frontiers,* J. Pearn and M. Cobcroft (eds), (Brisbane: 1991), 146; B. Gandevia, *Modern Methods in the History of Medicine,* E. Clarke (ed.), (London: 1971), 90; B. Gandevia, *Tears Often Shed. Child Health and Welfare in Australia From 1788,* (New South Wales: 1978), 37, 89; R. E. Wright-St Clair, 'Causes of Death in Colonial Doctors', *New Zealand Medical Journal,* 88 (1978), 49–51.

21. Quoted in Garton, *op. cit.* (note 12), 1. See also R. Watts, 'As Cold as Charity', *Making a Life. A People's History of Australia Since 1788,* V. Burgmann and J. Lee (eds), (Victoria: 1988), 92–3.
22. M. Lewis and R. MacLeod, 'A Workingman's Paradise? Reflections on Urban Mortality in Colonial Australia 1860–1900', *Medical History,* 31, 4 (1987), 392.
23. Mein Smith, *op. cit.* (note 3), 44.
24. Garton, *op. cit.* (note 12), 39, 41; Lewis & MacLeod, *op. cit.* (note 22), 388, 389.
25. Lewis & MacLeod, *op. cit.* (note 22), 398.
26. Garton, *op. cit.* (note 12), 23; Lewis and MacLeod, *op. cit.* (note 22), 394.
27. Garton, *op. cit.* (note 12), 41.
28. Dunstan, *op. cit.* (note 15), 124, 125; D. Dunstan, 'Health Officers of the City of Melbourne', *Patients, Practitioners and Techniques. Second National Conference on Medicine and Healtb in Australia 1984,* H. Attwood and R.W. Home (eds), (Melbourne: 1985), 130.
29. V. Whittington, *Gold and Typhoid. Two Fevers. A Social History of Western Australia 1891–1900* (Nedlands, Western Australia: 1988), 9.
30. Garton, *op. cit.* (note 12), 41.
31. Lewis & MacLeod, *op. cit.* (note 22), 395; see also Curson & McCracken, *op. cit.* (note 7), 9.
32. M. Fairburn, *The Ideal Society and Its Enemies. The Foundations of Modern New Zealand Society. 1850–1900,* (Auckland: 1989), 12, 269.
33. Garton, *op. cit.* (note 12), 41.
34. See Fairburn, *op. cit.* (note 32), Part I; see also Woolcock, *op. cit.* (note 16), 187.
35. Curson & McCracken, *op. cit.* (note 7), 187, 194, 198; see also P. H. Curson, *Epidemics in Sydney 1788–1900. Times of Crisis* (Sydney: 1985), 137.
36. I. Hay, *The Caring Commodity. The Provision of Health Care in New Zealand* (Auckland: 1989), 41.
37. Maclean, *op. cit.* (note 13), 16.
38. *Ibid.*, 20.
39. See S. Garton, 'Sir Charles Mackellar: Psychiatry, Eugenics and Child Welfare in New South Wales, 1900–1914', *Historical Studies,* 2, 86 (1986), 21–34.
40. Garton, *op. cit.* (note 12), 105; see also M. Lewis, Lewis, 'The "Health of the Race"', and Infant Welfare in New South Wales: Perspectives on Medicine and Empire', *Disease, Medicine and Empire,* 304.
41. Mein Smith, *op. cit.* (note 3), 60; W. Selby, 'Maternity Hospitals and Baby Clinics', *Fevers and Frontiers,* 203.
42. Lewis, *op. cit.* (note 2), 4.
43. P. Mein Smith, 'Truby King in Australia', *NZJH,* 22, 1 (1988).

23–43; see also E. Olssen, 'Truby King and the Plunket Society: An Analysis of a Prescriptive Ideology', *NZJH,* 15, 1 (1981), 3–23.

44. Mein Smith, *op. cit.* (note 3), 97.
45. See F. T. King, *From the Pen of F. Truby King,* R. F. Snowden and H. Deem (eds), (Auckland: 1951).
46. Mein Smith, *op. cit.* (note 3), 112–14.
47. Moral clauses were still generally a part of social policy. This scheme was possibly inspired by that in Huddersfield, England, see D. Dwork, *War is Good for Babies and Other Young Children. A History of the Infant and Child Welfare Movement in England 1898–1918* (London & New York: 1987), 137.
48. Lewis, 'The "Health of the Race"', *Disease, Medicine and Empire,* 308.
49. M. Roe, *Nine Australian Progressives: Vitalism and Bourgeois Social Thought 1890–1960* (Queensland: 1984), 98; Gandevia, *op. cit.* (note 20), 71.
50. G. Gray, *Federalism and Health Policy. The Development of Health Systems in Canada and Australia* (Toronto: 1991), 60–1; M. Tennant, '"Missionaries of health": The School Medical Service During the Inter-war Period', *A Healthy Country,* 128–48.
51. Mein Smith, *op. cit.* (note 3), 141.
52. P. Baker, *King and Country Call. New Zealanders, Conscription and the Great War* (Auckland: 1988), 224; J. M. Winter, *The Great War and the British People* (Basingstoke: 1985), 55–9.
53. Bryder, *op. cit.* (note 9), 109–127.
54. Walker, *op. cit.* (note 9), 439–61.
55. This was transferred to the Education Department in 1923.
56. Lewis, *op. cit.* (note 2), 9 & 10.
57. D. Denoon, with K. Dugan and L. Marshall, *Public Health in Papua New Guinea: Medical Possibility and Social Constraint 1884–1984* (Cambridge & New York: 1989), 43. Australia was given a League of Nations Mandate over New Guinea after the First World War; Papua had been an Australian colony since 1906 (and British since 1884).
58. M. Roe, 'The Establishment of the Australian Department of Health: its Background and Significance', *Historical Studies,* 17 (1976–77), 188–9.
59. *Ibid.,* 44.
60. Lewis, *op. cit.* (note 2), 11 and 12.
61. Roe, *op. cit.* (note 49), 128.
62. Lewis, *op. cit.* (note 2), 13.
63. J. Dewdney, 'The Australian Health Care System: An Overview', *Sociology of Health and Illness. Australian Readings,* G. M. Lupton, J. M. Najman (eds), (Melbourne: 1989), 72–3; Thame, *op. cit.* (note 1), iv.
64. M. J. Thearle, 'Dr Alfred Jefferis Turner - "A Man before His

Time"', *Patients, Practitioners and Techniques,* 100; Selby, *op. cit.* (note 41), 197–212.

65. *Ibid.,* 198.
66. Olssen, *op. cit.* (note 43), 11.
67. See A. H. McKegg, '"Ministering Angels". The Government Backblock Nursing Service and the Maori Health Nurses, 1909–1939' (unpublished MA thesis, Auckland, 1991).
68. P. Davis, 'Jurisdictional Disputes in New Zealand Dentistry: Controlling Access to the Mouth and Entry to the Market', *A Healthy Country,* 26; T. W. H. Brooking, *A History of Dentistry in New Zealand,* (Dunedin: 1980), 102–6.
69. On Britain, see J. Lewis, *The Politics of Motherhood . Child and Maternal Welfare in England, 1900–1939* (London: 1980).
70. Lewis, *op. cit.* (note 2), 14.
71. See P. Mein Smith, *Maternity in Dispute, New Zealand 1920–35,* (Wellington: 1986).
72. M. Lewis, 'Doctors, Midwives, Puerperal Infection', *Occasional Papers on Medical History Australia,* H. Attwood, F. Forster and B. Gandevia (eds), (Melbourne: 1984), 98. E. Hanson, *The Politics of Social Security: The 1938 Act and Some Later Developments* (Auckland: 1980).
73. Lewis, *op. cit.* (note 72), 98.
74. MacLeod, 'Introduction', *op. cit.* (note 16), 9.
75. *Ibid.,* 9. This chapter does not explore the health of the indigenous population of Papua New Guinea, but for an excellent account of the history of its public health care, see Denoon, *Public Health in Papua New Guinea;* see also A. J. Radford, 'Papua New Guinea's Barefoot Doctors', *Patients, Practitioners and Techniques,* 115–28.
76. Originally stated in relation to the Maori population of New Zealand by Dr Isaac Featherston, Superintendent of Wellington Province in 1856, it was often quoted subsequently; see I. Pool, *The Maori Population of New Zealand 1769–1971* (Auckland: 1976), 191; see also Archdeacon Walsh, 'The Passing of the Maori: An Inquiry into the Principal Causes of the Decay of the Race', *Transactions and Proceedings of the New Zealand Institute,* 40 (1907), 154–75; R. Lange, 'The Revival of a Dying Race: a Study of Maori Health Reform, 1900–1918, and its Nineteenth Century Background', (unpublished MA thesis, Auckland University, 1972).
77. *The Queenslander,* 4 September, 1880, 306, quoted in S. Stone, *Aborigines in White Australia. A Documentary History of the Attitudes Affecting Official Policy and the Australian Aborigine 1697–1973* (Victoria & London: 1974), 96. See also H. Reynolds, *With the White People. The Crucial Role of Aborigines in the Exploration and Development of Australia* (Victoria: 1990), 127.
78. 'Aborigines', *Australians 1888,* G. Davison, J. W. McCarty and A. McLeary (eds), (New South Wales: 1987), 129–30.

79. A. Markus, 'Aborigines: Under the Act', *Australians 1938,* B. Gammage and P. Spearritt (eds), (New South Wales: 1987), 47.
80. *Historical Records of New South Wales,* (Government Printer, 1897), Vol.1, Part 2, 308, cited in Stone, *op. cit.* (note 77), 24.
81. F. L. Jones, *The Structure and Growth of Australia's Aboriginal Population,* (Canberra: 1970); H. Middleton, 'Aborigines', *Australian Society, A Sociological Introduction,* A. F. Davies, S. Encel and M. J. Berry (eds), third edn, (Victoria: 1977), 365.
82. Middleton, *op. cit.* (note 81), 365,
83. A. Gray, P. Trompf and S. Houston, 'The Decline and Rise of Aboriginal Families', *The Health of Aboriginal Australia.* J. Reid and P. Trompf (eds), (Sydney: 1991), 93.
84. A. Markus, *op. cit.* (note 79), 52.
85. Reynolds, *op. cit.* (note 77), 154; M. Franklin and I. White, 'The History and Politics of Aboriginal Health', *The Health of Aboriginal Australia,* 10–18.
86. T. Rowse, 'Aboriginal Australians: The Centre: A Limited Colonisation', *Australians from 1939,* A. Curthoys, A. W. Martin and T. Rowse (eds), (New South Wales: 1987), 151.
87. Franklin & White, *op. cit.* (note 85), 22.
88. S. Saggers and D. Gray, 'Policy and Practice in Aboriginal Health', in *The Health of Aboriginal Australia,* 389.
89. E. G. Whitlam, *Commonwealth Parliamentary Debates,* 1968, quoted in *Aborigines in White Australia,* 213. See also Senator Keefe, *Commonwealth Parliamentary Debates,* 4 November 1970, quoted in *Aborigines in White Australia,* 226; Dr H. C. Coombes, Chairman of the Commonwealth Office of Aboriginal Affairs, 'Aboriginal Health 1969', *Aborigines in White Australia,* 216–7; Middleton, *op. cit.* (note 81), 375.
90. Saggers & Gray, *op. cit.* (note 88), 389.
91. See G. Cowlishaw, *Black, White or Brindle. Race in Rural Australia* (Cambridge: 1988), 188; Franklin & White, *op. cit.* (note 85), 30, 31.
92. See, for example, *Body, Land and Spirit. Health and Healing in Aboriginal Society,* J. Reid (ed.), (Queensland: 1982), 8, 10, 11, 15, 22, 31.
93. J. Powles, 'Keeping the Doctor Away', Burgmann & Lee (eds), *op. cit.* (note 21), 84.
94. MacLeod, 'Introduction', *op. cit.* (note 16), 9.
95. H. B. Turbott, *Tuberculosis in the Maori, East Coast, New Zealand,* (Wellington: 1935).
96. I. Pool, *Te Iwi Maori. A New Zealand Population Past, Present and Projected* (Auckland: 1991), 133–214.
97. See E.W. Pomare, *Maori Standards of Health. A study of the 20 Year Period 1955–1975,* Medical Research Council of New Zealand, Special Report Series No.7 (Wellington: 1980); E.W. Pomare and G. M. de Boer, *Hauora, Maori Standards of Health. A Study of the Years 1970–1984,* Medical Research Council of New Zealand, Special

Report Series 78, (Wellington: 1988).

98. Franklin & White, *op. cit.* (note 85), 27–33; G. Salmond and J. V. Hodge, in Pomare and de Boer, *op. cit.* (note 97), 'Foreword'.

9

Crisis and Contradiction in India's Public Health

David Arnold

The origins of public health, whether in India or anywhere else, raise a number of questions not just about the relationship between disease and medical or administrative responses but also about the relationship between the state and the people. Who, for instance, decides what constitutes 'the public' and where its health needs and priorities lie? Are public health systems imposed by the state, or do they in effect emerge as a result of pressure from below, in response to the needs and demands of the community itself? What kinds of crises – whether social, political or epidemiological in nature – precipitate the formation of a system of public health, or bring about its reform and reconstruction?

These may be issues that concern scholars who investigate the rise and growth of public health systems in Western societies; but in colonial India, where the cultural, social and political gap between the rulers and the ruled was exceptionally wide and enduring, they have an additional significance. In a country where the institutional legacies of colonialism have been profound and long-lasting, the origins and orientation of public health are matters of more than simply historical interest.

Although other causes have undoubtedly contributed to the many problems that confront the health services in India today, such as the extent of poverty and under-nutrition and rapid demographic growth, one influential factor often cited even now, more than 40 years after Independence, is the misfit between a colonially-derived model of public health and the actual health needs of the mass of the population.

One way of trying to understand the contradictory elements in Indian public health today is thus to examine the historical context in which the system emerged under colonialism and in particular to identify those moments of crisis which helped to shape its character. If a series of epidemiological and political crises provided the dynamics of change, then the underlying contradictions between state priorities and public needs also help to explain the restricted or distorted nature of the policies and practices that followed.

Health and Medicine under Colonial Rule

On the face of it the history of public health in India has many similarities and parallels with that of Britain itself. As a colonial territory, ideas of public health and state medicine moved quickly from Britain to India, and with a medical élite (the Indian Medical Service) trained and recruited in Britain, it is not surprising that India's public health measures were often directly derived from British precedents. From the introduction of vaccination against smallpox (taken up by the colonial health authorities in India within a decade of Jenner's discovery), through the dispensary movement of the mid nineteenth century to the vaccination and contagious diseases acts, sanitation, water and sewage schemes, factory acts and municipal health legislation of the latter part of the century, British India appeared to follow closely the approved metropolitan mode .

But India was not Britain, and both the forms and functions of public health often differed significantly from British precedents. There have been various, often conflicting, explanations why this was so. It has sometimes been argued that colonial rule and the colonial economy actively contributed to India's health problems (by impoverishing the rural population or exposing it to harmful environmental changes), while doing little to protect or improve the people's health in return. Contrary to the claims made on behalf of British rule, it has been asserted that the colonial state failed to promote sanitation and public health in India during the nineteenth century because it was basically unconcerned about the well-being of its Indian subjects. The colonial regime was preoccupied with the economic exploitation and control of Indian trade, land and labour, and, so long as these yielded reasonably returns, there was no incentive to invest in the people's health and material welfare. A *laissez-faire* philosophy of government, still influential in India on the eve of the First World War, seemingly condoned a very limited view of the state's obligations towards its subjects even when in the second half of the nineteenth-century they were racked by famine and swept by successive epidemics of smallpox, cholera, malaria and plague.[1]

It has been said that before about 1900 the colonial regime felt directly responsible only for the health of the army (especially for its large European contingent) and for white officials and residents. It was the perceived task of the state and its doctors to make India 'liveable for the British', not to attend to the health needs of the population. Only in this small white 'enclave sector', Radhika Ramasubban has suggested, did the 'colonial mode of health care ... keep pace with metropolitan developments in sanitary and medical science'. Health provisions of the kind to be found in Britain's municipal acts were applied only to Indian cantonments (military stations) and adjacent bazaars, while the rest even of the urban population was largely ignored. According to Ramasubban, the country 'missed going through the period of sanitary reform which swept through most of Europe in the nineteenth and twentieth centuries', and 'Colonial health policy never really came to grips with the problem of public health in India.' The virtual absence of an effective public health system before 1900, and its slow, faltering growth thereafter, is thus directly attributed to the self-interested and 'enclavist' nature of colonial rule.[2]

It is not hard to find in colonial, and even post-colonial, writers a riposte to this argument which shifts the burden of responsibility from the British and on to the Indian population itself. Some writers have taken the view that the hazardous nature of India's disease environment was something intrinsic to such a poor and populous society and owed little to the impact of colonialism. On the contrary, the effects of British rule were broadly beneficial, resulting in improved material conditions and economic opportunities, and even eventually freeing India from the curse of famine.[3] Hugh Tinker, in his account of local self-government in South Asia written in the 1950s, is certainly not uncritical of many aspects of colonial health policy and administration, but he sees Indians as contributing in no small measure to their own misery by obstructing or ignoring well-intentioned British attempts to improve municipal health and welfare. In India, Tinker remarks, 'the public was not much interested in the promotion of public works and sanitation'. 'Unfamiliar western methods seemed to be opposed to all the teachings of religion and custom', and, in consequence, 'public health services developed only because officials fostered them. Almost the whole range of municipal services was evolved in response to pressure from British officials rather than as a result of the desires of the people'. He sees the 'barrier of custom' as standing in the way of the wholesale adoption of health care and sanitation and Asian cultural beliefs and social attitudes forming an almost insurmountable obstacle to Western innovation. There was, in his view, a 'lack of harmony between [Indian] social habits and the techniques of the West'. Tinker also cites some more specific factors to explain the backward state of public health in South Asia by the time of Independence.

He points, for instance, to the distraction of nationalist politics in the 1920s and 1930s, which turned municipal councils and big-city corporations into political battlegrounds to the apparent neglect of more practical matters like sanitation and sewage disposal. Indian inefficiency and nepotism are also invoked.[4] To be sure, Tinker does not go as far in this direction as many colonial writers who took the view that Indians were so sunk in 'ignorance, apathy and prejudice' that only an authoritarian sanitary regime under direct European supervision – or a very slow and arduous process of educating Indian opinion in 'modern ideas of sanitation' – would bring about the necessary change in Indian attitudes and behaviour.[5] Nonetheless, his argument still hinges heavily upon India's failure rather than Britain's culpable unconcern.

Was, then, the development of a more extensive system of public health in India before 1900, or even 1947 (the year of India's independence), undermined by indigenous opposition and disinterest or was it sabotaged by colonial neglect and blinkered self-interest? Was there, indeed, a fatal combination of the two which thwarted the emergence of a more effective and publicly acceptable health system?

Military Medicine

Ramasubban and other nationalist or left-wing critics are surely right to stress the restricted nature of colonial health interests, especially in the period before 1900, but the point cannot be accepted without qualification. The connection between the military and medicine was an intimate and long-standing one in India, as it was in many other parts of the colonial world, and this provided a very different basis for the development of health services than in Britain. In part this was a reflection of the powerful position occupied by the army in colonial society compared with its more marginal and politically circumscribed role in post-Cromwellian Britain. The first responsibility of the Indian Medical Service, the origins of which lay in mid-eighteenth-century Bengal, was to provide professional medical assistance for the armies of the English East India Company. With the take-over of the Company by the Crown following the Mutiny and Rebellion of 1857–8, the IMS was entrusted with the health of the Indian Army while soldiers of the British Army stationed in India were placed under the Army Medical Department (later the Royal Army Medical Corps). In peacetime, IMS officers were employed in a wide range of civilian as well as military duties: they ran hospitals, supervised jails, presided over provincial sanitation and vaccination departments. In times of war, however, the army again took priority and many IMS officers were drafted back to military duties.[6]

The military connection had far-reaching consequences for the nature of state medicine and public health in India. For much of the nineteenth century the army (along with the jails) was the primary site of clinical observation and for the collection of statistics on morbidity and mortality (William Farr's work as Registrar-General in London was an influential model here). At a time when Indian society was largely inaccessible to Western medical scrutiny, the army served as an observation post and a laboratory for medical ideas and techniques which might subsequently be expanded to embrace civilian society. The primacy of military medicine was further emphasized by the extent to which for most of the nineteenth century Western medicine in India remained a state preserve. Apart from the limited inroads of missionary medicine, an independent medical profession (whether European or Indian in composition) was slow to develop outside of a few major cities like Calcutta and Bombay. The active survival of indigenous medicine, ranging from various forms of folk practice to the complex systems of Ayurveda and Yunani, restricted the demand for Western medicine and limited the scope for a rival medical profession. Considering the perceived importance of the military to British rule in India, the size of the army (approximately a quarter of a million men by the 1830s, roughly 40,000 of whom were Europeans) and the military responsibilities of the IMS, it is not surprising that there was such a strong emphasis upon the health of the army and its white soldiery.

The Cholera Crisis

It was against this background that the first major crisis of public health occurred in the middle years of the nineteenth century. In a sense it was not a 'public' health crisis at all, but a crisis of health within the colonial order and specific to the army itself. The proximate cause was cholera, though the disease had appeared many times in epidemic form over the previous 40 years and had caused tens of thousands of civilian deaths without provoking a comparable crisis. As the statistical record of army sickness and death grew from decade to decade there was accumulating evidence of the heavy mortality caused by cholera, especially among European soldiers and their families: between 1818 and 1854 more than 8,500 British soldiers reportedly died of the disease in India. The cholera problem swelled to crisis proportions in 1861 with a fresh outbreak of the disease in northern India: nearly two thousand British soldiers, their wives and children were attacked, and of these 64 per cent perished. In one cantonment alone (Mian Mir just outside Lahore) a third of the 2,452 soldiers and their families were struck by cholera and 61 per cent of them died. The shock of this mortality (declared by the investigating committee to have had few parallels 'in modern times and among civilised men') was enhanced by the severe attrition of cholera mortality experienced by the army during the recent Mutiny campaigns and by the increased reliance upon British troops in the aftermath of revolt. That Indian soldiers suffered proportionately far fewer casualties (probably due to differences in housing and messing) only added further weight to alarm over European vulnerability.[7]

Even before the epidemic of 1861 had struck, high mortality among British troops had caused concern in India and London. A parliamentary commission was appointed in 1859, partly as a result of vigorous lobbying by Florence Nightingale, to enquire into the Sanitary State of the Army in India. Farr was one of its members. Significantly the commission did not visit India, but it took evidence from several 'old India hands', notably James Ranald Martin, until recently an East India Company surgeon in Calcutta. The transference of India from the Company to the Crown in 1858 strengthened administrative ties with London and left India more exposed to metropolitan scrutiny but not all the reforming influences came directly from London. Ideas of 'public health', 'sanitary reform' and 'state medicine' were in the air in India in the 1850s and 1860s, and held out the possibility of a system of state medicine that was not confined to the army alone. Some medical officers were beginning to regard improved public health as one of the basic duties of a civilized government; others, more pragmatically, stressed the benefits to the state of presiding over a healthier and hence more productive population. In a work outwardly concerned only with European health, J. R. Martin, taking his inspiration from Farr, called for a system of 'state medicine' that would, firstly

> ... direct public attention to the increased security of life and property, which must result from a sustained and organised investigation, by competent persons, of all those agencies and circumstances, moral and physical, which deteriorate, through local or general influences, the public health.

and which, secondly, would

> ... disseminate knowledge amongst all classes of the community, on the most obvious and well-ascertained causes of injury to public

> health, and ... the most effective and economical measures of sanitary improvement, both in town and country.[8]

When the Sanitary Commission reported in 1863, though it gave priority to improving the health of soldiers, it also maintained that Britain had certain moral and sanitary obligations to the people of India and anyway accepted that measures intended to protect the health of soldiers, if they were to be effective, could not simply stop short at the barrack gates.[9] The commission called for major improvements in civilian as well as military health, and in 1864, following further prompting from London, sanitary commissioners were duly appointed to each major province of British India. Technically, this was an important moment in the dawning of state responsibility for a wider, public health constituency. The success in reducing mortality among white soldiers over the next 20 years, partly as a result of sanitary measures recommended by the commission, was hailed not only as a triumph for military medicine but also as a demonstration of what could be done to transform civilian health as well.[10]

And yet, despite the enthusiasm of men like Martin, and several acts pertaining to public health introduced between the 1860s and the 1890s, there was an obvious reticence on the part of the government in India (as opposed to Parliament or the India Office in London) to implement such far-ranging proposals and pursue a more energetic health policy. As the form and content of the sanitary commissioners' annual reports aptly reveal, the health of the army remained the greatest priority, while the commissioners were denied the financial resources and technical staff that would have enabled them to develop a more effective public health administration.[11]

Adherence to an ideology of *laissez-faire* only partly explains this bureaucratic inertia, though it superficially accounts for opposition to such pivotal measures as quarantines and sanitary cordons. More influential were, firstly, the parsimony of the colonial state when it came to matters relating to Indian welfare and, secondly, the state's political 'reading' of public health and its reception by Indian society. In the aftermath of the Mutiny of 1857 the British were wary of provoking fresh waves of resistance and it was felt that interventionist sanitary and medical measures were likely to offend one section or other of the Indian population. Despite the great mortality it continued to cause, and despite pressure from other European powers to do more to control the disease in its country of origin, attitudes towards epidemic cholera as it affected the civilian population of India, were notably cautious and voluntaristic, partly because cholera epidemics had come to be closely identified with Hindu fairs and pilgrimages.[12] It could be said that the colonial state was unduly sensitive to the possibility of a political and cultural backlash and that its caution and conservatism were simply a front for its basic unwillingness to spend any of the profits of empire on Indian health. But the readiness to 'Orientalize', to see India as a time-bound, caste-ridden society, innately opposed to all rationality and progress, was itself a powerful ideological block to a more interventionist policy.

In some respects the limited progress made in public health in the second half of the nineteenth century suggest that one could push the idea of a medical 'enclave' rather further than Ramasubban does. As medical ideas and sanitary practices developed during the course of the century, especially as the germ theory of disease gained gradual acceptance, immense efforts were made to isolate cantonments from their surrounding environment and transform them into sanitary havens or 'oases'. State medicine was called upon to police the boundary between military and civilian society, and the military motivation behind even many notionally public health measures is readily apparent. One of the earliest pieces of medical legislation in India, the Contagious Diseases Act of 1866 (modelled on similar legislation in Britain), authorized the setting-up of lock hospitals to inspect and treat Indian prostitutes infected with venereal diseases. But this was solely intended to protect the health of British soldiers: the act did not address the considerable (and growing) problem of venereal disease among the civilians.[13] Again, one of the first uses of the provincial and India-wide Vaccination Acts of the 1870s and 1880s was to protect cantonments from the fearful scourge of smallpox. Only gradually were the acts extended to cover other urban and, eventually, rural localities: as late as 1946 primary vaccination was compulsory in no more than 81 per cent of the towns and cities of India and 62 per cent of rural circles.[14] Although never the subject of similar 'public health' measures, typhoid was another disease that figured prominently in the military medicine of the late nineteenth century. It was identified as a major cause of death among young white soldiers, but for several decades was thought to be a disease to which Indians were largely immune. In this case, too, intensive medical and sanitary measures, including anti-typhoid inoculations, were used specifically to protect British soldiers.[15]

The narrow focus on soldiers' health thus resulted in a series of localized, disease-specific measures designed to keep disease away from the army rather than to tackle the health problems of a wider civilian constituency. As the main site of state medical enquiry and practice, the army directed attention to diseases like cholera, typhoid, and syphilis which seemed most menacing to the health of the army, though these were not necessarily the most important causes of civilian ill-health and mortality. Further, the army, was essentially an adult male constituency (though the wives and children of many Indian and some European soldiers lived with them in the cantonments), and this encouraged a neglect of health problems and disorders more characteristic of female and infant populations, just as the IMS, until partly supplemented by the Women's Medical Service in 1914, consisted entirely of male medical practitioners. The male/adult bias evident in colonial medicine, exacerbated by those social, cultural and environmental factors which anyway discriminate against the health of women and children in India, has remained a characteristic feature of the country's public health administration.

The Plague Crisis

In the summer of 1896 an epidemic of bubonic plague erupted in the city of Bombay and within 12 years had spread to large areas of western and northern India, causing a mortality of at least six million people. The plague epidemic of the 1890s and early 1900s represented a second major crisis in the history of Indian public health.[16] Like the cholera crisis 40 years earlier, British control over India was a critical underlying issue. On this occasion, however, the health of the army was not at risk, and there were remarkably few plague cases and deaths among British and Indian soldiers. The significance of the army on this occasion was not as privileged victim, nor model sanitary enclave, but as an *ad hoc* agency for enforcing unpopular health measures, such as house searches and the compulsory hospitalization of the sick. The use of the army in this coercive role was short-lived in India, partly because it was the source of such bitter resentment, but it remained a familiar feature of public health campaigns in other parts of the colonial world.[17]

Instead of the army, the plague crisis centred around an unprecedented degree of state medical and sanitary intervention, triggered by fears that the commercial, industrial and administrative life of major cities like Bombay and Calcutta would be paralysed and that India's export economy would be crippled by international embargoes on its goods. The 1890s was also a period of new-found confidence in the capacity of medical and sanitary science to defeat an 'invading' disease. If the cholera crisis of the mid nineteenth century was an occasion for the partial or attempted introduction into India of sanitary and public health ideas that were gaining ground in Britain at the time, the plague episode 40 years later registered the emergence of a new and more assertive form of 'tropical medicine'. This scientific assertiveness found administrative force and legislative form in the far-reaching powers arrogated by the state under the Epidemic Diseases Act of 1897, only to be swiftly countered by a wave of Indian hostility and resistance, amounting at times to a violent confrontation between the state and the people. The state's lack of sanitary preparedness was exacerbated by the technical ineptitude and cultural insensitivity of many of the measures employed, some of which served more to spread the plague than to curb it. The strength of the public reaction was provoked by the brusqueness of the state's sanitary policy and the general failure to consult Indians over measures, like house-searches, that trespassed on their homes and privacy, or, like post-mortems, were culturally repugnant. Having at first suspended the policy of caution it had long followed towards epidemic cholera, the Government of India soon saw in the upsurge of public hostility to its anti-plague measures a persuasive case for urgently returning to a more accommodating and culturally circumspect approach.[18]

The plague epidemic has, however, also been seen as causing a significant advance in the development of public health in India. Arguably it was plague in the 1890s, rather than (as in Britain) the earlier epidemics of cholera, which prompted the state to at last take on practical responsibility for public health, and which, indeed, made the public more receptive to the very idea of public health. The inadequacy of existing sanitary services and the failure to respond effectively to the epidemiological crisis, was highlighted by the findings of the Plague Commission in 1904, and acknowledged in the Government of India's sanitary resolution of 1912. As a result, provincial governments strengthened their staff of trained sanitary officers while the Government of India set up a Medical Research Department and promoted a series of state-funded laboratories to conduct bacteriological research and prepare vaccines for public use. India, previously something of a backwater in terms of research in bacteriology and parasitology, was brought into line with recent advances in Europe. The sanitary resolution of 1912 was thus seen as 'the first concrete step' taken by the government to ensure that 'an effective machinery was provided to look into the sanitary problems [of the country] and to take preventive measures against the spread of disease'.[19] But, significantly, the emphasis was still upon curative rather than preventive medicine, and the creation of prestigious institutes in remote places like Kasauli and Coonoor directed the attention of the IMS towards the rewards of laboratory research and led it still further away from the street-level needs and practicalities of public health.

No less contradictory in its effects was the manner in which part of the responsibility for public health was transferred to municipal councils and district boards. This move was initiated more than a decade before the plague epidemic, in the early 1880s, by the Liberal Viceroy, Lord Ripon, who sought to give Indians a greater share in running their own affairs through greater representation and influence in local government. In practice, however, shifting responsibility to local boards seemed to reflect the low priority the state attached to public health, for they were poorly provided with the sanitary staff and medical expertise required to carry out their allotted tasks. Elected councillors were seldom willing to court unpopularity among rate-payers by raising taxes for costly health and sanitation schemes, even if they were convinced (and many were not) that these were desirable. Indeed, India's merchant, trading and landlord classes were among those most opposed, whether on cultural or financial grounds, to the expansion of public health. Over all, the attempted liberalization of local government seemed to show the limited utility of the British model of urban government and municipal health for India, especially when small towns were expected to cope with massive problems of sanitation, intensified by the plague epidemic of the 1890s and 1900s, without adequate financial resources and administrative powers, and when nine-tenths of the people lived in the countryside, far away from the facilities of urban hospitals, doctors and dispensaries.

A similar delegation of responsibility for public health was made under the Government of India Act of 1919. In this latest round of constitutional reform elected Indian ministers in the provinces were given charge of health and local government while control of finance remained in the hands of British civil servants. Again there was a conflict between a formal commitment to public health, seemingly restated by retitling the former sanitary commissioners as directors of public health, and the powers and resources actually at the disposal of health ministers and their directors.[20] Only with the advent of 'provincial autonomy' in 1937, barely ten years before Independence, were Indian ministers in a position to control provincial budgets and, if they chose to do so, divert a more substantial share of public funds to health programmes. The low priority given by the colonial regime to public health (as opposed to 'law and order', the security of the army, and the extraction of revenue) helped to create a political and administrative environment that was unconducive to the development of a more effective, publicly responsive health system.

Health and Hegemony

It is ironic, in view of this general record of colonial neglect, that medicine and sanitation occupied such a prominent place in the colonial rhetoric of the nineteenth and early twentieth centuries. Promoting health and curbing disease were goals repeatedly presented as part of Britain's larger imperial purpose in India, just as they were integral to the colonial denunciation of Indian society as backward and primitive. Far from being some kind of neutral or objective statement of scientific ideas, the health rhetoric of the period articulated many of the deepest assumptions and most hegemonic ambitions of colonial rule. Medicine and public health were seen as clear and indisputable evidence of Britain's humanitarian and benevolent intentions towards a benighted India, proof of the practical superiority of Western civilization over India's arcane social order.

In a speech he made in 1899, the Viceroy of the day, Lord Curzon, confidently asserted that the British had come to India not only as conquerors but also as benefactors, bringing the gift of their religion, law, literature and science with them. There might, he conceded, be some who questioned the benefits of Britain's laws and religion, but about science – especially medical science – 'no two opinions can possibly be entertained'. Medicine alone, he claimed, was justification enough for British rule.

> For what [he asked] is this medical science we bring you? It is no mere collection of pragmatical experimental rules. It is built on the bed-rock of pure, irrefutable science; it is a boon which is offered to all, rich and poor, Hindu and Mahommedan, woman and man. It lifts the purdah without irreverence. So far as I know, it is the only dissolvent which breaks down the barriers of caste without sacrilege. Medical science, indeed, is the most cosmopolitan of all sciences because it embraces in its merciful appeal every suffering human being in the world.[21]

Despite Curzon's proud boast, there was a great gulf between colonial rhetoric and reality, between what Western medicine and public health might promise and what it actually delivered to the people of India. The British were in the paradoxical position of needing to project an image of Indian backwardness and resistance to bolster their claims to imperial authority while at the same time freeing themselves from actual responsibility for the chronic state of Indian ill health. This is not to deny that there was opposition to Western medicine in India – indeed it was a more critical part of the unfolding history of Indian public health than writers like Ramasubban have allowed – but to stress the excessive importance it assumed in colonial ideology and administrative practice. However, whether state medicine and indigenous concepts of health and healing should be represented in such crudely oppositional terms – as they commonly were in Curzon's day and as they appear in Tinker's account – is questionable. It is clear, for instance, that there was a two-way traffic between Western and indigenous medical ideas and practice, particularly through the European investigation of India's rich *materia medica* and the infiltration of Western concepts and therapies into the Ayurvedic and Yunani systems. What is clear, though, is that the distance between Western and indigenous medicine, already large during the early phase of colonial rule, grew greater as the nineteenth century progressed, as Western medicine shed the humoural pathology that continued to characterize the indigenous systems and became more convinced of its unique rationality and therapeutic powers. Viewed from the other side, however, the methods and ambitions of state medicine could appear particularly disturbing and intrusive.

For instance, the indigenous practice of variolation (smallpox inoculation) was widespread in many parts of India in the early nineteenth century, especially in Bengal where as many as 70 per cent of the population may have been inoculated in childhood. Although usually performed by an itinerant specialist (a *tikadar* or 'markmaker'), the practice of variolation and the dietary and social precautions that accompanied it involved a degree of mutual cooperation among families or whole villages. Through long usage it had become a trusted and culturally acceptable prophylaxis. It was, in effect, a form of community medicine, dependent upon local participation and support, not state supervision or control. The British, however, reversed this situation by seeking to outlaw variolation (as an obsolete and dangerous practice) and substituting state-funded vaccination. Quite apart from doubts about the efficacy of vaccination compared to variolation, this change caused religious offence, aroused suspicion about the state's motives in wanting to put its 'mark' upon the people, and produced evasion and even conflict whenever state vaccinators arrived in a village and began searching for children to vaccinate. Only gradually, and partly through the exercise of sheer coercive power, did the British succeed in replacing variolation with vaccination.[22]

Opposition of the kind encountered by state vaccination during the nineteenth century encouraged the government and its medical practitioners to believe that improvements in public health could only come about as a result of their activity and not as a result of any indigenous initiatives. However, by the end of the century public health was becoming a significant factor in indigenous networks of power and in the emerging struggle for political authority in India. In a style of philanthropy that went back far beyond the advent of colonial rule, Indian princes and commercial magnates became patrons of medical institutions, in some instances donating considerable sums of money to establish dispensaries, hospital and medical schools. The Calcutta School of Hygiene and Tropical Medicine which opened in 1922 owed a large part of its funding to donations from Indian princes, landlords and businessmen (as well as European entrepreneurs and business houses).[23] Long used as assistant surgeons, apothecaries and vaccinators, Indians were also becoming active in medical research and administration by the 1920s and 1930s and beginning to breach the racially exclusive preserve of the IMS.[24]

Elite patronage and professional participation were not the only Indian responses. From the 1890s onwards there also developed a vigorous political critique of colonial public health policies and practices, a critique which reversed the old Orientalist shibboleths about Indian fatalism, superstition and inertia and instead attacked the colonialists for failing to do enough to tackle the urgent health needs of the country. This critique came mainly from the growing forces of middle-class nationalists, who through the press, public platforms, local boards and legislatures, called for medical and public health facilities to be made freely available to the people of India. But even within the ranks of the middle classes there were divergent trends. One feature of the period from the 1890s onwards was a revival of the traditional systems of Ayurvedic and Yunani medicine, in part in conscious reaction to the cultural imperialism of colonial rule, in part because they (like homeopathy, a flourishing European importation that quickly became naturalized in India) represented a more culturally sympathetic and holistic approach to the body and its ills. Although the IMS was most unwilling to make any compromise with indigenous medicine, whose claims it had so long disputed, political pressure eventually forced provincial governments to give some recognition to the practitioners of Ayurvedic and Yunani medicine, though without allowing them to undermine the dominance Western medicine had established for itself.[25] A more genuinely pluralistic system of state medicine and public health might have better reflected the cultural diversity of India and helped to compensate for the deficiencies of Western medicine, with its élitism, and its strong urban, curative and technological bias. Governments in India since Independence have carried the compromise with indigenous medicine rather further than the British did, but the lion's share of state funding in India still goes to 'allopathic' medicine.

Another example of the varied paths public health might have travelled in India is M. K. Gandhi's rejection of Western medicine and his desire for a form of health care in keeping with the needs, resources and traditions of the Indian people. Gandhi's views were most forcefully expressed in his tract *Hind Swaraj*, written in 1909, which saw the study and pursuit of European medicine as part of India's slavish dependence on the decadent civilization of the West, castigated hospitals as 'institutions for propagating sin', and portrayed doctors as individuals with private profit rather than public welfare uppermost in their minds. In his view Western medicine encouraged self-indulgence and vice; it tempted Indians to neglect the care of their own bodies through self-discipline and moral restraint.[26] Gandhi's hostility to Western medicine was sharpened by its close association with the power of the state. He wanted responsibility for health to be given back to the individual and to the local community, decentralized to India's many thousands of villages. But Gandhi's voice did not prevail, and though since Independence the Government of India has tried periodically to develop community health programmes, these have failed to realize Gandhi's aims and have tended to remain a form of external imposition. By contrast, the main thrust of health policy has been to incorporate public health into government planning programmes along the lines of Soviet state socialism. Gandhi failed to break the dependence of public health on state power and the tendency to override local needs and initiatives.[27]

The Crisis of Legitimation

By the end of the Second World War, as colonial rule in India was tottering to its close, there were attempts to refashion the existing system of public health to tackle persisting health problems and to align the health services more closely with the needs of an independent nation state. Unlike those precipitated by cholera and plague in earlier times, this was not an epidemiological crisis, though mortality did rise sharply during the war as a result of the Bengal famine of 1943–4, high prices and shortages in India generally, and wartime disruption to the medical services. Rather this was a crisis of political legitimation, defining the positive contribution Western medicine had to make to the material progress of the new India and distancing the medical services from the failures of the colonial past. As the main nationalist party, the Congress prepared its own plans to revitalize India's public health after Independence, but the clearest expression of this crisis of legitimation was the Bhore Committee, which was set up in 1943 but reported only in 1946, a year before the British departure from India.

The Health Survey and Development Committee, headed by Sir Joseph Bhore and numbering senior medical officers as well as a few selected politicians among its members, criticized the poor record of public health in British India and demonstrated the urgency for a system of public health that was directed to meet the present and future needs of the Indian people rather than those of the dying colonial state. It clearly identified the nation as the health constituency that needed to be addressed. Health, it insisted, should be available to all members of the community 'irrespective of their ability to pay for it' and not confined to any privileged group. The Bhore Committee pointed out that the death rate in British India was nearly twice that in England and Wales in the 1930s; that infant mortality was almost three times as high; and that life expectation at birth was less than half what it was in England and Wales. The report was especially scathing about the poor state of maternal and infant health and estimated that maternal deaths alone amounted to 200,000 a year: 'any plan for improving the health of the community must pay special attention to the development of measures for adequate health protection to mothers and children'. It attributed India's massive health problems partly to a physical and sanitary environment that was unconducive to 'healthful living', but also severe deficiencies in the existing health services which it found 'altogether inadequate to meet the needs of the people'.[28] In the United Provinces, to cite an extreme instance, there were only 456 rural hospitals and dispensaries or one medical institution for every 105,626 people. Other provinces were better served, but even in the more favoured Madras there were 28,496 people for every urban hospital or dispensary and 42,672 for every rural one. In the whole of British India, there were only 47,400 Western-style doctors for a population of 300 million – one for every 6,300 people – and only 7,000 nurses and 5,000 trained midwives.[29] The report concluded that:

> the present low state of the public health in India is reflected in the wide prevalence of disease and the consequent high rates of mortality in the community as a whole and, in particular, among such vulnerable groups as children and women in the reproductive period. It is considered that at least 50 per cent. of the existing mortality in the country is preventable and should therefore be prevented.[30]

The task of redirecting India's health services to meet the needs of the people, and especially its more vulnerable or neglected sectors, was too massive for the departing colonial power to consider undertaking. Indeed, the report of the Bhore Committee reads like an epitaph for colonialism's imminent demise. It offered instead a blueprint for an expanded health service in an independent India: significantly, in this reaffirmation of Western medicine's continuing role in India, the report showed little sympathy for either indigenous medicine or a more Gandhian approach to health, but then India's independence, though long fought for and hard won, represented no more than a partial revolution in government and society. It was a 'transfer of power' from a departing British élite to an incoming Indian one, unaccompanied by any radical overhaul of existing institutions or even a major shift in attitudes and personnel. The Indians who took over from British medical officers in 1947 had served such a long period of colonial apprenticeship that 'their socialisation into the model of Western medicine was already complete'.[31] And in the years since Independence, the Government of India (like its neighbours and fellow successor states in Pakistan, Bangladesh and Sri Lanka) has had only limited success in resolving the contradictions inherent in the colonial health system.

In keeping with the aspirations of the time, India's new constitution declared its commitment to the task of eliminating 'poverty, ignorance and ill-health' and recognized improving health and nutrition as among the 'primary duties' of the state to its people.[32] It was perhaps only at this late stage that public health in India reached the position identified by George Rosen when he remarked that 'The protection and promotion of the health and welfare of its citizens is considered to be one of the most important functions of the modern state.'[33] But the Indian constitution failed to recognize health as a legally enforceable, 'fundamental' right. It also allowed responsibility for public health to be divided (much as it had been shared in colonial times between the central and provincial administrations) between the Government of India and the constituent states of the Indian Union. One result of this has been a lack of coordination over health policy between the Centre and the states, which for financial and political reasons of their own, have often failed to endorse initiatives and directives emanating from Delhi. This problem of divided responsibility was reflected in the failure shortly after Independence to introduce a 'model public health act' that would be acceptable to all the states. On the other hand, the Government of India has sometimes found it hard to maintain an appropriate and acceptable balance between state power and civil liberties. During Mrs Gandhi's Emergency of 1975–7 attempts to implement family planning objectives, especially through a vasectomy campaign, were coercive, even dictatorial. The reaction that followed was not very different from that provoked by the British anti-plague measures of the 1890s, and the part this played in Mrs Gandhi's fall from power in 1977 has perhaps made subsequent governments even more wary about embarking on similar medical and health crusades.[34]

While there has been a proliferation of specialist bodies at the Centre and special campaigns which have targeted particular diseases, there has been a reluctance to tackle the broad spectrum of ill health and its underlying socio-economic causes. Nevertheless, a more resolute political will and new technological resources brought some notable advances in public health in the first post-Independence decades, and these were duly reflected in the substantial fall in the death rate between the early 1950s and late 1970s. There were major campaigns against smallpox (launched in 1962 and supported by the World Health Organisation from 1966), against malaria (begun in 1953 and intensified in 1958), and filaria (1955). The smallpox eradication programme proved effective, but early success against malaria has been followed by a tragic resurgence of the disease. Levels of mortality among women and children still remain unacceptably high, while a host of fatal or incapacitating diseases continue to plague India and to cast doubt upon the government's ability to achieve its declared aim of 'health for all' in the foreseeable future.[35] The hospital-based, curative approach to health, inherited from the colonial period and powerfully entrenched among the medical élite has failed to meet the challenge of India's massive health needs, especially in rural areas and among the nation's poor. In 1980 a joint report drawn up by the Indian Council for Medical Research and the Indian Council for Social Science Research concluded that:

> The imported and inappropriate model of health services is top-heavy, over-centralised, heavily curative in its approach, urban and elite oriented, costly and dependency creating. The serious shortcomings of the model cannot be cured by small tinkerings or well-meant reform.[36]

And two years later, in 1982, the Government of India's own statement of 'National Health Policy' voiced similar reservations, admitting, in effect, that many of the fundamental problems of health in India in the 1980s remained not very different from those which had been described by the Bhore Committee 40 years earlier.[37]

Conclusion

Many (though by no means all) of the characteristics of the present-day system of public health in India can be traced back to the way in which the system developed under colonial rule. Geared to the priorities of the state rather than the needs of the people, and more a consequence of colonial imposition than of public demand, the Indian system of public health was slow to adapt itself to the country's own requirements. A series of crises, spaced 40 to 50 years apart, marked significant stages in the progression from a state-centred system of health focusing on the needs of the army, to a health system formally dedicated to serving the needs of an independent and developing nation. But, although other possible and arguably more suitable public health models have been available in India, the country remains formally attached to a system of public health that is all too remote from the mass of the population and appears inappropriate or irresponsive to their specific needs.

Notes

1. For example, Prafulla Chandra Ray, *Life and Experiences of a Bengali Chemist,* II (Calcutta: 1935), 137–55; Ira Klein, 'Malaria and mortality in Bengal, 1840–1921', *Indian Economic and Social History Review,* IX (1972), 132–60; *idem,* 'Death in India, 1871–1921', *Journal of Asian Studies,* XXXII (1973), 639–59; and for the general critique of colonialism, Rajani Palme Dutt, *India Today* (revised edn, Bombay: 1949).
2. Radhika Ramasubban, 'The Development of Health Policy in India', in Tim Dyson and Nigel Crook (eds), *India's Demography: Essays on the Contemporary Population* (New Delhi: 1984), *idem,* 'Imperial Health in British India, 1857–1900', in Roy MacLeod and Milton Lewis (eds), *Disease, Medicine, and Empire: Perspectives on Western Medicine and the Experience of European Expansion* (London: 1988), 38–60.
3. Notably, Morris D. Morris, 'Towards a Reinterpretation of Nineteenth-century Indian Economic History', *Journal of Economic History,* XXIII (1963), 608–18; Michelle Burge McAlpin, *Subject to Famine: Food Crises and Economic Change in Western India, 1860–1920* (Princeton: 1983).
4. Hugh Tinker, *The Foundations of Local Self-Government in India, Pakistan and Burma* (2nd edn, London: 1968), 73, 287–9.
5. Surgeon-Colonel R. Harvey, IMS, cited in A. E. Grant, *The Indian Manual of Hygiene,* I (Madras: 1894), ciii–civ.
6. The standard history of the IMS remains D. G. Crawford, *History of the Indian Medical Service, 1600–1913,* 2 vols (London: 1914).
7. *Report of the Commissioners Appointed to Inquire into the Cholera*

Epidemic of 1861 in Northern India (Calcutta: 1862), ii, 6, 248–50, 254.

8. James Ranald Martin, *The Influence of Tropical Climates on European Constitutions* (London: 1856), 103–4; cf. C. MacNamara, 'Remarks on Cholera', *Indian Medical Gazette,* I, (1866), 178.
9. *Royal Commission on the Sanitary State of the Army in India,* (C. 3184) (London: 1863).
10. Sir Joseph Fayrer, *On the Climate and Fevers of India* (London: 1882), 24.
11. For the modest achievements of the period, see *Report of the Health Survey and Development Committee,* I (Delhi: 1946), 23 (hereafter cited as Bhore Committee *Report*); John Chandler Hume Jr., 'Colonialism and Sanitary Medicine: The Development of Preventive Health Policy in the Punjab, 1860 to 1900', *Modern Asian Studies,* XX (1986), 703–24; A. E. Roberts, 'Public Health and Vital Statistics', in *The Imperial Gazetteer of India, Volume I: Descriptive* (revised edn, Oxford: 1908), 500–35.
12. David Arnold, 'Çholera and Colonialism in British India', *Past and Present,* 113 (1986), 118–51.
13. Kenneth Ballhatchet, *Race, Sex and Class under the Raj: Imperial Attitudes and Policies and Their Critics, 1793–1905* (London: 1980).
14. Bhore Committee *Report,* I, 110.
15. See the *Annual Report of the Sanitary Commissioner with the Government of India for 1890,* 33; *1894,* 31; *1910,* 10–15; *1913,* 5.
16. For an account of the epidemic see L. Fabian Hirst, *The Conquest of Plague: A Study of the Evolution of Epidemiology* (Oxford: 1953); *Report of the Indian Plague Commission* (Cd. 810), (London: 1902).
17. See J. J. McKelvey, *Man against Tsetse: Struggle for Africa* (Ithaca: 1973); Reynaldo C. Ileto, 'Cholera and the Origins of the American Sanitary Order in the Philippines', in David Arnold (ed.), *Imperial Medicine and Indigenous Societies* (Manchester: 1988), 125–48.
18. See David Arnold, 'Touching the Body: Perspectives on the Indian Plague, 1896–1900', in Ranajit Guha (ed.), *Subaltern Studies V* (Delhi: 1987), 55–90; I. J. Catanach, 'Plague and the Tensions of Empire: India, 1896–1918', in Arnold *op. cit.* (note 17), 149–71.
19. O. P. Jaggi, *History of Science. Technology and Medicine in India: Volume 14: Public Health and Its Administration* (Delhi: 1979), 113. See also the account of these institutes in Bhore Committee *Report,* I, 23–4, 176–8.
20. For a critical account of health provision during this period, see V. R. Muraleedharan, 'Rural Health Care in Madras Presidency, 1919–39', *Indian Economic and Social History Review,* XXIV (1987), 323–34.
21. *Indian Medical Gazette,* XXXIV (1899), 134.
22. David Arnold, 'Smallpox and Colonial Medicine in Nineteenth Century India', in Arnold *op. cit.* (note 17), 45–65.

23. *An Appeal on Behalf of the Calcutta School of Tropical Medicine and Hygiene and the Carmichael Hospital for Tropical Diseases* (Calcutta: 1920), 1–2, 9–10.
24. Roger Jeffery, 'Recognising India's Doctors: The Establishment of Medical Dependency, 1918–39', *Modern Asian Studies,* XIII (1979), 301–26, *idem,* 'Doctors and Congress: The Role of Medical Men and Medical Politics in Indian Nationalism', in Mike Shepperdson and Colin Simmons (eds), *The Indian National Congress and the Political Economy of India, 1885–1985* (Aldershot: 1987), 163–6.
25. Charles Leslie, 'The Professionalising Ideology of Medical Revivalism', in Milton Singer (ed.), *Entrepreneurship and Modernisation of Occupational Cultures in South Asia* (Durham, N.C.: 1973), 691–708 and 'The Modernisation of Asian Medical Systems' in J. J. Poggie and R. N. Lynch (eds), *Rethinking Modernisation* (New York: 1974), 691–708, Roger Jeffery, *The Politics of Health in India* (Berkeley: 1988), ch. 2, and 'Policies Towards Indigenous Healers in Independent India', *Social Science and Medicine,* XVI (1982), 1835–42.
26. M. K. Gandhi, *Hind Swaraj* (Ahmedabad: 1938), ch. 12.
27. Meera Chatterjee, *Implementing Health Policy* (New Delhi: 1988), chs 5 & 9.
28. Bhore Committee *Report,* I, 8–11.
29. *Ibid.*, 37.
30. *Ibid.*, 11.
31. Jeffery, *op. cit.* (note 24), 325.
32. Chatterjee, *op. cit.* (note 27), 2 & 18.
33. George Rosen, *A History of Public Health* (New York: 1958), 17.
34. Marika Vicziany, 'Coercion in a Soft State: The Family Planning Programme of India', *Pacific Affairs,* LV (1982–3), 373–402, 557–92; Dilip Hiro, *Inside India Today* (revised edn, London: 1978), 270–3.
35. Chatterjee, *op. cit.* (note 27). ch. 3; Mike Shepperdson, 'The Political Economy of Health in India', in Shepperdson & Simmons *op. cit.* (note 24), 304–71.
36. Quoted in Jeffery, *op. cit.* (note 25), 116.
37. Chatterjee, *op. cit.* (note 27), ch. 1.

10

Public Health in Colonial Africa: The Belgian Congo

Maryinez Lyons

'Do no good; suffer no ingratitude.'
Confucius

The history of public health in Africa is located within the broader history of European imperialism and colonialism.[1] Relatively brief, the colonial period lasted roughly between 1885, when the Great Powers[2] divided the sub-continent among themselves, to the early 1960s, when most colonies achieved independence.[3]

Hegemonic Ideologies

In Africa, the introduction of Western material culture was accompanied by a set of powerful hegemonic ideologies.[4] Religious missionaries, representatives of the law, educators and health practitioners were all involved in the attempt to persuade Africans to accept new concepts and modes of behaviour. Rooted in the political economy of nineteenth-century Western Europe, ideas of public health found quite different expression in sub-Saharan African colonies. Lacking a resonance with African socio-economic and political conditions, public health ideology did not graft easily on to prevailing systems of health management. It has been argued that the long-term impact of European ideologies and systems was weak, even ephemeral, as 'authentic' African forms and systems reassert themselves today.[5] When in June 1960, the Belgian Congo gained independence after 75 years of domination, the departing colonialists were confident that the gift of medical and public health systems grounded in Western biomedicine was the best legacy bequeathed to the Congolese. However, we need to examine success of the graft of a public health ideology introduced under the conditions of colonial rule.

The colonial medical and public health services reflected patterns of social, scientific and medical thought prevailing in London, Paris, Berlin and Brussels. There was an important difference, however, for in the colonies administrators were free from many of the social and political constraints of a more informed public. Nor were they constrained by the climate of concern in Europe for individual rights and the humanistic obligations of the state. All colonial administrations were undemocratic but policies varied: the German,[6] Portuguese and Belgian systems were far more authoritarian and centralized than the British. But in general, Europeans were confident that the simple transfer of their ideology and technology to Africa would address the widespread ignorance, lack of sanitation and poor health. It is not surprising that nineteenth-century Europeans regarded their recent scientific and medical achievements as evidence not only of their ability to transform the world to suit their own ends but also, as irrefutable proof that European societies were superior in all respects to those recently discovered in other parts of the globe. Social Darwinism[7] was a powerful concept and early European colonizers rarely doubted their rights to invade, conquer, rule and exploit African societies. Through the process of colonization, Africans would be saved, cured and modernized[8] and the new biomedicine was among the foremost technologies which would help to accomplish this immense task.

Public Health and the State

African societies provided a quite different context for the new field of public health evolving in Europe and elsewhere. The concept of public health implies the notion of the state as benefactor and protector of its charges. In Europe the rich realized 'that if they neglected the poor it would be at their own peril'[9] and concerned citizens investigated the living conditions of the labouring classes. Reform and public health movements were gathering momentum. But while European states were becoming sensitive to the status of health among the poor at home, abroad they were seeking new lands and whole populations to exploit.

The colonial powers hoped to expand their influence to non-western regions through religion, industry and commerce, activities which were glossed with the rhetoric of 'mission'. The discourse changed over time but a central feature remained the professed concern for the diseased bodies and fallen souls of Africans. There was much anxiety about 'filthy and backward natives' who were perceived to be a potent source of contagion. The contradictory role of the state as protector and predator was clear in the colonies of sub-Saharan Africa. Nowhere was this more apparent than in the Belgian Congo.

Pre-Colonial African Ideas of Health

African societies had their own ideologies and practices for the preservation of well-being long before Europeans arrived. These were based on quite different conceptions of what constitutes and maintains well-being but they were rejected by Europeans who considered them to be backward, superstitious and even harmful. One former colonial physician explained that the Congolese 'perception of health problems was so irrational and preposterous according to our western approach, that no great efforts were made to understand their views'.[10] African modes of health preservation were closely allied to, and controlled by, religious and political authorities which sharpened the conflict with European systems. Covering more than 900,000 square miles, the Belgian Congo contained a number of distinct cultural zones and many hundreds of African societies, each with its own language and culture. The great variety of African methods of health management presented an enormous challenge to the imposition of a uniform, biomedical model of health.

African Political Structures and Well-Being

Public health, with its focus on the group rather than the individual, requires the sanction and organizing capabilities of a strong central authority. In Europe, the authority to implement and enforce broad public health measures resided within the emerging national states of the nineteenth century. The new African colonies bore no resemblance to nation states. Enclosed by artificial boundaries drawn at the convenience of Europeans, African societies often found themselves divided among several colonial powers. One large society, the Azande, estimated to number over a million, was divided among three colonial territories: French Equatorial Africa, British Sudan and the Belgian Congo. In colonial Africa where European political authority was often tenuous and contested in the early stages of colonial rule, public health initiatives sometimes resulted in confrontation as African authorities struggled to maintain their hegemony. Nineteenth-century Africa contained many complex state structures such as the kingdoms of the Hausa, Yoruba, Asante, Bakongo in the west and the Azande, Mangbetu, Luba, Lunda and Baganda of the east. There were, as well, many hundreds of smaller, non-centralized, self-governing lineages[11] in societies commonly referred to by Europeans as 'stateless'. In all social formations, however large or small, lineages provided individuals a degree of social security and assistance in times of need. All pre-colonial African societies acknowledged some form of religious or political authority and the well-being of society at large, the 'public', was traditionally a concern shared by political and religious authorities.

Among the Shambaa people of Tanzania, healers, in alliance with their political leaders had a much wider range of control over the social conditions of health before colonial rule than they have had ever since.[12] In northern Congo, Azande rulers resisted the incursions of alien medicines and practices, including European, and declared that their subjects should not seek healing from other than Azande sources.[13] African healers and leaders throughout the continent regularly supervised activities intended to protect and maintain the public well-being. Westerners would recognize some of these as falling under the rubric of 'public health' while others did not. Examples include instructions on variolation for smallpox, choice of location and construction of latrines, cleaning of areas of habitation, planting of certain crops and the maintenance of insect control measures. In addition to individual afflictions, healers were consulted for the most propitious times to plant crops, at times of drought or famine or for good luck in combat. A most common reason for consulting healers in most African societies has always been in reference to problems of infertility. In short, healers were consulted at times when either individuals or the society at large felt unwell or threatened.

Social Relations

Many illnesses are conceptualized by Africans as resulting, at least in part, from disturbed social relations. A powerful and widespread African notion of well-being concerns the reintegration of unwell individuals into the larger social fabric.[14] Since an individual's meaning and worth is located essentially within the web of his social relations, in most societies many conditions can be diagnosed and treated only within the context of family or kin.

Illness as Misfortune

Among many African societies, disease is included within the broader category of 'misfortune'. Other misfortunes might be droughts, famines, loss of a cow, a barren wife, a strained ankle or a cold. Help is more readily available for some misfortunes than it is for others. Thus a common cold, the cause of which might be associated with a chill sent by an angry neighbour, requires a visit to the specialist healer for an incantation accompanied by a substance to be rubbed on the skin. Barrenness might require the propitiation of a disgruntled ancestor. An epidemic disease however, say smallpox, which was believed by many African societies in the past to be causally linked with a more distant source, a god, which would be more difficult to appease, might require flight from the region in which it occurred or isolation of the afflicted.

The aetiology of a disease thus would include disrupted social relations as well as those features more easily recognized in the West as diagnostic signs such as skin eruptions and gastroenteric disturbances. An individual will seek a therapy for the latter and concurrently seek to redress the ultimate cause for the misfortune which might reside within his social setting. That might require investigation into what we in the West might think of as sociological or psychological features. Does a neighbour harbour malice or anger, for instance? Has the individual either intentionally or inadvertently offended someone, living or dead? In this sense, all health is conceptualized as related to the public domain in spite of its individual manifestation. Diseases which result from the ill-will of members of one's own kin or social group can be prevented to a degree by means of particular rituals or protective medicines. The Western model of public health with its measures to protect the larger society would for most Congolese earlier this century only make sense in as much as the individual found protection from a wide range of misfortunes. Public health measures would have to fit into the African's much broader range of notions of misfortune, only one form of which fits the more limited European notion of disease.

Isolation or Quarantine?

I have mentioned the African practice of isolation of ill individuals which was recognizable by Europeans as a public health strategy. There were important conceptual differences, however, separating African from Western practice. The Azande of northern Zaire practised isolation of individuals. A local administrator reported how

> The Azande transport the patient to a shaded riverbank where they construct a habitation and the relatives care for him. Generally a village where a death occurred is abandoned until the next rainy season.[15]

Avoiding direct contact, yet still caring, kin left food for the ill on the path outside the isolation hut.[16] On the other hand, an unwell person might not be isolated alone in the forest but would be taken to distant kin relations in order to remove him from the possible harmful influence of closer relations or neighbours. The choice of isolation depended upon the diagnosis of the 'illness' which, as I have already pointed out, was often thought to be related to disturbed social relations. Thus preventive steps taken by Africans to protect the larger group or society were based upon quite different concepts of disease causality and therapy. From the African view, isolation of an individual away from close kin but in open contact with more distant kin was a form of disease prevention. Not understanding the complex interplay of physical and cultural notions involved in ideas of disease and therapy, western Europeans regarded such measures as examples of backward Africans.

In fact, the introduction during colonialism of the Western, biomedical model of medicine with its clinical emphasis,[17] diagnosis and treatment of individuals was adapted sometimes more easily to African concepts of disease [misfortune] and treatment [diviner/healer] than were European ideas of public health, those sets of precautions taken to prevent disease among the wider public, which were not as easily grafted on to existing African concepts.[18] A few Belgians appeared to understand the difficulty of imposing Western rationalism on non-Western systems of thought.[19] Professor P. G. Janssens who was in charge of public health at the Kilo-Moto Gold Mines in northern Zaire for many years explained that the

> acceptance of ... preventive measures implies an orientation to the future, in which wc indulge, with our ability to relate cause and effect, but unfamiliar to those fatalistic pupils of ours orientated towards the past and adhering to other explanations than a germ theory, malnutrition and the like.[20]

The conflict between master and subject was compounded further by the unfamiliar technology and alien, unwelcome colonial state which accompanied European public health.

Colonialism: The Example of Belgian Congo

The Motive

The Congo Free State,[21] an extreme example of imperialism, was the creation of the ambitious, entrepreneural King Léopold II of Belgium. Through the methodical exploitation of its natural and human capital, the King and a small circle of financial backers were substantially enriched. Blunt in his assessment, Léopold realized the potential human capital in his new state and even declared that the Congolese populations were the 'best of his riches'. Later colonialists more often tempered the economic reality with a moral gloss. For instance, nearly a century later, a former colonial physician observed that

> Colonization has been an ambiguous undertaking. It aimed at development, but such development was obviously more closely

> related to the interests of the colonizers than to those of the colonized. The latter had to be saved anyway from a primitive underdeveloped state, and for that particular purpose whatever was deemed good for Europeans was deemed all the more advisable for Africans.[22]

In 1908 the private Congo Free State was transferred to Belgian rule becoming a colony. In response to the concerted attacks of the international humanitarian community the new colonial administration attempted over time to temper the mode of commercial exploitation somewhat while the methods were modernized and expanded. Nevertheless, until 1960 and independence, the colony remained primarily a business enterprise with profit as the objective.

Profits were gained from agricultural products such as rubber, cotton, coffee, tea, tobacco, sugar, groundnuts and timber while mining of gold, diamonds, copper, lead, tin, uranium, zinc, tin and other minerals was a prime source of income for colonizers and investors. These enterprises required huge, sustainable amounts of labour which by the early 1920s had become increasingly difficult to obtain. The supply of labour remained a major issue during the entire colonial experience. The earliest instructions to state agents stressed the signficance of labour as the pivot of the Belgian's 'civilizing mission'.[23]

African Labourers

The reality of the Belgian 'civilizing mission' in the Congo was reduced nutritional status, damaged immune systems, increased disease and death. Belgian methods of profit extraction were harsh and destructive of Congolese populations. To begin with, time spent by Congolese working for the state meant a loss of productivity within their own societies. The new colonial rulers forced many thousands of Congolese to work as porters, paddlers, wood cutters, cultivators and miners far from their home regions for long periods of time. Separated from families and kin and subjected to new disease environments and diets Congolese labour suffered and sickened. In the villages, food production was seriously affected as people were siphoned off to perform tasks for the new colonial power and the reduction in nutrition exacerbated existing stresses. An important result was impaired resistance to endemic diseases such as sleeping sickness which in some instances became dramatically epidemic.

In the Congo, as in other African colonies, the earliest medical efforts were directed at protecting the health of Europeans and those Africans in their service.[24] New disease environments had resulted in high morbidity and mortality of Europeans which fully occupied the extremely limited numbers of medical staffs.[25] The extraction of profit, however, depended upon the uninterrupted supply of African labour. Thus in spite of the lack of medical staff, quite early on, the topics of African health and fertility became major colonial concerns. This was especially true when labour appeared to be under threat of extinction through the increased morbidity and mortality resulting from epidemic diseases.

> Despite frequent appearances to the contrary, the colonial administration did not attempt to kill the milch-cow which Africans represented.[26]

Whereas the initial rhetoric of empire had dwelt upon the fallen state of the native soul, very soon the need for strong productive labour meant that the rhetoric reflected increasing concern for the native body.

The Rationalization

In 1949 the Colonial Minister, Pierre Wigny, introducing the new ten-year plan for development, clearly articulated the economic motive of Belgian colonization of the Congo.

> *L'amélioration des conditions d'existence des indigènes est la justification de notre présence et la récompense morale de notre effort. Mais, répatons-le une fois de plus, cette politique s'impose aussi pour des raisons d'ordre économique.*[27]

Belgians were in Africa for economic reasons, their method was brutal and destructive but their rationalization was clear and often repeated. Belgian colonial ideology was a mixture of moralizing theories and scientific discourse. Belgians were 'improving the natives' or 'civilizing the savages' with the aid of medicine and hygiene. Labour was conceptualized as an important means for improving African societies in much the same way it was believed by Protestants in Europe that salvation lay in part in good, honest labour. 'Civilization and progress were synonymous with the arrival of industrial and agrarian capitalism and the social order they implied'.[28] Civilization could be achieved through labour; it provided the lesson while improved health would be a significant portion of the reward. In contrast to earlier visitors to the continent, nineteenth-century Europeans tended to regard Africans as dirty, diseased, contagious and dangerous and in need of cleansing. Thus, in addition to protecting the health of Europeans, the introduction of Western notions of hygiene would help African societies to evolve towards more civilized status.[29] The Colonial Minister explained in 1949 that the authorities in the Congo were responsible for the tutelage of more than ten million natives. These, he continued

> *sont incapables d'assurer par eux-mêmes une évolution suffisament rapide de leurs méthodes de production et une élévation progressive de leur niveau de vie. Ils comptent sur nous.*[30]

Thirteen years later, a leading Belgian medical specialist still claimed that

> It is an obligation of the authorities who have taken charge of the evolution of a population toward civilization and progress, to actively intervene to break the vicious circle of sickness and poverty on one hand and to introduce better labour techniques as well as raise the level of health in a way to render individuals more apt for physical and intellectual effort.[31]

'Civilizing the savage' remained a central tenet of Belgian colonial ideology throughout the period of their control,[32] clearly articulated in the area of public health. The civilizing process would be enhanced through the implantation of Western, bourgeois values which were considered a necessary corollary to the successful grafting of bio-medical ideology and systems.[33]

Public Health in the Belgian Congo
The Beginning: Segregation

In 1908 when the Congo Free State passed to the administration of the Belgian Parliament, a new colonial charter included provision for the 'conservation of the native populations and the amelioration of their moral and material conditions of existence'.[34] The Charter's explicit provision for the health of the Congolese was in contrast to earlier public health initiatives, a good number of which aimed at protecting European residents from African pollution. An 1887 contagious diseases decree resembled contemporary European efforts to regulate population movements at frontiers and ports. The first of many public health decrees in the Congo, the 1887 decree reflected fear of contagion and focused especially upon sanitation measures in areas of white settlement such as administrative posts and military camps. Fear of contagion resulting from the intermingling of races in population centres led as early as 1892 to a ruling which detailed sanitary measures for residents of *centres extra-coutumiers* [CEC], or native quarters. In Belgian Congo well before the turn of the century there were clear moves to segregate the races and the 1898 decree firmly established the separation of European and African residential zones.[35] Smallpox vaccination had been obligatory since 1894 for urban residents and a vaccine institute had been established in the capital, Boma. In 1899 special, three-man Hygiene Commissions were founded in each of the major trading centres, Boma, Matadi and Léopoldville.[36] Their brief was to oversee sanitary conditions, enforce hygiene decrees and report quarterly to the provincial medical officers but for the most part, they remained a dead letter.

Sleeping Sickness and Cordon Sanitaire

The epidemic outbreak of sleeping sickness in Uganda which killed nearly 300,000 Africans by 1905 compelled some colonial administrations to take seriously for the first time the public health of all residents, black and white, and programmes to control and eradicate epidemic sleeping sickness were in fact the earliest 'vertical' health campaigns in Africa.[37] King Léopold invited scientists from the Liverpool School of Tropical Medicine to assess the situation in his State. In 1904 the experts declared that there was a widespread epidemic throughout the Congo basin.[38] In the Belgian Congo, sleeping sickness was the single most important factor responsible for the early provision of a medical service which eventually resulted in a broader public health policy and programme.[39] 'The idea of social medicine was born in the sleeping sickness campaigns' explained Dr Jacques Schwetz.[40]

Initially, the campaign against the disease endeavoured to identify and isolate all infected individuals in special centres, or lazarets and to create a sanitary cordon around zones deemed uninfected. After the development of the first effective chemotherapy, atoxyl, in 1905, the campaign aimed to achieve the 'sterilization' or 'atoxylization' of all people suspected of harbouring the parasite which causes the disease. The examinations and isolation were never voluntary and throughout most of the colonial period, Africans were frightened by these procedures and very often attempted to flee the medical teams. Some Belgians disagreed with the roughshod methods of public health in the colony. Some, like Dr Zerbini who was employed in the Colonial Medical Service, spoke out on behalf of African's rights. Zerbini said he could not approve the 'radical measure' of 'involuntary isolation' of all Africans suspected to be infected with sleeping sickness.[41] Referring to public health practice in Europe, he reminded the governor general of the Congo Free State that 'in Europe, tubercular patients, a constant danger to all, are allowed their individual liberty'. He believed that to isolate all Congolese simply suspected of infection showed the arbitrary nature of public health policy in the colony.[42]

Employing the model developed by Eugene Jamot in French colonies, from 1916 the Belgians attempted systematically to examine the entire population. Of course, with the limited staff available that was not accomplished until nearly 1960 but by 1931, the Belgians claimed to be examining over five million Congolese annually in a total population of some ten million. This was the *prophylaxie médicale.* The campaigns included a second important aspect, *prophylaxie biologique,* or the sanitation and social engineering aspects of public health. Thus coterminus with the increasing medicalization of the Congolese were strategies aimed at preventing disease and introducing hygiene. As mentioned earlier, it was the second aspect, social engineering, which occasioned the greatest misunderstanding and resistance to Western concepts of health. The annual sleeping sickness surveys, over time, evolved towards public health surveys taking note of other endemic diseases such as yaws, malaria and measles.

Sleeping Sickness Legislation

Epidemics occasion lively interest in broader social issues. In the Belgian Congo, the sleeping sickness epidemic provided the impulse for a proliferation of public health legislation over time. Halfway through the colonial period, in 1934, there were already over 125 rules concerning this one disease alone. Many of the health regulations inconvenienced and disrupted African societies considerably, even to the extent of destroying important economic resources. The tsetse-fly which transmits the form of the disease found throughout the Belgian Congo lives along secondary, slower-moving rivers and streams, thus it made sense to the Belgians to prohibit Africans from waterways designated to be unsafe. They were forbidden to wash, collect water, fish or travel on certain waterways. Nor were they allowed to harvest the salt-bearing grasses which grew on the banks of such forbidden waters.[43] Colonial administrators were empowered to confiscate and destroy the large canoes used for fishing and transport. The manufacture of the canoes represented many man-hours and much expense. Another feature of the public health policy abhorrent to the Congolese was the regrouping and resiting of entire populations in order to remove them from regions thought to be contaminated with sleeping sickness. Oblivious of the deep psychic harm involved in removing Africans from lands with ritual associations, the Belgians proceeded to implement what was in their eyes a logical public health policy. Public health regulations had wide-ranging effects on Congolese social, economic and political life and in those areas where enforcement was attempted, tensions between Europeans and Africans were constant.

Inter-war Period: Urbanization and Labour Needs

In 1922 a Colonial Hygiene Service was established marking a new direction in public health in the Congo. Independent of the colonial Medical Service, established in 1909, Hygiene was responsible for urban sanitation, potable water supply, port hygiene, campaigns against insect vectors, and the overall health of African labourers. Laboratories were opened and posts for medical hygienists established in the provincial capitals, Léopoldville, Elisabethville and Bukavu as well as the ports of Banana, Boma, Matadi, Jadotville and Albertville.[44]

Rapid urbanization in the inter-war period accompanied by ever-increasing needs for African labourers were the two factors most responsible for the increasing attention given to matters of public health. Public health followed the pattern of other social services which in the Belgian Congo were shared among the state, the private sector including industrial, agricultural and commercial enterprises, and the religious missions. The state sector, described above, was staffed and financed by the Colonial Ministry and tended to operate in tandem with other health projects undertaken by private initiative. This resulted in patchy public health services with some regions benefiting while others were ignored.

Private Sector and Public Health: Mines, Plantations and Companies

Mining companies, commercial concerns and agricultural plantations were required to include public health among their activities.[45] The state required companies to employ one medical officer for each 1,000 employees and, that they 'be available for the treatment of the native population (in addition to labourers) within the concession areas'.[46] The widespread use of a much-enforced medical passport system in the Belgian Congo made possible the overall surveillance of population movements in addition to the assessment and control of individuals. All tax-paying Congolese, that is adult men, were compelled to carry medical passports. Developed by the sleeping sickness surveys, the medical passports formed an important aspect of the overall public health policy and were often admired by observers from other colonies.

> The compulsory possession by natives of certificates of health is a

> matter that might well be considered by the Union [South Africa] and British Governments for the more effective control of native diseases.[47]

Introduced in 1910, the medical passports soon took up much time and administrators complained. One overworked individual complained that passport administration took two hours each day.[48] Special 'observation posts' were established on the peripheries of zones thought to be free of sleeping sickness. But Africans successfully eluded detection while others forged passports. It proved difficult to obtain the cooperation of the many concessionary companies whose continual need for labour led them to overlook public health regulations. There were suggestions of other ways to enforce the public health legislation. In 1912, Dr Pulieri in Equateur District had several suggestions. Africans who had been treated for sleeping sickness could be given permanent 'marks on their bodies' in the form of tattoos. They could be injected for the disease in such a way as to leave a particular pattern of needle marks, or, they could be injected in a 'special place' on their bodies.[49] In 1914 one vice-governor suggested the adoption of the German colonial practice of metal bracelets, permanently welded on wrists.[50]

During typical recruitment of labour in villages, individuals who did not already possess a medical passport which included, in addition to personal details, a record of his infectivity status, were issued such passports which they were then required to carry for life. Without these documents, individuals were not allowed to travel more than very short distances from their home territories. In this way, a public health document became a useful means of controlling African mobility.

Recruiting for *Union Minière* in the mid-1920s was done by European agents accompanied by medical officers who visited villages where the first 'sorting' of candidates took place. Those Africans selected were then transferred to special camps where they were weighed, treated for intestinal parasites and given various protective vaccines. Following a short period of observation, the recruits were then moved to *Union Minière's* main camp at Lubumbashi where some might be re-vaccinated and finally the men were assigned to various mining camps to work out their three-year contracts.

Permanent white settlement was not encouraged in Belgian Congo and with the exception of a small number of residents in eastern Kivu Province, the majority of Europeans present in the colony were employed by the state, the missions or one of the many companies. The large numbers of labourers required in these concerns caused a lively interest in issues of public health. As mentioned earlier, the problem of labour supply reached crisis proportion in the early decades of this century and many firms like the Kilo-Moto Gold Mines in northern Congo attempted to solve it through the implementation of programmes designed to assist the reproduction, rather than the constant replacement, of labour.[51]

Mining Companies

By the mid-colonial period, the public health programmes of most of the major mining and concessionary companies in Belgian Congo had taken as their model the Transvaal gold mines in South Africa. The public health programmes of other major concessionary companies such as Huileries Congo Belge, Forminière, Unilever, Symétrain and Kilo-Moto Gold Mines followed the lead of the major mining concession, Union Minière de Haut Katanga. William Gorgas had proved the worth of his public health ideas in relation to labour supply in the tropical conditions of Panama while working on yellow fever. The major feature of his plan was the screening and maintenance of labour. He discovered that selected workers fared better and lived longer when a stabilized labour force was permanently established consisting of men with their families residing near the site of employment. Adapted to tropical African conditions, many of Gorgas' ideas were employed in the Belgian Congo. Health provisions for women and children were gradually included. By the 1920s Kilo-Moto had exhausted the local supply of labour and was recruiting hundreds of miles distant in Uele, Kivu, Rwanda and Burundi. The management complained that Uelians were sickly and died too soon. It is clear from this distance in time, that men recruited from Uele, hundreds of miles from the mines, and who, in the early days, had to walk the whole distance, succumbed to a new disease environment. Their lack of resistance was undoubtedly exacerbated by a combination of stresses induced by back-breaking work (hand-sluicing for gold), poor and new diet, and lack of access to kin relations for care when in need. The mine management, like others in Africa, was eventually compelled to do something about health conditions. At Kilo-Moto a public health scheme gradually evolved which included by the 1950s free medical care, maternity and out-patient services for the surrounding villages as well as the workers inside the mines. Water management, waste disposal, malaria control, housing and health problems specific to mines such as dust control and miners' phthisis surveillance involved the action of technicians, engineers, accountants and managers as well as medical staff.[52]

Mining compounds were carefully constructed according to European conceptions of order and hygiene and provisioned with safe water, sewage disposal and latrines. Africans were not consulted.[53] 'To sum up, the employer tried to provide the native workers with a life centred more upon European conceptions than upon theirs.'[54] The result was that Africans intensely disliked the uniform and impersonal blocks of habitations, avoided use and cleansing of latrines which they had not helped to build and were often indifferent to the potable water supply preferring closer sources. Hygiene measures imposed by an uninvited and unwelcome authority, without local consultation, made little headway. Nevertheless, the mining and commercial companies prided themselves on the provision of public health programmes. Strongly motivated by economic necessity, the commercial sector provided an example to government health services which often followed their lead.

Maternal and Child Health

As we have seen, by the mid-colonial period the reproduction of labour had become a great concern and attention turned to Congolese women, their practices of infant and child care and more generally to the broader issue of fertility. There were increasing reports from local administrators and health personnel of 'diminishing populations' which was thought to result mainly from reduced fertility coupled with high infant mortality. This was an area which had been left traditionally to the missionaries who provided a substantial portion of all health services. Throughout colonial Africa, missionaries provided medical assistance which varied greatly depending on the religious order and the particular circumstances. In the Belgian Congo the state depended heavily upon missionary medicine. In the early decades Protestant missions[55] had far exceeded their Catholic counterparts in the provision of medicine but from the 1930s the latter were urged by the colonial ministry to increase health services.

The state encouraged the creation of *maternités,* special centres which provided rudimentary services and education for Congolese mothers of young children, which were often attached to local hospitals or dispensaries and most often staffed by female missionary orders. Attendance at the *maternités* was encouraged in the hope of persuading women to deliver under supervision of Western style midwives rather than the traditional African birth attendants. It was estimated in 1947 that 43 per cent of all births had been at *maternités,* which meant that 189,383 babies had been delivered under medical supervision.[56] By 1956, in addition to the *maternités,* there were 884 consultations de nourissons, or baby clinics, with attendances of 342, 621 babies.

Parastatal Organizations and Health

Independent health organizations, some funded in part by central government, contributed significantly to public health efforts in the Belgian Congo. Health provision was provided by a combination of the government medical service, philanthropic medical organizations, concessionary companies and a few private practitioners. There was a greater development of parastatals, semi-official health organizations, in the Belgian Congo than in French or British colonies, a situation similar to that in Belgium where preventive services were often in the hands of voluntary associations.[57] Unofficial organizations included: *Service Auxiliare de l'Assistance Médicale aux Indigène* (SAMI) which included numerous medical missions and religious infirmaries; the *Croix-Rouge du Congo* which focused on a small region of northern Congo; the *Fondation Médicale de l'Université de Louvain au Congo* (FOMULAC) which aimed to bring medical assistance direct to villages; *Le Centre Médical et Scientifique de l'Université de Bruxelles au Congo* (CEMUBAC) which functioned in eastern areas of the colony; *La Fondation Père Damien pour la lutte contre la lèpre* (FOPERDA); and *l'Assistance aux Maternités et Dispensaires du Congo* (AMDC)[58].

Foreami

A good example of such associations was the *Fondation Reine Elisabeth pour l'Assistance Médicale aux Indigènes* (Foreami), which was established in 1930 with a combination of funding from the Belgian and Congo governments, the Queen of Belgium and a permanent endowment fund.[59] By the late 1930s Foreami employed 27 Belgian doctors, 20 sanitary agents[60] and a large number of African assistants[61] maintained permanently in the field. Foreami was the conceived by Dr G. Trolli, who had been Chief Medical Officer of the Congo Free State Service. It was his idea to launch an 'intensive, methodical, systematic, exhaustive and simultaneous campaign against all the diseases of a specified area' which should take four or five years after which the team would move on to a new area leaving the 'cleansed' area to regular medical care.[62] The impact of this cleansing on African health was superficial, but the experiment was important because of its impact on the policy of 'planning and perfection of preventive medicine'. This particularly Belgian 'dynamic', in contrast to 'static', medicine was a direct outgrowth of the large, mobile sleeping sickness surveys with their impressive teams of physicians, sanitary agents and

African helpers. Medicine, together with preventive measures, was taken to the people, a 'revolutionary act' according to one observer.[63]

In 1958, after decades of concentrating on western districts of the colony, Foreami began a new project in Uele District in northern Congo. Just two years before independence swept the unprepared Belgians from the Congo, Foreami initiated its comprehensive programme aimed at understanding and responding to the demographic regression believed to exist in the Uele District of northern Congo. The administration estimated a birth rate for the dominant ethnic group, the Azande to be 10 to 13/1000 where as in the western district of Kwango the rate oscillated around 40/1000. This fact, coupled with high rates of miscarriage and infant mortality, meant that the Azande were 'disappearing'.[64]

The brief of Foreami reached far beyond curative medicine combined with a few preventive measures and a closer look at some of the assumptions and research goals elucidates the paternalistic nature of public health policy at the end of the colonial period. It also reveals the continuing strength of the evolutionist strategy and the belief in the civilizing and modernizing influence of the superior, rational medicine and health policy of the European. Foreami's plan extended to basic African social and political relations which lay at the heart of their social structure. Factors to be investigated included nutrition, endemic diseases such as leprosy which was thought to afflict seven per cent of the population, widespread thyroid deficiency and sexually transmitted diseases. Far more than purely medical matters would be studied. For instance, Foreami planned to study what were believed to be the deleterious effects of 'degenerate nocturnal orgies' and the practice of polygamy which led to widespread endogamy and 'racial degeneration'. Sexual licence was thought to have resulted in prostitution, anti-conception and abortion practices and amorality. African social organizations in which 'superstition and divining ceremonies' took place would also be scrutinized. The 'therapeutic arsenal'

> would be accompanied by a policy to ameliorate hygiene conditions in vast regions by proceeding with the regrouping of fragmented hamlets and families isolated in villages.[65]

Relocating Populations

Insensitive to African patterns of cultivation and social relations the colonial rulers felt that without the stability of village locations, it would be foolish to dream of replacing huts made of perishable materials with solid constructions which alone would permit 'rational organization' of homes.[66] This policy had been vigorously pursued in the early days of the sleeping sickness campaigns and was based on much the same pragmatic need of the colonial power to group and situate African populations more conveniently for reasons extending far beyond the bounds of public health concerns. For instance, in the earliest sleeping sickness survey of 1915 in northern Congo, Uele District, the doctor was accompanied by local administrators who took advantage of the medical surveys to impose new tax regulations. It was observed then that the scattered settlement pattern of the Azande-speaking peoples was a great inconvenience for administrative purposes.

By 1960, over half a million Congolese had been moved from their home regions and reorganized into *paysannats agricoles,* an involuntary system of 'rational exploitation of the soil by groups of families under the direction of an agricultural technician'. Implemented in the 1950s, this system of government-sponsored settlements did bring some benefits through investment in infrastructure and hygiene. However, 'To many, the *paysannat* seemed to be little more than a sophisticated form of agricultural bondage'.[67] *Paysannats* were permitted to construct their homes according to the 'norms of hygiene' and were to be provided with community services of potable water and waste removal. The administration announced that the result would be 'complete enlightenment of rural life'.[68]

To the end of their colonial rule, the Belgians retained their strong penchant to restructure African societies by appointing new political leaders, to impose new sets of social regulations and even to reorganize populations and then to move them far from ritually and historically important home areas to regions many miles away in the cause of 'social medicine'.

Post WWII: Demography, Urbanization and Health

The Belgian Congo was vast and public health programmes patchy both in terms of time and space affected. There are some general indicators for the overall health status of the population. Mortality rates, widely accepted as the most fundamental measure of the health status of populations,[69] varied from place to place and at different periods. Health statistics must be analysed with great care and consideration given to their political as well as their objective purposes. By the late colonial period, for instance, it was politically, as well as economically, expedient, that the large mining companies be seen to take seriously the welfare of their labourers. The population of the colony was 10,761,353 in 1947 with 9,083,910 Congolese residing in the rural sector and 1,677,443 in urban centres. The post-war birth-rate was 31 per 1,000 and the overall mortality rate was 25 per 1,000. Life expectancy at five was 39 for males and 45 for women.[70] The author of the 1950 *Ten Year Development Plan* explained that with an average population density of 4.6 persons per square kilometre, the colony was in the midst of a demographic crisis.[71] The low fertility was thought to be the result of a combination of factors, the major one of which was the 'disturbing' degree of exodus of rural dwellers into the urban centres which is discussed below. It was calculated that 16 per cent [21 per cent males and 14 per cent females aged 15 to 30] of the total population had already left the countryside. It was believed that the sexual imbalance of the sexually productive in the towns together with their freedom from traditional legal, religious and cultural sanctions resulted in unstable unions, prostitution and widespread venereal diseases.[72] The colonial administration believed that the Congo, with its slowly increasing population, was suffering a demographic regression. Aberrant African behaviour was the administration's explanation for the low rate of increase. Africans moved about too freely and congregated in urban centres where they escaped their own cultural constraints. Africans were said to be out of control.

Urbanization

The colonial administration was motivated by two factors to act in the interest of public health for Africans. The first was the need for a stable and capable labour supply and the second was the growing concern about rapid urbanization. Several urban studies in the 1960s[73] provide us with useful data. I shall take the example of Léopoldville which at independence contained nearly 400,000 people. From the earliest days there had been an attempt throughout the colony to regulate and control the migration of rural Africans away from their 'traditional' milieu. The 1898 decree mentioned earlier which established CECs was followed for decades by a rather more informal policy to keep Africans out of towns. This urban policy was completely revised in the 1930s and the 1931 *Décret sur les Centres Extra-coutumiers* formulated a much stricter control of African movement. As a result, by 1935 there were 21 legally designated CECs in the major population centres of the colony. Semi-autonomous units, CECs had their own administrations which remained under the firm control of central government. There were strict regulations concerning housing, sanitation and hygiene; for instance, housing was to be laid out in orderly 'avenues' in the form of multiple-family compounds. Each compound was to have its own latrine behind while many in Léopoldville had their own wells. The European zone of the city was separated from the *Cité Africaine* as it was called by a sanitary cordon of uninhabited ground consisting of a golf course, botanical gardens and a zoo. 'This arrangement was designed to prevent the spread of African disease into the white area.'[74] Between 9 p.m. and 6 a.m. no Congolese were allowed in the white area without a special pass with the exception of the tiny number of *immatriculés*, Africans who had proven themselves to be civilized and therefore worthy to be adjudged by Belgian rather than their own customary law.[75]

In 1962–3 Léopoldville, like other cities in the Congo, was a magnet to rural Africans who pitched together habitations on the peripheries of the CECs in unauthorized squatter settlements known as *quartiers satellites*. One area of about 12,500 acres was estimated to accomodate about 300,000 people most of whom lived in

> the merest shacks of saplings and mud, with thatched roofs... There is, of course, no public lighting system or garbage disposal, and no water supply, except for the polluted and meagre streams which dry up in the hot season.[76]

For nearly a century it had been Belgian policy to control Congolese mobility. The result was that with Independence in June 1960 and the breakdown of control over movement, Congolese, long denied access, flocked to urban areas where the vast majority lived in squalor.

Colonization: 'Modernization' and Public Health? *Mens Sana in Corpore Sano*[77]

The polemical view of Walter Rodney that the 'African peasant entered the colonial period with the hoe, and he came out of it with the hoe' deserves examination in relation to the history of public health in Zaire.[78] Discussing Papua New Guinea, Donald Denoon asserted that colonialism had been a health hazard.[79] How should we interpret the Belgian view that one of the most important factors in their efforts to civilize the Congolese was the introduction of Western medicine and public health strategies? Public health provision related directly to a deeply paternalistic notion of African development, expressed in a discourse of evolution towards civilization. The evolution was to be carefully monitored at a pace which reflected the requirements of the state.

The rationalization for Belgian public health policy was firmly located in their 'evolutionist, civilizing model' of colonial rule. One colonial physician explained proudly that

> when the umbilical cord with Belgium was cut off the Congo Republic, renamed Zaire, had well-organized and well-equipped health services available on the whole even to people living in the remotest regions. The health infrastructure was solid, in fact strong enough to survive many years of turmoil.[80]

It is true that when the colonial rulers abruptly departed from the Congo there was an extensive medical infrastructure consisting of over 3,000 hospitals, clinics, dispensaries, nearly 100 specialized health facilities, two medical training schools, a nursing school and thousands of low-level Congolese medical auxiliaries though not a single Congolese physician.[81] There were three schools to train sanitary guards and four for midwives which in 1956 had over 50 students each.[82]

The mortality rate that year was 22 per 1,000 while fertility had reached 35 per 1,000.[83] However, and more important for the success of a public health programme,

> since civilization was a threat with hygiene as its punishment during colonial rule, it is hardly surprising that with independence, people often did not fulfill demands that they were earlier forced to meet.[84]

The Collapse of the Civil State

I mentioned at the beginning of this chapter that public health is related to the state in its role as protector and benefactor. The colonial state, while weak in many respects, in the Belgian Congo was pervasive enough to affect the lives of millions of people and this was exemplified in the huge campaigns to combat sleeping sickness. By 1960, very few Congolese could avoid some form of contact with the health infrastructure and the many health regulations. But since 1960, the civil state has disintegrated in Zaire.

Between 1960 and 1965, Zaire experienced a series of violent upheavals and civil wars culminating in the coup which brought to power Mobutu. A decade later a survey of health revealed that

> in contrast to the generally linear progression of the health system in most less developed countries, Zaire has since 1960 actually gone backwards.[85]

Another decade later, a Zairean political scientist concluded,

> Zaire is a country in crisis. After 25 years of independence, including 20 years of relative political stability under the authoritarian rule of President Mobutu Sese Seko, there is virtually no improvement in

> the quality of life of ordinary men, women and children.[86]

By the 1970s, spiralling inflation and prodigious neglect had resulted in the overall disintegration of the economy with dire implications for the overall health status of the Zaireans.[87]

The 1975 health survey revealed a grim scenario. Infant mortality was estimated to be 150 to 200 per 1,000, while cumulative child mortality (under age five) was circa 500/1,000. Women who traditionally wanted five living children would have to have ten to fifteen pregnancies. Malnutrition was widespread.[88] In early 1974, one in four urban residents had access to piped water while the vast majority of the rural areas were completely unserved by potable water. An estimated 75 per cent of the population had no access to a formal health care delivery system and relied totally upon traditional medicine.

> The almost complete destruction of the health infrastructure in the immediate post-independence period and its slow redevelopment, coupled with rapid population increase, significantly impeded adequate health care coverage.[89]

Zaire, like many other ex-colonial countries, had continued after independence the pattern of heavier concentration upon curative medicine with all the implications of financial burden entailed in such a policy. In 1975 there was no truly 'national' health sector and the government relied almost entirely, as had its colonial predecessor, on the philanthropic and uncoordinated activities of private organizations.

By 1991, a per capita income of $150 ranked Zaire as one of the poorest countries on the continent with one of the larger populations, 32,604,000.[90] The under-five mortality rate remained at an estimated 150 to 200 per 1,000 live births while life expectancy in western Zaire is estimated to be 42.8 years according to recent studies.[91]

Conclusion

At the beginning of this chapter I said that public health, more than a medical system, requires a viable state structure and a policy of care for its citizens. Given the policy of social medicine which evolved in the colony, it might appear that the Congolese enjoyed improved health. More importantly, it might appear that Africans, armed with new hygienic concepts, changed their behaviour, an outcome required for the success of any public health programme. In reviewing the history of public health in the colony, it is abundantly clear that the colonial state was indeed paternalistic and in spite of budgetary and staffing constraints, it was able to control a massive territory and a large number of Africans.

There are numerous reasons, however, why this argument fails. Let us return to the question of the 'graft' of public health and its success in Belgian Congo/Zaire. Belgian paternalism differed considerably from the government of a caring and consultative state. The Congolese were not citizens. They were colonial subjects in a harsh, exploitative economic system and they were not in a position to freely cooperate with public health policy, a necessary precondition for the success of any programme. They were not consulted about their own ideas, beliefs and practices on topics as varied as the construction of dwellings, the disposal of sewage or child-rearing. Western public health ideology is intimately tied to a wide range of cultural beliefs and practices. Its application often requires sweeping changes on the level of social engineering. Lacking sufficient relation to African cultural and social factors, the conceptual basis of the new ideology could not be adequately internalized by the mass of Congolese, the 'public'. Independent in 1960, the Congolese were able for the first time this century to decide for themselves which elements of the Western health model to retain, adapt or jettison. Unfortunately, the post-independence period has been one of such economic and political stress that the very basis for a successful public health programme, the state, has to all intents and purposes, collapsed. Public health provision in Zaire is now almost entirely in the hands of the private and philanthropic sector.

The Future

Finally, Zaire like many African states at the end of the twentieth century, faces a new public health crisis occasioned by the AIDS epidemic. Epidemics are testing times in which deeper societal tensions as well as social relations are illuminated. Epidemics, perhaps more than any other single health factor, require well established and comprehensive authority structures through which to implement control and prevention measures. AIDS is occurring at a momentous period in the history of sub-Saharan Africa, which like other regions of the globe, have been pressured by international forces to adapt democratic forms of government. It remains to be seen how smoothly the transition to more representative government will be and what impact that will have on the creation of an effective and culturally relevant public health programme.

Notes

1. For collected essays on the subject of colonialism, imperialism and medicine see: Roy MacLeod and Milton Lewis (eds), *Disease, Medicine and Empire: Perspectives on Western Medicine and the Experience of European Expansion* (London: Routledge, 1988); David Arnold (ed.), *Imperial Medicine and Indigenous Societies* (Manchester: Manchester University Press, 1988). See also M. Lyons, *The Colonial Disease: a Social History of Sleeping Sickness in Northern Zaire, 1900–1940* (Cambridge: Cambridge University Press: 1992).
2. The Conference of Berlin from November 1884 to February 1885 was an occasion for the European Powers (the United States was represented as well) to formalize their respective 'spheres of influence' in Africa. King Léopold II of Belgium's claim to the vast Congo Basin was accepted and with the permission of the Belgian Parliament, he was named 'Sovereign' of the new state.
3. Zimbabwe [Southern Rhodesia], Angola, Mozambique, Guinea Bissau and Namibia [Southwest Africa] gained their independence many years later following protracted wars.
4. See Shula Marks and Dagmar Engels, *Contesting Colonial Hegemony: State and Society in Africa and India, 1858 until Independence* (Oxford: Oxford University Press, forthcoming).
5. 1 May, 1991, Columbia University, Center of African Studies, public lecture by Professor Ali Mazrui.
6. The German colonies in Africa, Tanganyika, German Southwest Africa, Togo and Kamerun, were redistributed among the British and French following the defeat of Germany in the First World War.
7. Charles Darwin's *Origin of Species* (1859), was a watershed in the history of biological determinism.
8. It has been suggested that 'modernization', for example, the adoption of the biomedical model, means 'Westernization' and that without the ideological underpinning of the latter, European technologies and systems cannot be successfully implanted in less developed areas. See John Caldwell, 'Old and new factors in Third World health transitions', unpublished paper presented at British Society for Population Studies Annual Conference, Southampton, 11–13 September, 1991.
9. Anthony S. Wohl, *Endangered Lives: Public Health in Victorian Britain* (London: Methuen, 1984), 6.
10. P. G. Janssens, 'Old and New Dimensions in Medical Aid', *Transactions of the Royal Society of Tropical Medicine and Hygiene,* 65 (1971), *Supplement* 1–15: 9.
11. 'In a lineage, the reckoning of kin starts from a single dead ancestor and includes all his or her descendants either through male links (in which case the system is patrilineal) or through female links (matrilineal), rather than starting from a living individual and working back to multiple

ancestors'. Philip Curtin, Steven Feierman, Leonard Thompson and Jan Vansina, *African History* (Harlow, Essex: Longman, 1978), 157–8.
12. *Ibid.*
13. Lyons, *op. cit.* (note 1), ch. 9.
14. John M. Janzen, *The Quest for Therapy in Lower Zaire,* (Berkeley: University of California Press, 1978).
15. Brussels, Ministère des Affaires Entrangères, Archives Africaines (MAEAA) 831.383 20 Février 1912. Chef de zone, Ermingen, Uere. Service Médical et de l'Hygiène, *Rapport annuel:* Uere-Bili.
16. Interviews with Mboli André (Azande) and Ngbato Gilbert (Babua) at Tongerloo Abbey, Belgium, 20 and 21 August, 1982; Larken 'Azande Background', 32; Armand Hutereau, *Histoire des Peuplades de l'Uele et l'Ubangi* (Brussels: 1922), 74, relates an Abandyia tradition.
17. See Michel Foucault, *The Birth of the Clinic: and the Archaeology of Medical Perception* (London: Routledge, 1989), ch. 6 for a discussion of the clinical diagnosis in the West.
18. For a good discussion of this, see Robin Horton, 'African Traditional Thought and Western Science', *Africa,* 37 (1967), 50–72.
19. *Ibid.,* 50–72; 155–87.
20. Janssens, *op. cit.* (note 10), 2–15: 9.
21. Originally the private empire of King Léopold II of Belgium, the Congo Free State [1885–1910] became the Belgian Congo [1910–60] when it came under the administration of the Belgian Parliament. In 1974 President Mobutu renamed the country Zaire in his effort to impose *authenticité.*
22. P. G. Janssens, 'Comparative Aspects: The Belgian Congo', in *Health in Tropical Africa During the Colonial Period,* E. E. Sabben-Clare, D. J. Bradley and K. Kirkwood (eds), (Oxford: Clarendon Press, 1980), 221.
23. J. Wauters, *Le Congo au Travail* (Brussels: 1924); A. Bertrand, *Le Problème de la Main d'Oeuvre au Congo Belge: Province Orientale* (Brussels: 1931); F. A. Lemaire, *Au Congo: Comment Les Noirs Travillent* (Brussels: 1895); Dr Daco, 'Le problème de la main d'oeuvre indigène au Congo belge', *Bruxelles-Médical,* 21; 22; 23 (Mars-Avril 1929).
24. Dr A. Broden, 'l'Hygiène coloniale et les principales maladies tropicales', in *Compte Rendu de la IIIème Congrès International Colonial,* (Gand: 1922), Tome I, 43–56.
25. Philip D. Curtin, *Death by Migration: Europe's Encounter With the Tropical World in the Nineteenth Century* (Cambridge: Cambridge University Press, 1989). Dennis G. Carlson, *African Fever: a Study of British Science, Technology, and Politics in West Africa, 1787–1864* (Canton: MA, Science History Publications, 1984).
26. Bogumil Jewsiewicki, 'Rural Society and the Belgian Colonial Economy', in David Birmingham and Phyllis M. Martin (eds),

History of Central Africa, Vol. 2, 95–125, 106.

27. Ministère des Colonies, *Plan Decennal pour le Développement Economique et Social de Congo Belge* (Bruxelles: Eds. de Vissher, 1949), xxi.
28. Jean Comaroff and John Comaroff, *Of Revelation and Revolution: Christianity, Colonialism, and Consciousness in South Africa*, Vol. 1 (Chicago: University of Chicago Press, 1991), 70.
29. R. Mouchet, 'Medical Assistance to Natives, with Special Reference to the Belgian Congo', *The East African Medical Journal*, 9 (1932), 246–57.
30. Ministère des Colonies, *op. cit.* (note 27), xii.
31. M. Kivits, 'Hygiène et santé publique', in *Livre Blanc*, 1962, Vol. Two, 273.
32. Jewsiewicki, *op. cit.* (note 26), 117.
33. M. Lyons, 'The Power to Heal: African Medical Auxiliaries in Colonial Belgian Congo and Uganda', *op. cit.* (note 4).
34. MAEAA 4389.1090. 9 December, 1943, Brussels. Colonial Minister of Health, Dr A. Duren to M. Leemans, Régie des Distributions d'Eau.
35. Decree of 14 September, 1898. For a discussion of this topic in another colony, see Maynard Swanson, 'The Sanitation Syndrome: Bubonic Plague and Urban Native Policy in the Cape Colony, 1900–1909', *Journal of African History*, 18 (1977), 387–410.
36. Ministère des Affaires Etrangères, Brussels. African Archives. [MAEAA] Service de l'Inspecteur général de l'Hygiène, 4395.414. 9 Février 1928, Inspecteur Général to Secrétaire Général, 'Fonctionnement des commissions d'Hygiène. Leur utilité'.
37. Vertical health care delivery systems had become so entrenched across sub-Saharan Africa by the 1970s that the World Health Organization focused effort on expanding them to 'horizontal', or more comprehensive public health programmes.
38. Lyons, *op. cit.* (note 1).
39. This was equally true in other colonies which experienced epidemic sleeping sickness such as Uganda.
40. Jacques Schwetz, *l'Evolution de la Médecine au Congo Belge* (Brussels: Institut du Sociologie Solvay, 1946).
41. The most common diagnostic technique being employed at the time was the palpation of swollen cervical glands which should be followed ideally by a microscopic examination of blood for trypanosomes, the pathogenic parasite. For many decades, however, diagnosis very often rested upon palpation alone and misdiagnosis was estimated by some specialists to be in the range of 30–50 per cent. Dr Robert Dumont, 'Le conflit des conceptions médicales au Congo', *l'Avenir Colonial Belge* (1934).
42. MAEAA 847.112 , 28 November, 1905. Dr Zerbini, Boma to Governor-General.
43. Salt deposits are lacking throughout large regions of the Congo Basin and Africans had learned to process crucial potassium salts from

certain plants.

44. Kivits, *op. cit.* (note 31), 900–1. The 19 July, 1926 Decree on Hygiene and Public Health formed the basis of most legislation to follow by making provision for (1) taking necessary measures at frontiers to prevent introduction of contagious disease; and (2) taking measures necessary to protect the public health of the colony. This included the sanction to isolate individuals involuntarily; administer medical examinations; to enter and inspect homes; and to either disinfect or destroy suspect material objects.
45. A. Pearson and R. Mouchet, *The Practical Hygiene of Native Compounds in Tropical Africa* (London: Tindall-Cox, 1923); Dr H. Gillet, 'Que font les sociétés minières pour l'hygiène des noirs au Congo Belge?' *Bulletin de l'Association pour le Perfectionnement du Matériel Colonial Bruxelles* (Avril 1929); Major A. Cayen, 'l'Effort sanitaire des sociétés industrielles', l'Essor Economique Belge. *Expansion Coloniale,* I (1932), 177–8; J. Van Riel, *Le service médical de la Campagnie Minière des Grands Lacs Africains et la situation sanitaire de la main-d'oeuvre (*Bruxelles: G. van Campenhout, 1939).
46. W. B. Johnson, 'Notes Upon a Journey Through Certain Belgian, French and British African dependencies to Observe General Medical Organisation and Methods of Trypanosomiasis Control', *Lagos, Government Printer* (1929), 3.
47. S. V. Humphries, 'The Control of Native Diseases in the Belgian Congo', *South African Medical Journal* (9 September, 1939), 640.
48. MAEAA 849.291 15 Mai 1911, Buta, Uele District. Dr Van der Sloten to Governor-General.
49. MAEAA 849.355, 23 November, 1912. Dr Pulieri, Coquilhatville, District of Equateur to Governor-General.
50. MAEAA 850.1 12 Avril 1914, Stanleyville, Vice-Governor-General Malfeyt to Governor-General.
51. Janssens, *op. cit.* (note 22), 209–27.
52. *Ibid.,* 209–27, 218.
53. A. Pearson and R. Mouchet, *The Practical Hygiene of Native Compounds in Tropical Africa* (London: Tindall-Cox, 1923).
54. P. G. Janssens, 'La mortalite infantile', *Bulletin de ARSO,* (1952), 105–19, 110.
55. Most Protestant sects present in the Belgian Congo were foreign, that is, not home-based in Belgium. Of over 60 missions, only one or two were Belgian. The remainder were mainly from the United States while others were Norwegian, Swedish, South African and British.
56. Ministère du Congo Belge, *La Santé en Afrique Belge* (Bruxelles: InforCongo, 1958), 55. Calculated on fertility rate of 35/1000 which meant approximately 437,500 births per annum.
57. E. B. Worthington, *Science in Africa: a Review of Scientific Research Relating to Tropical and Southern Africa* (London: Oxford University Press, 1938), 499. For instance, in 1933 in the Congo there were

129 doctors employed by the state and 143 employed in the private sector. [Foreami – 17; Croix-Rouge – 4; companies – 66; religious missions – 56]. 'Combien de médecins y a-t-il au Congo?' *L'Aide Médicale aux Missions,* 2 (15 Avril 1933), 35–7.

58. Ministère de Congo Belge, *op. cit.* (note 56), 15; Dr Marchand, 'Les réalisations de la "Fomulac"', *L'Aide Médicale aux Missions,* 4 (15 October, 1933), 95–7.
59. R. Mouchet, 'The Foreami', *Transactions of the Royal Society of Tropical Medicine and Hygiene,* 44 (1951), 483–500.
60. A class of European public health auxiliaries used in the Congo after a four month theoretical course in Belgium and two months' practical course in the Congo.
61. MAEAA 4389.1020, Congo Belge. Ordonnance du 10 Fèvrier 1930, No. 18, Hygiene, créant le cadre des gardes sanitaires indigènes. Congolese sanitary guards were supervised by medical hygienists. Their duties included surveillance of water sources and testing of larvae, rat control, disinfection and vaccinations.
62. P. G. Janssens, 'Cooperation Belge au Zaire: le FOREAMI', *Afrique Médicale,* 12 (1973), 621–4, 621.
63. *Ibid.*
64. Brussels, Foreami, *Rapport Annuel, 1958,* 77.
65. *Ibid.,* 79.
66. Kivits, *op. cit.* (note 31), 899–916 in *Livre Blanc: Apport Scientifique de la Belgique au Développement de l'Afrique Centrale* (Brussels: Académie Royal des Sciences d'Outre-Mer, 1962).
67. Jewsiewicki, *op. cit.* (note 26), 95–125, 116.
68. Kivits, *op. cit.* (note 31), 909.
69. Richard G. Feachem and Dean T. Jamison, *Disease and Mortality in Sub-Saharan Africa,* (Oxford University Press [for the World Bank], 1991).
70. Jacques Lefebvre, *Structures Economiques du Congo Belge et du Ruanda-Urundi* (Bruxelles: Editions de Treurenberg, 1955), 16.
71. *Ministère des Colonies, op. cit.* (note 27), 10–12.
72. By 1950, sexually transmitted diseases were, after malaria, the most important endemic diseases. *Ibid.,* 41.
73. Valdo Pons, *Stanleyville: an African Urban Community Under Belgium Administration* (London: Oxford University Press, 1967) Bruce Fetter, *The Creation of Elizabethville 1910–1946* (Stanford, Hoover Institution Press, 1976). J. S. La Fontaine, *City Politics: a Study of Léopoldville 1962–63* (Cambridge: The University Press, 1970).
74. La Fontaine, *op. cit.* (note 73), 19.
75. Immatriculés were granted the status of 'quasi-Europeans' after careful selection which involved rigorous inspection of their homes, their education level and their private lives.
76. La Fontaine, *op. cit.* (note 73), 25.
77. R. Mouchet, 'Medical Assistance to Natives, with Special Reference to the Belgian Congo', *The East African Medical Journal,* 9 (1932),

245–7, 246.

78. Walter Rodney, *How Europe Underdeveloped Africa* (London: 1972), 239.
79. Donald Denoon, *Public Health in Papua New Guinea: Medical Possibility and Social Constraint, 1884–1984* (Cambridge: Cambridge University Press, 1989), 32.
80. Janssens, *op. cit.* (note 22), 223.
81. Willy de Craemer and Renée C. Fox, *The Emerging Physician: a Sociological Approach to the Development of a Congolese Medical Profession* (Palo Alto: Stanford University Press, 1968).
82. Ministère des Affaires Etrangères et Africaines, Archives. R/CB 151. 31 March, 1932 Dr Fontana, Report on Hygiene Service in Province Orientale for 1931. Ministère du Congo Belge, *La Santé du Afrique Congo* (Bruxelles: InforCongo, 1958).
83. Ministère du Congo Belge, *La Santé en Afrique Belge* (Bruxelles: InforCongo, 1958), 8.
84. J. Janzen, *Quest for Therapy in Lower Zaire*, 43.
85. K. E. Lashman, *Syncrisis: the Dynamics of Health: SIV: Zaire* (Washington D.C.: U.S. Department of Health, Education and Welfare, 1975), 85.
86. Nzongola-Ntalaja (ed.), *The Crisis in Zaire: Myths and Realities* (Trenton, New Jersey: Africa World Press, Inc., 1986), 'Introduction', 3.
87. Janet MacGaffey, *Entrepreneurs and Parasites: the Struggle for Indigenous Capitalism in Zaire* (Cambridge: Cambridge University Press, 1987). 'Health services in rural areas are almost non-existent', 189. See also Michael G. Schatzberg, *The Dialectics of Oppression in Zaire* (Bloomington: Indiana University Press, 1988).
    In 1987 the GNP per capita was $150 US and the average inflation between 1980–7 was 53.5 per cent. The World Bank, *Sub-Saharan Africa: From Crisis to Sustainable Growth* (1989).
88. The average daily intake of protein was 33 to 43 grams, half the amount recommended by the United Nations' Food and Agricultural [FAO] Organization while caloric intake was estimated at 85 per cent of the FAO requirement.
89. Lashman, *op. cit.* (note 85), 1–27 passim.
90. Feachem, 7.
91. John G. C. Blacker, 'Infant and Child Mortality: Development, Environment, and Custom', 75–86; 77 and Ian M. Timaeus, 'Adult mortality: levels, trends, and data sources', 87–100; 93 *op. cit.* (note 69). It should be noted that population and health statistics for Zaire are lacking with very little reliable data since the early 1970s.

11

Public Health in Modern Japan: From Regimen to Hygiene

Mahito H. Fukuda

Historical Background

This essay examines the history of public health in Japan from the Edo Era (1603–1868) governed by the Tokugawa Shogunate (feudal and military dictatorship) through to the Showa Era (1926–89). From 1868 until the end of the Second World War in 1945, the Japanese Empire was governed by three emperors, namely the Emperors of Meiji, Taisho and Showa.

Nagayo Sensai, the first director of the Board of Public Health in the Interior Ministry, came across the German idea of Hygiene or *Gesundheitpflege* during his journey in Europe as a member of the Iwakura Mission (1871–3) to the Western countries. He translated these words into Japanese as *eisei* (hygiene) when the Department of Medical Affairs, the Ministry of Education (first established in 1872), became a board in the Interior Ministry in 1875. When searching for an appropriate name for this new department, Dr Nagayo discovered the word *eisei* in a text written by the Chinese thinker Soshi (*Chang–tze, Zhuang Zi*).[1]

This little episode about the coinage of *eisei* shows very clearly that the Japanese had almost no notion of collective sanitation or hygiene before the Meiji Era except for the idea of individual 'wholeness' or health interest in general terms. Naturally they wanted to be happy and healthy as other nations did, but they didn't form a concept of being hygienic or sanitary in a medical sense. While some thinkers and philosophers tried to deal with individual health, it was not until the nineteenth century that the problem of protecting and promoting community health became a matter of national concern which would lead to various health measures taken over the following course of years.

As far as individual health is concerned, people had practised many holistic regimens such as tea-drinking, martial arts and other habits believed to promote good health. Also, Chinese medications like acupuncture and moxibustion together with herbal therapy, *Inyou-do* (yin and yang) therapy and *Ki* (vital energy) therapy had been practised. Some books such as *Kissa-yojoki (The Regimen of Tea-Drinking,* (1211) by Eisai (1141–1215) and *Yojokun (Maxims of Regimen,* (1713), by Kaibara Ekiken (1630–1714) were widely read and were used mainly by those of the warrior and merchant classes. In particular, *Yojokun* became quite popular due to its simplicity and diverse advice covering everything from diet, breathing, and sexual activities, to application for herbal medicine and acupuncture.

Japan has a long history of medicine greatly influenced by Chinese and Korean medicine dating back to the sixth and seventh centuries; this influence lasted more than a thousand years until the introduction of Western medicine in 1549, together with Christianity. As early as 723, two institutions, *Seyaku-in* (Medication Centre) and *Hiden-in* (Philanthropy Centre) provided medicine and shelter for the sick and poor. In the sixteenth and seventeenth centuries, two Japanese medical schools were founded after Western medicine was introduced by the Portuguese and Spanish missionaries in 1549. At this time the Dutch, who continued to teach and introduce updated medicine to the Japanese, remained the only traders with the Japanese at a restricted area in Nagasaki under the National Seclusion Policy adopted by the Tokugawa Shogunate in 1639. This policy persisted until 1853 when four American battleships paid an unwelcome visit to Japan after 219 years of isolation.

During this period, many Dutch physicians and surgeons, as well as some from other nationalities, visited Nagasaki and had a profound influence on the development of medicine and science in Japan. At the same time in the West, advances were being made in medical knowledge upon which the bases of modern public health was founded.[2]

Before the Meiji Era (1868–1912) Japanese thinking about health was dominated by concern for individual well-being. If, for example, one was afflicted with a certain disease, especially in the countryside, what he or she might do was to go to a shrine or temple to pray to a god, or he practised *Zen* (religious meditation), or took some herbal medicine, or applied acupuncture or moxibustion. It was rather rare for them to go and see a doctor. Therefore, it was well known that drug merchants from Toyama Prefecture prospered and in each district there were many shrines and temples that specialized in protection against certain diseases and injuries such as eye diseases, stiff shoulders and even for stillborn babies.

In 1722 *Koishikawa Yojosho* (Infirmary) was opened in Edo (now Tokyo) to offer medical care to the sick poor, but the first Western-style hospital was built in Fuani (now Oita) by the Portuguese clergyman and surgeon Luis de Almeida in 1577. The concept and understanding of a need for social assistance in case of sickness or other kinds of misfortunes, however, still wasn't highly developed during the Edo period. Even when Buddhist medicine was pre-eminent, religion did not play an important role in providing medical relief work or philanthropic activities. In fact religion was often a barrier to the development of community action on health.

Vaccination against smallpox in 1798 was one of the most important and early contributions of the nineteenth century to public health. In 1801 Jenner's theory of vaccination for smallpox reached Japan just a few years after its discovery, and in 1848 the Dutch doctor Otto G. Mohnike introduced Jennerian vaccination to Japan.

Due to recurrent epidemics of smallpox, the government established the *Shutojo* (Vaccination Place for Smallpox) in 1858, which became *Seiyo-igakusho* (Western Medical School), in 1861. In 1869 it became *Daigaku Toko* (University East School), and in 1874 *Tokyo Igakko* (Tokyo Medical School) which later became the Faculty of Medicine, University of Tokyo.

Unfortunately, Japan did not undergo the cultural and economic changes experienced in the West during the Enlightenment and the Industrial Revolution. Japan would have to wait until her own enlightenment period, represented in the Meiji Restoration of 1868. At the end of the Tokugawa Shogunate and the beginning of the Meiji Era was a time of transition, and it was at this time that Japan experienced her period of great scientific outburst, enabling medical doctors and researchers to understand the nature of diseases more precisely and correctly.

It is not clear what sort of diseases were prevalent before 1868, but according to the medical historian Fujikawa Yu, there were 507 episodes of epidemics between 552 and 1867, among which 65.1 per cent was due to *ekibyo* (epidemics which may include various infectious diseases), 13.2 per cent was smallpox, 8.3 per cent was influenza, and 7.5 per cent was measles.[3] Further insight can be gained from the birth and death record found at a temple in a remote countryside village in Hida district with a population of 3,000. These show that in the ten years between 1841–50 the most common cause of death was infant death, the number of these was 307 out of 778 in total, followed by smallpox (94 deaths), respiratory diseases (37), acute infectious intestinal diseases including cholera (34), intestinal diseases (34), icterus (26), apoplexy (21), tuberculosis (16), nervous system disorder (16), death related to delivery (15), accident (14), others (46) and unknown cause (118).[4] The preventive and curative measures taken were in the form of prayer to the gods, bathing, attention to daily regimen, room fumigation and isolation. There were probably further various healing rituals observed by common people, which certainly had questionable results.

Meiji Restoration and the New System

The Meiji policies of *Shokusan-kogyo* (Increase in Production and Promotion in Industry) and *Fukoku-kyohei* (Enrich the Country and Strengthen the Army) aimed to increase national power and wealth. Securing a large healthy population for the factories and the army became a government priority and thus stimulated the development of policies on national public health.

The new government established the Department of Medical Affairs in the Ministry of Education, in order to institutionalize medical care, medical education and public health administration and services. *Tokyo Iggako* (Tokyo Medical School) was created in 1874 and became the model for many medical schools subsequently established throughout Japan. In the same year, an epoch-making decree, *Isei* (Medical Order), was promulgated. Though it was not a formal act and many of its sections were not actually implemented, it gave a good start to public health administration in Japan. It was drafted by Nagayo Sensai, who had visited the United States and Europe and came to realize the vital necessity of the nationwide public health service and sanitation system. He aimed to design a system which would institutionalize public health, medical education and the foundation of hospitals, as well as regulate medication and the distribution of pharmaceuticals, namely, doctors, nurses, midwives and pharmacists.

In 1875 the examination system for issuing a medical doctor's licence began in Tokyo, and later this was extended to the whole country. In 1874 the total number of doctors in Japan was 28,262, of whom 23,015 were traditional Chinese-style and 5,274 Western-style. However, as Western medicine was officially adopted by the Meiji government, and since the medical examination system itself was designed for it, the number of medical practitioners of traditional Chinese-style began to decrease, and by 1925 more than

95 per cent of the doctors studied Western medicine. The number of the medical schools increased accordingly from 9 in 1874 to 20 in 1900 and 50 in 1970. The number of nurses also increased from 11,574 in 1910 to 138,346 in 1940 and 273,572 in 1970.

In 1871 the *Koseki-ho* (Household Act) was passed which, together with *Isei*, established nationwide registration offices and made a population census possible. The *Eiseikyoku-Nenpo (Annual Report of the Board of Hygiene)* was first published in 1877 and *Tokei-Nenkann (The Statistical Almanac)* first appeared in 1882.

The population in Japan prior to the Meiji Era has been estimated to be between 30–32 million and it is believed that this figure remained roughly constant throughout the Edo Era. Population growth was restricted due to recurrent epidemics, famines and the practice of infanticide but poverty was the main cause for keeping the infant survival rate low. However, even without this, the population could not increase dramatically because of the high infant mortality rate and low birth-rate among the peasants and farmers.

The new Meiji government began to take various public health measures which included some environmental improvements following the epidemics of cholera and typhoid in the 1870s. People began to realize the vital necessity for cleanliness, and the word *eisei* became popular among the learned and the common people alike. The first step was the construction of wholesome water supplies and creation of hygienic provisions for sewerage. In 1878 the Drinking Water Caution Regulations Act was passed followed by the Regulation for Street Sweeping, the Regulations for Lavatory Structure and Excrements Removal and the Regulation for Bath Houses of 1879, the Regulations of Theatres of 1882, and the Regulations of Graveyard and the Burial of the Dead of 1884. The first water supply system was completed in Yokohama in 1887, and in 1890 the Water Supply Act was passed. The first Pharmacopoeia of Japan was set in 1886, and in 1889 the Regulations for Drug Trade and Management was enacted to control pharmacists and their dispensation.

In 1899 Japan experienced its first attack of plague which was imported from Hong Kong. Although only 45 people died, it aroused great public fear exacerbated by the government encouraging the eradication of rats by purchasing them from the citizens. The epidemic originally appeared in Hong Kong and Canton in 1894, the same year that the cause of the plague, *Pasteurella pestis*, was identified by Yersin and Kitasato. In the next ten years from 1900 to 1909, there were 2,406 incidents of plague and 1,155 deaths in

Japan. As the result of the modern system of quarantine and other public health measures it was never as devastating as it was in the West, in India or China. In 1900 many new public hygiene laws and regulations were introduced including the Nuisances Removal Act, the Sewerage Act, the Regulations of Food and Drink, the Milk Selling Regulations, the Regulations of Poisonous Colouring, the Regulations of Soft Drinks, the Regulations of Utensils for Food and Drink and the Regulations of Ice Selling.

Infectious Diseases and the Government

As early as 1822, even before the opening of the country, an epidemic of cholera caused severe devastation throughout Japan. In 1857 cholera returned when an American battleship, the Mississippi, imported infected patients which led to a massive epidemic throughout the country that killed over 100,000 people in Edo alone over the next three years. But this did not change the course of the Tokugawa Shogunate, because by this time it had already lost its power and administrative capacity. Later, as had happened in Britain, recurrent epidemics of cholera, smallpox, dysentery, typhoid and typhus created the necessity for effective public health measures and organization. (See Table 1) After the opening of the ports to foreign countries, cholera continued to invade. Many people believed that with each ship a new epidemic occurred, when ships came and went without any quarantine procedure. This led to a new public demand for the revision of unequal treaties with foreign countries. Under the new treaty Japan implemented quarantine at certain ports of entry, which decreased the number of patients and deaths from infectious diseases. The numbers of patients and deaths in the cholera epidemic in 1877, the first attack in the Meiji Era, were 13,816 and 8,027, respectively, 163,637 and 105,786 in 1879, and 155,923 and 108,405 in 1886.[5]

The Interior Ministry issued guidelines for the 'Prevention of Cholera' in 1877. In 1879 the Central Sanitary Committee was established in the Interior Ministry to deal with cholera epidemics and this led to the establishment of the Local Sanitary Committee, *eisei-ka* (Department of Hygiene) and the appointment of *eisei-iin* (Sanitary Officer) in each town. In 1880 the Regulations for the Prevention of Infectious Diseases were issued, which made six infectious diseases notifiable, namely, cholera, typhoid fever, dysentery, diphtheria, typhus and smallpox.

Table 1: Infectious Diseases in Meiji Era

	Cholera		Dysentery		Typhus		Smallpox	
Year	No. of Patients	No. of Deaths	No. of Patients	No. of Deaths	No. of Patients	No. of Deaths	No. of Patients	No. of Deaths
1876			976	76	869	108	318	145
1877	13,816	8,027	349	38	1,964	141	3,441	653
1878	902	275	1,078	181	4,902	558	2,896	685
1879	162,637	105,786	8,167	1,477	10,652	2,530	4,799	1,295
1880	1,580	618	5,047	1,305	17,140	4,177	3,415	1,731
1881	9,378	6,237	6,827	1,802	16,999	4,203	342	34
1882	51,631	33,784	433,20,1	1,313	17,308	5,231	1,106	197
1883	669	434	72	5,066	18,769	5,043	1,271	295
1884	904	417	22,702	6,036	23,279	5,969	1,703	410
1885	13,824	9,329	47,307	10,690	29,504	6,672	12,759	3,329
1886	155,923	108,405	24,326	6,839	66,224	13,807	73,337	18,678
1887	1,228	654	16,147	4,257	47,449	9,813	39,779	9,967
1888	810	410	26,815	6,576	43,600	9,211	4,052	853
1889	751	431	22,873	5,970	35,849	8,623	1,324	328
1890	46,019	35,227	42,633	8,706	34,736	8,164	296	25
1891	11,142	7,760	46,358	11,208	43,967	9,614	3,608	721
1892	874	497	70,842	16,844	35,636	8,529	33,779	8,409
1893	633	364	167,305	41,284	34,069	8,183	41,898	11,852
1894	546	314	155,140	38,094	36,667	8,054	12,418	3,342
1895	55,144	40,154	52,711	12,959	37,015	8,401	1,284	268
1896	1,481	907	85,876	22,356	42,505	9,174	10,704	3,388
1897	891	488	91,077	23,763	26,998	5,697	41,946	12,276
1898	655	374	90,976	22,392	25,297	5,697	1,752	362
1899	829	487	108,713	23,763	27,673	6,452	1,215	245

from MHW, *Isei Hyakunen Shi*; 544–5

The public health machinery was transferred from the Board of Internal Affairs to the Board of Police, Interior Ministry, in 1893. Unfortunately this meant that more emphasis was placed upon administration and strict regulation than on implementing the effective measures of prevention and treatment. This oppressive attitude of the medical police did more harm than good especially in 1882 when Tokyo was attacked severely by a cholera epidemic. Then the Tokyo Metropolitan Police enforced an isolation policy which forcibly separated infected people from the healthy but did not provide any treatment. Furthermore, deep-rooted and widespread popular fears of the police together with superstitions concerning the disease probably resulted in a much smaller number of notified patients of infectious diseases recorded than actually existed. For example, the numbers of notified patients and deaths of tuberculosis were 22,827 and 153,154 respectively in Japan in 1940. This meant that only 14.9 per cent of the deaths due to tuberculosis were notified annually by the early twentieth century whereas, 71,745 and 38,173 in England and Wales were notified in 1927 (187.9 per cent), 44,051 and 21,400 in Prussia

(Germany) in 1930 (205.8 per cent) and 3,163 and 3,439 in Austria in 1927 (92 per cent).[6]

As is clearly seen in Table 1, there were many infectious diseases prevalent in the Meiji Era, such as dysentery, typhoid fever, typhus, smallpox and diphtheria. Due to sporadic epidemics of smallpox, the government issued a notice to all the prefectures to promote vaccination in 1870. The Regulations for Smallpox Prevention made the vaccination of smallpox compulsory in 1876.

Deaths from infectious diseases increased drastically in 1946 just after the Second World War; 1,245 from cholera, 13,409 from dysentery, 5,446 from typhoid, 3,351 from typhus, and 3,029 from smallpox. In particular, the number of deaths from dysentery did not decrease until well into the 1950s.

Venereal diseases (VD) received much attention from the viewpoint of public health. Mainly these were syphilis and gonorrhoea which were widespread and caused much illness, both physical and mental. Syphilis attacked Japan for the first time by way of China in 1512, 31 years before the first Europeans, the Portuguese, visited Japan in 1543. In 1867, just one year prior to the Meiji Restoration, the first medical examination of the prostitutes was carried out under the advice of the British Minister to Japan, Sir Harry Smith Parks. Inspection took place firstly in Yokohama and later in Nagasaki and Kobe, but with the main purpose of protecting the health of the British Army stationed in Japan.

The first government regulations on venereal diseases were issued in 1871 which established *Kenbaisho* (Syphilis Inspection Centre) in various places throughout the country. The number of hospitals specializing in venereal diseases increased from 3 in 1875 to 135 in 1881.[7] In 1876 the Interior Ministry issued further regulations which established syphilis inspection sites in areas containing houses of ill repute which led to the nationwide inspection of all prostitutes. All inspections were accompanied by the police but their presence often promoted an atmosphere of fear making many of those being inspected uncooperative.

In 1900, the Regulations of Prostitutes legalized registered prostitution. Anyone who was not registered in the list of prostitutes was prohibited from practising their trade. In 1905, the Japanese Association for the Prevention of Venereal Diseases was established in the private sector to promote health education concerning the prevention and treatment of the venereal diseases. In 1927, the Venereal Disease Prevention Act was promulgated which required municipal authorities to provide for the setting up of treatment clinics.

After the Second World War the number of the venereal diseases patients almost doubled in 1947 to 391,811 patients. In 1948, the Venereal Disease Prevention Act was passed which made it compulsory to notify and submit to examination and, if necessary, treatment. Finally, in 1958, the Prohibition of Prostitution Act was promulgated. However, though official prostitution itself was prohibited, many prostitutes went underground without taking any inspection or treatment. Even today, the real number of the patients is not known, for venereal diseases are usually spread as the result of promiscuity which is a problem of ethical standards, considered outside the scope of preventive medicine.

Combat Against Diseases: Tuberculosis – a Case Study

Of all the diseases in nineteenth- and early twentieth-century Japan tuberculosis was the greatest threat to national prosperity and power. Especially since issues of health and disease were viewed by the Meiji government chiefly in terms of maintaining and augmenting a population that could be economically productive and provide stout soldiers.

Devastating epidemics of infectious diseases were the initial impetus to early Japanese sanitary reform. However, there were some pioneer health reformers in Japan who, at the same time, observed that high levels of endemic and epidemic diseases followed industrialization, as in Britain, Germany, France or the United States. Japan began to face similar consequences of industrial and economic development and began to urgently need similar cures. Premature death and ill health were common among workers and their families, partly due to the bad working conditions, and partly due to congested and insanitary urban communities.

This is clearly reflected in the governmental survey report entitled *Shokko-Jijo (The Conditions of the Workers)* in 1902 compiled and published by the Ministry of Agriculture and Commerce. Furthermore a lecture given by Dr Ishihara Osamu after completing a long survey gave an even greater shock to the government and the industrial world as well. The lecture *Joko-to-Kekkaku (Female Mill Hands and Tuberculosis)* in 1913 inspired the Factory Legislation in 1911 and its enforcement in 1916. In this Act people under 12 years of age were prohibited from working and further restrictions were set regarding working conditions.

Consumption, or tuberculosis, was the common disease amongst workers and was considered to be the most devastating one. Despite the fact that the government began to pay attention to the rising mortality from tuberculosis from 1884, it was not until 1901 that the Act of Prevention of Cattle Tuberculosis was passed. In 1904 the Interior Ministry issued its first decree on the Prevention of Pulmonary Tuberculosis. This decree, however, is often called the 'sputum pot' decree, because it only ordered pots to be set up in public places and had no penal regulations for those who broke the law.

The effects of harsh working conditions upon the high mortality rate from tuberculosis among female workers in textile mills was documented in *Joko-aishi (A Tragic History of Female Workers)* by Hosoi Wakizo in 1925. It should be noted that until 1933 more than half of the work-force consisted of young farm girls. Between 1910 and 1914, 71 per cent of all labourers and about 90 per cent of all textile workers were women.[8] Substantial improvement in working conditions did not occur, however, until the end of the Second World War in 1945.

Koch's discovery of the *tubercular bacillus* in 1882 was quickly accepted by the Japanese medical community but it took decades before it received general recognition amongst the broader population. On the one hand this meant that the failure of tuberculin did not affect the Japanese people in general. On the contrary, its newly developed fluid was in use as late as 1940. On the other hand, however, its failure set back general acceptance of any specific anti-bacterial cure for years. Resistance to bacteriology strengthened a belief in open-air treatment for tuberculosis together with diet therapy.

Before the advent of effective antibiotics such as streptomycin in 1944, a change of air and sanatorium treatment were believed to be the only curative treatments. However, due to its drastic propagation and a widespread belief that tuberculosis was not infectious but hereditary, tuberculous patients and their families tended to conceal the fact and to resort to a wide variety of alternative cures, medical and non-medical alike. Thus medical quackery and imitation drugs became enormously popular. Only wealthy people could afford to take sanatorium treatment or spend the long period necessary for the 'change of air'. For example, the number of deaths from all forms of tuberculosis was 123,409 in 1934, but in that year there were only 13,334 beds for the tuberculous patients.[9]

In 1908 the German bacteriologist Robert Koch visited Japan and received an enthusiastic welcome throughout the country. Thus, together with the Emperor's campaign for the promotion of welfare for the destitute in 1911, the prevention of tuberculosis attracted new social attention and public support. The Japanese Association for the Prevention of Tuberculosis was formed to facilitate sanitary education and combat tuberculosis. The Association ran the Site for Early Tuberculosis Diagnosis, which identified 1,208 in 1926.[10]

Despite widespread and energetic activities by voluntary organizations such as the Association and the Salvation Army, which opened a sanatorium in 1916, the mortality and morbidity rates from tuberculosis continued to increase. In 1918 the mortality rate from tuberculosis reached its highest 257.1 per 100,000 population with total deaths of 140,747. (It is probable that at the end of the Second World War it reached its highest level, but due to the chaotic circumstances of the times no survey on health and hygiene was done.) During the Taisho Period (1912–26), the mortality rate and the number of death per annum continued to exceed 200.0 and 100,000 respectively, and showed a rising tendency. In response to this undesirable situation, the Tuberculosis Prevention Act was passed in 1919, which finally included penalties for those who broke the laws on public hygiene. Following this, new legislation introduced a general system of health insurance. The Health Insurance Act, modelled on that designed by the German Chancellor Otto von Bismarck, was passed in 1922 and came into effect in 1926. The Japanese system covered medical care, sickness allowance and funeral fees, as well as the cost of and allowance for childbirth, which relieved the difficulties of the workers to a certain extent. In the same year, the Tuberculosis Society was founded under the guidance of the Tokyo Municipal Dispensary and played an important role in medical research of the disease.

In 1926, the Army set up the Committee for Pleurisy in order to promote prevention and treatment for increasing numbers of tuberculous soldiers. The number of patients also began to increase in the formerly tuberculosis-free areas such as the farming countryside and mountainous places, especially in Ishikawa Prefecture.[11] In 1928, the Department of Hygiene set up a Tuberculosis Counselling Centre and in 1931, together with the Tokyo Metropolitan Police, it created the first Municipal Health Counselling Centre (later Koishikawa Health Centre), at Koishikawa in Tokyo.[12] Under the 1937 Public Health Centre Act the government planned to establish 650 centres for health counselling. The priority of eradicating tuberculosis also stimulated the creation of *Koseisho* (the Ministry of Health and Welfare, MHW) in 1938. Various functions formerly controlled by the Interior Ministry, the Ministry of Education and some other ministries were now synthesized into one department.

In 1939 the Foundation for the Prevention of Tuberculosis was established by the request of the Empress. In the same year, the

Department of Tuberculosis was formed in the Prevention Bureau, MHW. Under these two institutions, mass medical examination by X-ray filming, tuberculin testing, percussion and auscultation were carried out extensively and intensively, and those who had not yet been infected with tuberculosis received inoculation by BCG vaccine. However, owing to the war and the resulting social uncertainty, the number of patients and deaths from tuberculosis did not diminish. Since the end of the Second World War, the development of streptomycin and gradual improvements in medical services and technology (and perhaps owing to further unexplained factors) the mortality and morbidity rates finally began to decrease. It has been constantly declining from 187.2 in 1947 to 3.2 in 1988 (mortality rate per 100,000 population). (See Table 2)

Present Picture of Public Health and the Future

The basic problem of public health in Japan was the urgent need to create a strong and effective administrative machinery. For this purpose, the government established the Department of Medical Affairs followed by the Board of Hygiene in the Interior Ministry. Unfortunately, this board functioned not as a preventive and sanitary machine, but instead was an oppressive body limited to policing infectious and hereditary diseases. Today, the Ministry of Health and Welfare is responsible for all aspects of the health services in Japan. The district health department of each prefecture, city and town, is responsible for the planning and operational administration of all health services in their areas. They coordinate the provision of services by doctors, nurses, medical technicians, pharmacists and dentists.

Basically, the Japanese Government has long been concerned with the prevention and treatment of diseases that threaten society. However, less attention has been paid to the promotion and maintenance of health in general and this continues to be the case. One particular reason for this is the drastic change in the picture of disease and health. It is widely believed that all sorts of acute infectious diseases have been subdued and that the scope of public health has been widened enormously. Meanwhile, the development of medical science and technology has enabled people to receive medical care of higher quality and more diverse fields. However, Japan still keeps its unique disease characteristics; after the 1950s, the most common cause of death has been cerebral apoplexy, while cardiac disorders continue to dominate the West. Another example is cancer. In Japan the most common type of cancer of the digestive tract is stomach cancer, whereas in the West intestinal cancer is most predominant.

Table 2: Number of Deaths and Mortality Rate from Tuberculosis

Year	No. of Deaths	Mortality Rate	Year	No. of Deaths	Mortality Rate
1883	13,808	73.5	1929	123,490	194.6
1884	29,269	77.1	1930	119,635	185.6
1885	—	—	1931	121,875	186.2
1886	36,138	93.1	1932	119,196	179.4
1887	36,369	92.0	1933	126,703	187.9
1888	39,687	99.0	1934	131,525	192.5
1889	42,452	104.3	1935	132,151	190.8
1890	46,025	112.3	1936	145,160	207.0
1891	54,505	132.1	1937	144,620	204.8
1892	57,292	132.6	1938	148,827	209.6
1893	57,798	137.4	1939	154,371	216.3
1894	52,888	122.3	1940	153,154	212.9
1895	58,992	137.0	1941	154,344	215.3
1896	62,790	144.3	1942	161,484	223.1
1897	—	—	1943	171,473	235.3
1898	—	—	1944	—	—
1899	—	—	1945	—	—
1900	71,771	163.7	1946	—	—
1901	76,614	172.7	1947	146,241	187.2
1902	82,559	183.6	1948	143,909	179.9
1903	85,132	186.9	1949	138,113	168.8
1904	87,260	189.1	1950	121,769	146.4
1905	96,030	206.0	1951	93,307	110.3
1906	96,069	204.2	1952	70,558	82.2
1907	96,584	203.7	1953	57,849	66.5
1908	98,871	206.1	1954	55,124	62.4
1909	113,622	234.0	1955	46,735	52.3
1910	113,203	230.2	1956	43,874	48.6
1911	110,722	222.1	1957	42,718	46.9
1912	114,197	225.8	1958	36,274	39.4
1913	110,753	215.9	1959	32,992	35.5
1914	113,341	217.8	1960	31,959	34.2
1915	115,913	219.7	1961	27,916	29.6
1916	121,810	227.7	1962	27,852	29.3
1917	124,787	230.5	1963	23,302	24.2
1918	140,747	257.1	1964	22,929	23.6
1919	132,565	240.9	1965	22,366	22.8
1920	125,165	223.7	1966	20,064	20.3
1921	120,719	213.0	1967	17,708	17.8
1922	125,506	218.7	1968	16,922	16.8
1923	118,216	203.4	1969	16,392	16.1
1924	114,229	194.0	1970	15,899	15.4
1925	115,956	194.1	1971	13,608	13.0
1926	113,045	186.1	1972	12,565	11.9
1927	119,439	193.7	1973	11,965	11.1
1928	119,632	191.1			

Imperial Statistical Almanac

With regard to population, high mortality rate together with high birth-rate has been replaced by low mortality and low birth-rate. The early pattern maintained an average population of about 30 million throughout the Edo period. Then as health measures began to be effective and the government encouraged large families, the population increased continuously from 36.7 million in 1880 to 72 million in 1940 and 103.1 million in 1970. Today, Japan has a new picture of population structure consisting of fewer children and more aged people. Modern Japanese demographics now has the world's longest life expectancy (75.2 years for male and 80.93 for female in 1986) but also has a high ratio of aged people (older than 65 years of age), 12.5 per cent, which is expected to reach its highest point by 2005, exceeding even that of Sweden.[13] In view of this exploding population, it is desirable that fewer children are born. However, the Japanese population will soon begin a decreasing trend which may result in the many aged people being supported by fewer younger generations. If so, the present health insurance system may certainly be in grave danger of collapsing. Therefore, a new medical insurance system and improved technology for taking care of the aged should be widely researched and constructed as soon as possible. The community should concern itself with the health problems that plague the aged population. These diseases are diabetes, cancer, cardiovascular conditions, musculoskeletal diseases, as well as mental changes associated with ageing.

Since the end of the Second World War, Japan developed dramatically in terms of industrial production and international trade, but at the cost of environmental beauty and healthy living conditions. More attention should be paid to the rapidly deteriorating environment. The once dominant problems of impure water supply, dirty air without ventilation and food adulteration have been replaced by modern contaminations. Water and air pollution has been caused by industrial and economic growth; poisonous or dangerous food additives exist in our diet; some people suffer from mental problems such as stress due to the pressures of modern urban living and new technology.

The modern era has new public health problems, for example, arsenic in Morinaga powered milk for babies in 1955; *Minamata-byo* (Minamata Disease) in Kumamto Prefecture due to the eating of fish with organic methyl mercury exhausted from the Chisso Company; *Yokkaichi Asthma* due to air pollution by the petro-chemical industry in Mie Prefecture. Consequently in 1971 the Environment Agency was established to deal with environmental problems and public nuisances. This agency established limitation on exhaust fumes and enforced penalties.

Since the 1980s a new health consciousness has been growing in Japan. For example, positive attitudes have developed toward sports and physical training such as aerobics, jogging and jazz-dance. Also, an increase in taking various kinds of vitamin tablets by 'health-conscious' people or drinking a bottle of the widely distributed 'stamina drink'. However, this doesn't mean that people really understand the seriousness of the unsolved health problems or ensure that people are really living a healthy life in a healthy environment. The reality seems to be to the contrary. Here are some examples revealed by recent surveys; For example, only 8 per cent of the Japanese feel that AIDS is threatening, whereas 74 per cent of the people in Greece, where there is about the same rate of incidence occurring, consider it to be a great threat (the official numbers of the infected and death due to AIDS in Japan are 1,852 and 202, respectively in 1990)[14]; secondly, more than 40 per cent of the patients with cerebrovascular disorder are overdosed with drugs and some are medicated with up to seven drugs, some of which provide the exact same effect.[15] It is true that people in Japan depend on drugs excessively and many are, in fact, overdosed. The reason for this is that normally doctors in Japan dispense drugs directly from their offices, and secondly, a doctor's income depends to a certain extent on the amount of drugs he prescribes. Under these circumstances, there exists competition within the drug industry to promote their products to doctors.

Therefore, there is an urgent need for the re-evaluation of the medical system as well as the insurance system. Health education is also needed to enlighten people regarding the doctor–patient relationship, physical exercise for health and the problem of excessive drug dependency. Some other problems come into the scope of public health such as the increasing trend of mental disorders in Japan; the problems of services in remote areas without any doctors; the lack of experienced nurses together with their poor working conditions; the mental stress of the workers and people living in urban areas; the problem of ageing; the quality of medical education; the organization of hospitals and their function and facilities; a review of a comprehensive emergency medical care system; and the issue of drug misuse and abuse. The demand for personal social services will rise in the next few decades and owing to the increasing number of the aged in Japan and the changing attitude towards the pattern of care for mental and chronic illness as well as the attention to the care of handicapped people.

With regard to drug abuse or narcotic drugs, the number of violations of the law has been increasing at a constant rate recently. As this cannot be solved only within the country, international co-operation is required not only in the field of criminal inquiry but also public health. International cooperation is equally necessary for the fight against AIDS. It cannot be either prevented or cured without a working international information network. In order to cope with these problems, nationwide reassessment of our medical care system as well as health care services at the local level is required. Traditionally, central government exercises authority over a locality, therefore any health programme that has been formulated on a state basis can be carried out. Nevertheless, each political level has its own public health responsibilities and functions. At the moment there are about 850 public health centres throughout Japan, whose aims should be re-examined and whose workers should be re-educated.

Japan would then be in a much better position to fulfil its role in the world health care system. Japan should acknowledge its responsibilities to the international community not only because it is economically strong but because it has been asked to take part in an international enterprise of health and welfare. It has enormous potential to make a major contribution both through manpower and specialized knowledge and skills to the World Health Organization.

Notes

1. Nagayo, Sensai (Ogawa, T. and Sakai, S. (eds), *Shoko-Shishi (Shoko Private Journal*), 133
2. Two of those Dutch medical doctors and teachers were Pompe van Meedervoort (1829–1908) and Antonius Francis Bauduin (1822–?). Pompe published his memoire, *Vijf Jaren in Japan (Five Years in Japan) (1857–1863)* and this contains lots of explanations concerning disease and doctors in Edo period Japan.
3. Fujikawa, Y., *Nihon Igakushi* (*A Medical History of Japan*), 345–7.
4. Suda, K., *Hida O-Jiin Kakocho no Kenkyu* (*A Survey of the Death Register in O-Temple in Hida District*), Vol. 2 (Basic Material Sources), 163–81.
5. Koseisho, Imukyoku (Board of Medical Affairs, Ministry of Health and Welfare), *Isei Hyakunenshi* (*A History of One Hundred Years since the Medical Order*), Vol. 2, 545.
6. Kondo, K., *Kekkaku no Yobo to Sono Taisaku* (*Prevention and Counter-Measure for Tuberculosis*), 217.
7. Koseisho, *op cit.* (note 5), Vol. 2, 565.
8. Kazahaya, I., *Nihon Shakai-Seisakushi* (*A History of Social Policy in Japan*), Vol. 1, 80.
9. Mitsui Hoonkai, *Eikoku ni okeru Kekkahu Taisaku oyobi sono Jigyo* (*Anti-Tuberculosis Measures and Scheme in Britain*), 26.
10. Koseisho, *op cit.* (note 5), Vol. 1, 235. There were 1,360 sites for the diagnosis of and treatment for TB throughout Japan including some other organizations.

11. From 1922 until 1942, Ishikawa Prefecture remained the worst in terms of the mortality rate from TB: 293.6 (national average, 191.1 per 100,000 living people) between 1922–6, 306.8 (191.7) between 1932–6, 344.1 (203.0) in 1937. Kondo, *op. cit.* (note 6), 156.
12. Koseisho, *op. cit.* (note 5), 235. From 1932, a certain amount of money was drawn from the revenue of Nihon Hoso Kyokai (NHK, Japanese Broadcasting Corporation) in order to establish anti-TB programme and centres for counselling TB patients and their families, medication and arrange treatment through proper institutions, In 1932, 26 centres were built.
13. *Asahi Shinbun* (*The Asahi Newspaper*), 15 September, 1991 issue. According to the Agency of General Affairs, the ratios of the aged over 65 are 17.8 per cent in Sweden, 15.6 per cent in Britain and Denmark and 12.3 per cent in the USA. Interesting statistics are that the ratio of working-age people is 24.3 per cent (3.6 million) in Japan, wherease 11.9 per cent in the USA, and in many industrial countries it is between 3 and 7per cent. The Japanese ratio is exceedingly high.
14. According to the questionnaire carried out by the Team for AIDS and its Immunity Survey, MHW, released the facts in *Mainichi Shinbun* (*The Mainichi Newspaper*) issued on 14 August, 1991.
15. *Asahi Shinbun*, 14 September, 1991. On average, 40.4 per cent of the patients are more or less overdosed with more than four drugs. 47 per cent of the patients older than 70 were dosed with various medicines, whereas, 28 per cent for under 70.

Bibliography

Abe, Koki. 'Meiji izen no Wagakuni no Koshu-Eisei (Public Health in Japan before the Meija Era)', *Minzoku Eisei (Human Ecology and Race Hygiene),* Vol. 42, No. 1, (Tokyo: 1976).

Fujii, Naohisa. *Igaku Bunkashi Nenpyo* (*Cultural Chronology of Medicine in Japan*) (Nisshinshoin, Tokyo: 1942).

Fujikawa, Yu, *Nihon Igakushi* (*Medical History of Japan*) (Heibonsha, Toyko: 1969).

Fujikawa, Yu, *Nihon Shippeishi (History of Epidemics in Japan)* (Heibonsha, Toyko: 1969).

Fujikawa, Yu, *Nihon Igakushi Yoko* (*Summary of Medical History of Japan*) (Heibonsha, Toyko: 1974).

Jannetta, Ann B., *Epidemics and Mortality in Early Modern Japan* (Princeton: Princeton University Press, 1987).

Kawakami, Takeshi, *Kindai Nihon Iryoshi* (*History of Medical Treatment in Modern Japan*) (Keiso-shobo, Tokyo: 1965).

Komatsu Yoshio, *Wagakuni no Kekkaku (Tuberculosis in Japan)* (Yakugyojihosha, Tokyo: 1973).

Koseisho, Imuka, (Board of Medical Affairs, MHW). *Isei Hyakunen-shi* (*One Hundred Years since the Medical Order*) (Gyosei, Tokyo: 1974).

Nagayo, Sensai (Ogata and Sakai, eds). *Shoko Shishi* (*Shoko Private Journal*) (Heibonsha, Tokyo: 1980).

Nohon Kagaku-shi Gakkai (Japanese Society for the History of Science), *Nihon Kagaku Gijutu-shi Taikei* (*Series of the History of Science and Technology in Japan*), Vol. 24, 25 (Medicine) (Daiichi Hoki Shuppan, Tokyo: 1965).

Ogawa, Teizo, *Igaku no Rekishi* (*History of Medicine*) (Chuokoronsha, Tokyo: 1964).

Ogawa, Teizo (ed.), *Tokyo Daigaku Igakubu 100-nen shi* (*History of 100 Years of the Faculty of Medicine, University of Tokyo*) (Tokyo: Tokyo University Press, 1967).

Okanishi Junjiro, *Kekkaku Zetsumetu eno Michi* (*Toward the Eradication of Tuberculosis*) (Yakugyojihosha, Tokyo: 1973).

Okanishi Junjiro, *Jinrui to Kekkaku* (*Mankind and Tuberculosis*) (Ishiyaku-Shuppan, Tokyo: 1973).

Sakai, Shizu, *Nihon no Iryoshi* (*History of Medical Treatment in Japan*) (Tokyoshoseki, Tokyo: 1982).

Tanami Yukio (ed.), *Koshu-Eisei no Hattatsu* (*Development of Public Health*) (Nohon Koshu-Eisei Kyokai, Tokyo: 1967).

Tatsukawa, Shoji, *Igaku no Shakaishi* (*Social History of Medicine*) (NHK Press, Tokyo: 1971).

Yamamoto, Shunichi, *Nihon Korerashi* (*History of Cholera in Japan*) (Tokyo: Tokyo University Press, 1982).

12

Internationalism in Medicine and Public Health

Milton I. Roemer

As communications and trade have increased among nations in all parts of the world, people have come to recognize the interdependence of each country's health on the disease problems of all other countries. In its broadest sense, international health work concerns the many resultant health activities carried out across national boundaries.

Colonialism, Religious Missions and Philanthropy

The beginnings of internationalism in medicine or cross-national health work must be traced to colonial take-overs in Asia and Africa. In the sixteenth century, the Portuguese established settlements in China, India and the Malay Peninsula in southeast Asia. Later the Dutch and then the British became the principal European colonists in both Asia and Africa. Great Britain was the dominant imperial power in the eighteenth and nineteenth centuries. As colonial governments grew stronger and their military and civilian personnel increased, small garrison hospitals or medical stations were established for their care. Sometimes special wards would be set up for the 'natives'.

A customary course of events was illustrated by the British colonization of East Africa around 1890. The initial settlement was by the Imperial British East Africa Company (IBEA), which soon engaged British doctors to take care of its employees. In 1894, the British government's Foreign Office took control of this work, including the medical services. A few years later these services became a medical department in the British protectorate of Kenya and Uganda, but its resources were very small. In a book published in 1905 on *The East African Protectorate,* the medical services were considered necessary only to protect Europeans against tropical health hazards. Some attention was also given to workers imported from British India, but the health of native Africans was not considered a British responsibility. Colonial government medical services for the control of tropical diseases and for general medical care were generally not extended to the African population until after the First World War (1914–18).

The strategy of colonial health services was to provide support for the general objectives of colonial agriculture. This put the greatest emphasis on growth and export of cash crops, through transfer of male workers to areas of commercialized agriculture, with consequent reduction of traditional food crops at home. This led to extensive malnutrition, even while the income from foreign trade increased. This was evident under the German and later the British colonial policies in what is now Tanzania.

Recent historical research on European imperialism, however, has recognized a complex mixture of motives and strategies in the role of Western medicine in Asian and African colonies. In the early nineteenth century, the health protection of European military personnel and civilian settlers was clearly the main objective. Colonial medical services were largely confined to the main cities, where Europeans were concentrated. When quinine was used by Europeans in an African expedition of 1854, it was described as 'the prime factor in allowing the white man's conquest of Black Africa'. After the 1880s and the great breakthroughs in bacteriology, the discipline of 'tropical medicine' took shape, but its principal objective was to make tropical environments more congenial to European colonists.

In the late nineteenth and early twentieth centuries, the rationale of colonial medical services gradually changed. It was increasingly appreciated that the health of soldiers and other Europeans depended largely on the health of 'native populations' around them. As early as 1865 a British official in the Bengal region of India wrote: 'Even if we look no further than the protection of the health of the European soldiers, it will be evidently insufficient if we endeavour to improve the condition of our cantonments alone, and ignore the existence of the masses of the native population by which our troops are surrounded'. The Indian Medical Service, nevertheless, though started by the British in 1714, did not really begin to serve the Indian people until the twentieth century. In Africa, a Colonial Medical Service for the British colonies was started only in 1927.

In mining and agriculture, disease among indigenous workers was increasingly seen as an impediment to production. It was an obstacle, in later terminology, to economic development. Reduced output of commodities likewise meant lesser tax collections. Also, as the political consciousness of native populations rose, health services were recognized as useful in displaying benevolent and paternalistic intentions among the foreign masters. For all these reasons, by the First World War and even before the 'national liberations' after the Second World War, colonial health services had acquired a much broader meaning – that is, to apply scientific medicine as well as public health strategies to the needs of general colonial populations.

Medical services by religious missions were entirely separate from the colonial government, and these might help the Africans. A 70-bed hospital was built in 1897, for example, by the Church Missionary Society in Uganda, principally to serve African natives. The colonial government administration looked upon these mission services as a useful supplementation to the official programme.

In the nineteenth and early twentieth centuries, Christian missions came from Europe and North America to spread the doctrines of Christianity. As vehicles for their evangelism associated with humanitarianism, they developed hospitals or clinics in many small towns and villages. These facilities often provided the first contact of rural people with Western medicine. In Latin America hospitals, founded by religious groups (mostly Catholic) from Spain and Portugal, became the most numerous facilities in several countries. In the later twentieth century most of these *beneficencia* hospitals were subsidized and then taken over by governments.

In 1799, John Vanderkemp had been the first medical missionary in Africa. He was a Dutch physician whose work was sponsored by the London Missionary Society. Later in the mid nineteenth century a Scottish physician, David Livingstone (1813–73), served as a medical missionary in South Africa (what is now Botswana), and after 1850 he became a general explorer in central Africa. In the late nineteenth and early twentieth centuries, Albert Schweitzer (1875–1965) established the hospital at Lambaréné in French Equatorial Africa, eventually attracting world-wide attention.

Missionary work by physicians started in China at Canton around 1840. These evangelical physicians brought to imperial, and later republican China, its first acquaintance with Western medical education. They introduced concepts of bacteriology and organ pathology, and demonstrated the role of nurses in caring for patients in hospitals. Several Western-type medical schools were founded, leading up to the Peking Union Medical College, started with support from the Rockefeller Foundation in 1914. After 1949 under the Communist government, Western religious missions were terminated in China, but the PUMC was continued as a high-level medical school.

International health work was carried out in many countries by the Rockefeller Foundation from the United States. The Rockefeller International Health Division (started in 1913) promoted health activities in Latin America and Asia involving (1) basic health research, (2) training health personnel through supporting graduate education and (3) setting up demonstrations of model health programmes. Among its more notable achievements, the Rockefeller Foundation developed an effective yellow fever vaccine, mounted a campaign against the mosquito vector, and trained health personnel to carry out this preventive work.

Specific enterprises for mining, agriculture, or other forms of production often established medical units for the care of their employees and their families. In the nineteenth and early twentieth centuries some colonial governments required business enterprises, with more than a certain number of workers, to establish units for medical care. This was the policy in India, for example, and in Egypt and Nigeria. After national independence was gained, such requirements usually became more rigorous.

Aside from direct colonial domination, overt military hostilities promoted by foreign governments have seriously impaired health services in certain newly independent countries. This has been evident recently in the support of counter-revolutionary *contras* by the United States to erode the health gains of the Sandinista government of Nicaragua in the 1980s. It is seen also in the insurrections supported by the government of South Africa against the FRELIMO independence movement that gained control over Mozambique in 1975.

On a non-religious and non-governmental basis, another sort of international health work was done by heroic figures such as Norman Bethune (1890–1939) of Canada. In support of the republican (Loyalist) cause in Spain, he performed surgery behind the battle lines in 1936, and then went to China in 1938 to work with the Red Army before its final victory in 1949. There can be little doubt that inspiration from religion or political conviction or a spirit of international goodwill has figured prominently in the extension of international health work.

International Sanitary Conferences

The first truly international collaborative work, involving 12 European countries (including Turkey), was a meeting in Paris in 1851. It was designated as an International Sanitary Conference. Although it lasted from July 1851 to January 1852, the discussion of different policies on quarantine regulations at national borders failed to lead to any agreement. There were unresolved disputes among the delegates about the contagiousness of the plague, yellow fever and cholera – whether these dreadful scourges were communicated from the sick to the well or whether they were due to certain atmospheric, climatic and soil conditions creating an 'epidemic constitution'. A majority of the delegates voted that cholera should be subject to quarantine regulations, but none of the participating governments acted to ratify such regulations. The only accomplishment of this six-month meeting was the basic experience of several countries in meeting together to discuss an international health problem.

After eight years, a second International Sanitary Conference was held in Paris in 1859. In that eight-year interval an Italian microscopist, Filippo Pacini (1812–83), described clearly the *cholera vibrio* as the pathogenic agent of the disease – a discovery overlooked for 30 years until it was reaffirmed by Robert Koch (1843–1910). Also in 1854, John Snow (1813–58) demonstrated the contagiousness of cholera through ingestion of fecally contaminated water in London from the River Thames. After five months, the Second Conference adjourned with no resolution of the dispute between the contagionists and the miasmatists, and no subsequent ratification of the 'draft convention' on quarantine of cholera by any country.

The third International Sanitary Conference was held in 1866 in Constantinople, followed by a Fourth Conference in Vienna in 1874. Still no effective agreements could be reached, despite a fifth conference in Washington in 1881 and a sixth conference in Rome in 1885. It was only at the seventh International Sanitary Conference in Venice, held in 1892, that agreement was finally reached. It had taken 41 years of discussion to reach agreement of very limited scope on quarantine of westbound ships with a case of cholera on board. This first historic convention also provided that the Pan-Arab Quarantine Board of Health in Egypt should prepare compatible provisions regarding plague and yellow fever, although their aetiology and epidemiology were still quite unknown.

An eighth Sanitary Conference was held at Dresden in 1893, followed soon by a ninth one at Paris in 1894. At the tenth conference held in Venice in 1897, agreement was reached on a second international convention on plague (the spread of which by fleas on rats was to be discovered only some years later). This conference of 21 nations also decided that an international committee should be constituted to codify the sanitary conventions and conclusions of the conferences of 1892, 1893, 1894 and 1897.

International Sanitary Conferences continued to be held periodically until the fourteenth in 1938. This conference brought to an end the international work of the Health, Maritime and Quarantine Board, that had been functioning in Alexandria (although largely under the control of the Egyptian Ministry of Health) since 1881. Later the structure that housed this Alexandria agency became the site of the Eastern Mediterranean Regional Office of the World Health Organization. Another border quarantine agency, founded in 1838 at Constantinople (now Istanbul), with field offices throughout the Ottoman Empire, was completely terminated by the League of Nations (see below) in 1923.

In 1902, as a sequel to these international quarantine efforts, the republics of Latin America, along with the United States, established the Pan-American Sanitary Bureau (PASB), with offices in Washington, D.C. The strong voice of the United States in this body was reflected in its first several Directors, each of whom was a recently retired Surgeon-General of the US Public Health Service. Other leading US figures continued to occupy this post until 1958, when the first Latin American health leader was chosen – Dr Abraham Horwitz (1910–) of Chile. Since then several notable Latin American figures have served in this role, while a United States physician has always occupied a second place as Deputy-Director. In 1949 the PASB became the Regional Office for the Americas of the World Health Organization.

Aside from this long series of international conferences to halt the spread of infectious diseases, the nineteenth century spawned international congresses on other medical and related subjects. In 1867 the first general medical congress, with representatives from many nations, was held in Paris – followed every two years by similar meetings in Florence, Vienna and other European cities (except for 1887 in Washington) up to 1913 in London. International congresses on specialized health-related subjects had, in fact, been held earlier in Brussels – on statistics in 1851, demography and hygiene in 1852, and ophthalmology in 1857. Other international meetings were held in various European cities on veterinary medicine (1863), pharmacy (1865), tuberculosis (1888), dermatology (1889), psychology (1890), gynaecology and obstetrics (1892), alcoholism (1894), leprosy (1897), dentistry, 1900), surgery (1902), school hygiene (1904), physiotherapy (1905), cancer (1906), sleeping sickness (1907), epilepsy (1909), comparative pathology (1912), and the history of medicine (1920). These are only a sampling of the subjects of such international meetings – most of which seemed to be based on topics of interest to selected medical specialists.

The Red Cross and Geneva Conventions

Almost parallel with the International Sanitary Conferences and their development was another international initiative launched by private citizens. This was the Red Cross, founded by five leading citizens of Geneva in 1863. A Swiss philanthropist, J. Henri Dunant (1828–1910) had witnessed the bloody battle of Solferino (northern Italy) in 1859, and he formed the International Committee of the Red Cross – devoted to helping the wounded soldiers of any country. The impartial humanitarian spirit of the *Commitée Internationale de Croix Rouge* (CICR) was closely linked to traditional Swiss neutrality in international affairs; all members and employees of the CICR, therefore, had to be Swiss citizens.

Very soon several European nations formed their own national Red Cross societies, and they met in Geneva in 1864. This First Geneva Convention agreed that 'sick and wounded soldiers will be collected and cared for irrespective of nationality'. This remarkable impartiality was confirmed and extended at subsequent Geneva Conventions held in 1906 and 1929. The Third Convention in 1929 extended the Red Cross purposes to include help for prisoners of war and also for civilian victims of hostilities.

The several national Red Cross (and later in Muslim countries the Red Crescent) societies grew and developed during periods of peace after wars. In peacetime, they devoted their voluntary efforts to helping their own citizens in the event of various natural disasters, such as floods, hurricanes, earthquakes and fires; they also helped to care for people injured in domestic civil wars or other types of mass violence.

By the end of the First World War, the national Red Cross societies, while still non-governmental, had attained sufficient stability and recognition to be noted in the Covenant of the League of Nations (Article 25) in 1918. Then in 1919, under the leadership of the American Red Cross, there was formed, for the first time, an international League of Red Cross Societies. Initially there were member-societies from 26 countries, and this grew to 113 countries in 1970 and to 164 in 1987. The League of Red Cross Societies' headquarters is located in Geneva, but it is separate from the CICR, though obviously in close working relationship. The CICR is financed mainly by voluntary donations from the national societies.

The national members of the League meet every two years in Geneva, as a Board of Governors, with one vote per member (regardless of national population). In the Geneva secretariat there are several sections, most important of which are the Relief Bureau and the Health and Social Service Bureau. The latter has activities relating to 1) first-aid and accident prevention, 2) blood transfusion services, 3) standardization of medical equipment and 4) medical information and documentation. The League of Red Cross Societies as a whole is devoted to: 1) assisting national societies in their development of programmes and 2) coordinating collaborative international efforts of national societies. The League also maintains relationships with WHO and UNICEF.

OIHP and the League of Nations

Another milestone in international health was reached in 1907, when an agreement was reached in Rome among 23 European countries on the establishment of a permanent public health office in Europe. This was the *Office International d'Hygiène Publique* (OIHP), to be located in Paris. The functions of the 'Office' concerned the collection and dissemination of new knowledge on infectious diseases that should be embodied in international quarantine regulations. The principal focus initially was on cholera, plague, and yellow fever – three diseases that had occupied the attention of the International Sanitary Conferences. Eventually OIHP included nearly 60 countries in its membership, including Persia, India, Pakistan and the United States. French was the only official language.

Soon the concerns of OIHP were broadened to other communicable diseases, such as malaria, tuberculosis, typhoid fever, meningitis, sleeping sickness, and the overall suppression of insect vectors of disease. Interest was shown also in other public health subjects, such as food hygiene, the management of hospitals, and the hygiene of schools and factories. Although OIHP did not do any field work on these matters, it provided an international forum for their discussion among public health leaders of different nations. With the outbreak of the First World War in 1914, all OIHP discussions were suspended, except the publication of its *Bulletin*. Recommendations had been made to governments on environmental sanitation, notification of cases of tuberculosis, inoculation against typhoid fever and isolation of cases of leprosy. The dissemination and discussion of such ideas had some value, in spite of no national action being taken for their implementation.

After the First World War (1914–18), a world-wide desire for peace resulted in the organization of the League of Nations. To carry out the League's activities relating to the 'prevention and control of disease', it established a subdivision, known as the Health Organization of the League of Nations. The United States was not a member of the League, and – being a member of OIHP – it vetoed a proposal to move the Paris-based body into the League. Therefore, in 1921 there were three international agencies with very similar functions: the OIHP, the Pan American Sanitary Bureau and the League's Health Organization. Cooperative agreements among these were obviously necessary.

After the World War in 1919, typhus fever spread epidemically through Russia and Poland. Some 1,600,000 cases were reported in Russia; on top of this the unprecedented world pandemic of influenza arose, estimated to cause as many as 15,000,000 deaths by 1920. In this catastrophic situation, an International Health Conference met in London, but it was attended by only five countries – Great Britain, France, Italy, Japan and the United States. Eventually the Health Organization of the League of Nations became a Health Committee of the League, and of its eight members, four served also as members of the Permanent Committee of the *Office International d'Hygiène Publique.*

In spite of the diplomatic complexities of these relationships between the League's Health Committee and OIHP, several new international health activities were initiated by the League. Broadly speaking, these fell into two general categories: 1) international health studies, expert committees on selected subjects, and proposed international standards on certain issues; 2) field assistance to countries on special health problems.

With modest funding, most League health activities were of the first type. Studies were made and expert committees appointed on major diseases (malaria, syphilis, tuberculosis, leprosy, etc.), on aspects of health care (school health service, health centres, medical care administration, health insurance, medical education, etc.) and on other matters. International classification of the 'Causes of Death and Disease', the standardization of biological substances and potent drugs, and the methods of control of narcotics were solid achievements. Especially important studies were made and conferences were held on nutrition, the health aspects of housing, physical education and the general provision of public health services in rural areas. As part of its epidemiological intelligence work in 1925 the League Health Organization set up a field office in Singapore, to collect and disseminate reports on infectious diseases in the Far East.

The second main type of League health activities, on field

assistance to countries, was limited by insufficient funding. In 1928, Greece was assisted in reorganizing its public health services, followed by a similar service to Bolivia. In 1929, China was assisted in developing its public health service particularly for epidemic control. Smaller missions were sent to a few other countries and study-tours were made by health administrative officials from many countries to observe public health practices in selected European nations.

The Second World War

With the invasion of Poland by Nazi Germany in 1939, the League of Nations soon collapsed and, with it, the League's Health Committee. This gave a clear lesson to the group of public health leaders, who later set out to establish a 'World Health Organization' (WHO). The fate of WHO should not depend on the survival of its parent body, the United Nations. An Interim Commission was organized at an International Health Conference, held in New York in 1946. The WHO Constitution drawn up by the Commission was ratified and took effect on 7 April, 1948 with the signature of 26 member-states of the United Nations, but independent of the UN By 24 June, 1948, when the first World Health Assembly, held in Geneva, Switzerland, adjourned, the WHO Constitution had 55 national signatories.

In December 1946 the United Nations General Assembly established an International Children's Emergency Fund (UNICEF), to be supported by the voluntary contributions of governments. The Interim Commission to plan a 'World Health Organization' had just been formed, and the directors of the emergency Fund did not wish to encroach on its jurisdiction. From the outset, therefore, UNICEF worked in close cooperation with WHO, using its own money essentially for the provision of supplies (food and drugs) and equipment. UNICEF is governed by the Executive Board of members from 25 countries, and comes under the general supervision of the UN Economic and Social Council (ECOSOC). Although 'emergency' was soon deleted from the name of UNICEF, it was retained in the acronym, and the agency's robust performance has kept it alive to the present time.

In these Second World War years, other international orga nizations, with substantial health functions, were launched. To provide general relief, including health services, to the war-torn countries of Europe as well as to China, 43 nations formed the United Nations Relief and Rehabilitation Administration (UNRRA) in 1943. This was an intentionally temporary agency, in which representatives from the United States played a major role. The Health Division of UNRRA was transferred to WHO by a vote of its Council in 1946.

Another specialized agency of the United Nations, intended also to be temporary, was the International Refugee Organization (IRO) established in 1948. The former director of the displaced persons programme in the Health Division of UNRRA was taken on the IRO executive staff, based in Geneva. In January 1949, the United Nations Assembly terminated the IRO, but continued its important work through the UN High Commissioner for Refugees (UNHCR). The UNHCR had a relatively small staff, and did no international health work directly, but looked to WHO for technical advice. Health services to refugees were left in the hands of the host countries. The UNHCR still operates, with headquarters in Geneva, and works closely with WHO.

After the Second World War a new type of international work was developed through the initiative of the United States and several European countries – namely foreign aid from single industrialized countries to single developing countries. These 'bilateral assistance programmes' were designed to assist in many fields, including health service. By 1980 expenditures by most industrialized countries (principally the 17 member states of the Organization for Economic Cooperation and Development – OECD) were larger through bilateral than through multilateral programmes.

Out of a total of about US $30 billion for all types of foreign aid in general, about $3 billion or 10 per cent was earmarked for health projects. Of this amount, about one-third was spent through WHO and other United Nations affiliated agencies and two-thirds through bilateral aid programmes. The United States, for example, provided development assistance to 88 countries in 1980, of which health assistance applied to 60 countries. In the first post-war decades most bilateral US expenditures were focused on population control through family planning, but in the latter 1970s and the 1980s US policy shifted towards the support of the WHO strategy of emphasizing primary health care.

The World Health Organization and Its Work

In 1948, after its first World Health Assembly, the World Health Organization took action to form a Secretariat in Geneva. It was given space for its initial years in the Palais des Nations, which had been the last home of the League of Nations. As stated in Chapter I of its Constitution, WHO was 'to act as the directing and coordinating authority on international health work'. This was a much broader scope than any other international agency in the orbit of the United Nations.

WHO's structure and functions expanded rapidly. Its programme initially included activities acquired from the International Sanitary Conferences, the *Office International d'Hygiène Publique*, the Health Committee of the League of Nations and the Health Division of UNRRA, plus many new activities affecting the overall development of health systems in countries.

Soon after the establishment of WHO headquarters in Geneva, steps were taken to set up regional offices. The first was the South-East Asia Regional Office (SEARO), located in New Delhi, India, in January 1949. In July 1949 a second office for the Eastern Mediterranean Region (EMRO) was set up in Alexandria, Egypt, at the seat of the original pan-Arab Health, Maritime and Quarantine Board, established previously in Alexandria.

In the same month, July 1949, negotiations with the Pan-American Sanitary Bureau in Washington resulted in integration of the PASB with WHO, as the Regional Office for the Americas. In 1951 two more WHO Regional Offices were established for the Western Pacific Region, based in Manila, Philippines, and the African Region, based in Brazzaville, French Equatorial Africa – later the Republic of Congo. The last Regional Office, to be formed by the vote of a majority of its member states, was for Europe; located temporarily in Geneva in 1952, it was moved to its final location in Copenhagen (EURO) in 1957. The WHO Constitution provides for election of the Regional Office directors by a majority of the countries in each region.

Within WHO, the highest authority is the World Health Assembly, convened once each year for about three weeks in May. The Assembly includes representatives of all member states – some 166 countries in 1990 – with one vote each, regardless of size or financial contribution. Large countries, nevertheless, naturally have substantial influence. The Regional Boards in each of the six regions have a great deal of autonomy, since they are chosen by the countries in each region and they elect the Regional Director. In reality, the Regions tend to follow policy decisions of the global headquarters, but they are free to implement these in their own way.

Between assemblies, there are two meetings per year of an Executive Board, composed of 12 to 18 persons 'technically qualified in the field of health', but not representing their own countries. The Executive Board prepares the agenda for the World Health

Assemblies, and makes recommendations to the Assembly on all matters of world health policy.

For advice on almost every technical question, considered by WHO, the headquarters' Secretariat appoints Expert Panels, and from these are selected Expert Committees that recommend policies. In 1990, there were expert panels on 47 subjects – for example, malaria, maternal and child health, pharmaceuticals, environmental health, medical care organization, health manpower development, etc., – containing 2,600 persons from virtually all countries. The experts chosen for committee meetings are intended to represent all types of country concerned with the special problem discussed.

In its first decade, WHO focused major attention on specific infectious diseases afflicting millions of people in the developing countries. These included malaria, yaws, tuberculosis and venereal diseases. There was also a high priority for maternal and child health services, for environmental sanitation (especially safe water), and for standardization of drugs and vaccines. In these years WHO developed close working relationships with other UN agencies.

The second WHO decade (1958–68) was much influenced by the national liberation in Africa of several former colonies, which became voting members of the Organization. In 1960 the departure from the newly independent Democratic Republic of the Congo of nearly all foreign doctors, created a massive emergency. Working with the international Red Cross, WHO recruited 200 physicians and other health workers, and established a new fellowship programme to enable scores of Congolese 'medical assistants' to become fully qualified doctors. In this period, fellowships for health manpower development became a major WHO strategy in almost all countries.

WHO stimulated and even collaborated with the world chemical industry in the 1960s to develop new insecticides for fighting onchocerciasis ('river blindness') and for treating schistosomiasis, spread by snails. Demonstration that tuberculosis could be effectively treated, without expensive sanatorium care, was a great breakthrough of the late 1950s. Even the mundane standardization of the nomenclature of diseases and causes of death was an important contribution to international health communications.

The third WHO decade (1968–78) included the great world victory of eradicating smallpox from the earth. In 1967, smallpox was still endemic in 31 countries, afflicting 10 to 15 million people. The work was done by teams of public health workers in all the countries affected, with WHO serving as leader, coordinator, and inspiration. Millions of dollars were saved in countries by this achievement, which overcame various national rivalries and suspicions.

The momentum of this great campaign added strength to another drive, for expanding the immunization of the world's children against six once-ravaging diseases – diphtheria, tetanus, whooping cough, measles, poliomyelitis and tuberculosis (with BCG vaccine). After long hesitation for political reasons, in this period WHO finally entered the field of family planning (contraception) by promoting world-wide research and development on human reproduction. New efforts were also put into the control of malaria and leprosy. In this period WHO promoted the training of auxiliary health personnel, such as China's 'barefoot doctor' and India's traditional birth attendant. Such training was a sounder investment in most developing countries than preparing physicians for predominantly urban medical practice.

The fourth decade (1978–88) was ushered in by a great world conference of WHO and UNICEF in Alma Ata, a city in the Asiatic part of the Soviet Union. Thirty years after its birth, 134 member-states of WHO reaffirmed their commitment to equity – as embodied in the slogan 'Health for All'. In reaction against excessive attention to high technology, the Alma Ata Conference emphasized the great importance of primary health care, preventive and curative, as the best approach to national health policy. This approach, stressing community participation, appropriate technology, and intersectoral collaboration became the central pillar of world health policy (see below).

In this period, every country was encouraged to develop a list of 'essential drugs' for use in all public facilities, instead of the thousands of brand-name products sold in world markets. WHO's condemnation of the promotion of artificial infant formula products in developing countries also attracted world-wide attention. The control of world-wide infantile diarrhoea with simple oral rehydration therapy was another great advance, based on very simple principles.

Most of the estimated 500,000 maternal deaths each year are preventable through family planning – to avoid illegal abortions – and hygienic education of traditional birth attendants. WHO has also mounted increasing efforts against cancer, which now takes as many lives in the developing countries as in the affluent ones. The fight against tobacco – the largest single cause of preventable death in both men and women – is part of WHO effort in every country. Disseminating the simple rules of diet, exercise, not smoking, prudent use of alcohol and hygienic working conditions are major objectives of health education in WHO everywhere. The world-wide epidemic of AIDS (acquired immune deficiency syndrome) has presented another challenge to WHO in mounting global efforts to stem the spread of this lethal sexually transmitted virus disease. Underlying all these efforts is WHO's constant advisory activity to strengthen the official public health organization for health protection in all countries.

Interpreting the strategies of WHO work during its first four decades reveals a broad trend from the specific to the general. In its early years, the objectives were defined by specific diseases and conventional categories – such as preventive MCH services and environmental sanitation – within the established domain of public health. A massive crisis in the Congo led to a broader approach in one ex-colony of Africa, but the principal efforts went to the eradication of smallpox and the expanded programme of immunization. In the first two decades WHO was young, perhaps fragile, and dominated by a few Western industrialized countries. It was only in the third decade that the organization felt stable enough to explore the sensitive field of family planning (contraception) and even this was only to promote research in human reproduction.

It was not until the fourth decade that WHO felt strong enough to embrace a far-reaching objective of promoting world-wide equity for health. 'Health for all by the year 2000' was a slogan with the broadest possible political implications. The pathway to this goal was though 'primary health care', which included all principal strategies of prevention, as well as appropriate treatment of common diseases and injuries. The implications of this approach were not concealed, but called frankly for community participation and political commitment. No longer did WHO confine its interest to purely technical matters, but addressed openly the countless issues surrounding the organization of national health systems in every country.

In the fourth decade, after 1978, the great majority of WHO member-states were young developing countries. No longer were policies dictated by a handful of Western powers. The United Nations was firmly established and, even in the Security Council, veto power rested with the Soviet Union and the People's Republic of China, as well as with the United States and the United Kingdom. Among the several UN specialized agencies, WHO was probably the most universally respected. Its performance had won plaudits from countries of every political persuasion. Its Director-General was an unhesitant idealist, born in a small country (Denmark) from a missionary family. The Regional Committees had become an additional source of political expression, and five out of the six were dominated by developing countries. To these countries, dramatic national health problems were more important than the ideologies of

European or American medical associations.

Cooperation of WHO with other specialized agencies of the UN has been effective in avoiding jurisdictional disputes. Cooperation with the International Labour Office (located also in Geneva) has concerned activities in occupational health and in the health aspects of social security programmes. Regarding nutrition and control of animal diseases (*zoonoses*), there is substantial cooperation with the Food and Agriculture Organization (FAO), headquartered in Rome. School health programmes and the health education of teachers involve cooperative relations with the UN Educational, Scientific and Cultural Organization (UNESCO), based in Paris. Collaborative arrangements were even made with the International Civil Aviation Organization (ICAO) on the disinfection of aircraft landing across national borders.

Official relationships were also established between WHO and various international non-governmental organizations (NGOs). Important among these is the International Committee of the Red Cross and the League of Red Cross Societies, but there are hundreds of others in special fields. Under the sponsorship of WHO and UNESCO, an overall NGO was established for maintaining relationships with various scientific bodies. It is known as the Council for International Organizations of the Medical Sciences (CIOMS), and its headquarters, office is in the WHO building in Geneva. The 62 international members of the CIOMS are reviewed every two years by WHO officials. Members of CIOMS include such NGOs as the World Federation for Mental Health, the International Planned Parenthood Federation, the World Medical Association and the International Council of Nurses.

Alma Ata and Primary Health Care

The International Conference on Primary Health Care, held in Alma Ata, has been noted. Out of this conference there was issued the Declaration of Alma Ata, which states, among other things, that:

> A main social target of governments, international organizations and the whole world community in the coming decades should be the attainment by all peoples of the world by the year 2000 of a level of health that will permit them to lead a socially and economically productive life.

This 'primary health care' approach called for attention to major health promotive, preventive, and elementary treatment aspects of common disorders. Several overall strategies were emphasized, such as appropriate technology, community participation, and coordination of health work with other social sectors (education, agriculture, housing, etc.) or intersectoral collaboration. The governments of nearly all countries soon affirmed their support of this primary health care approach in their national health systems.

The Alma Ata Declaration reaffirmed the high priority that countries should give to at least eight well-established programmes of health promotion and protection. These were:

1. education on prevailing health problems and the methods of preventing and controlling them,
2. promotion of an adequate food supply and proper nutrition,
3. an adequate supply of safe water and basic sanitation (waste disposal),
4. maternal and child health care, including family planning,
5. immunization against the major infectious diseases,
6. prevention and control of locally endemic diseases,
7. appropriate treatment of common diseases and injuries, and
8. provision of essential drugs.

As this array of primary health care elements was discussed, an even broader range of health activities was encompassed. As back-up for PHC there had to be small general hospitals at the 'first referral level'. Community health workers, with training of only a few months, had to be prepared in large numbers for work in rural districts. In district hospitals or health centres for ambulatory care, appropriate simple laboratory and even X-ray equipment should be available. Even mental health problems should be identified by PHC workers, if only for appropriate referral to other resources.

General Principles of International Health Work

By the latter 1980s, several basic principles for international health work had become widely accepted by the World Health Organization and other agencies in the United Nations family. Abiding by these principles helps to explain the high respect accorded to WHO and UNICEF throughout the world and especially in the developing countries:

1. International health work in any country is done only at the invitation of the country. Multinational agencies are established by member states and have no supra-national authority.
2. All international civil servants must be devoted only to the agency in which they work, and not to their country of origin.
3. An international health agency must respond to requests for

help, without regard to the political ideology of the government in power. It must not pass judgment on the ethical values of that government. (An exception to this policy has been applied to South Africa, because of its extremely unjust racial policies embodied in 'apartheid'.)

4. The development of national health systems has become generally recognized as contributing to overall social and economic development. Healthy people are able to contribute more effectively to national productivity than people handicapped by disease and disability.
5. The health of a population is influenced by all social sectors, not only by the health services. Health objectives, therefore, demand the greatest possible emphasis on intersectoral collaboration.
6. In determining priorities among the countless health problems observed in all countries, the highest priority should be assigned to problems affecting the largest number of people. This criterion calls for lesser emphasis on high technology tertiary hospitals and greater emphasis on primary health care in all countries.
7. International health policies should promote national health systems that assure the most equitable distribution of health services – preventive and curative – to all people.
8. While motivated initially by the objective of stopping the spread of communicable diseases, international health work has become increasingly concerned with all aspects of health and health services in countries. The promotion of world health is recognized as being dependent on the prudent use of all types of health resources, the control of all types of disease and disability, and the provision of adequate economic support.

The heightened appreciation of international health work is matched, of course, by a greater recognition of the value of health services in virtually all countries. In the early decades of the twentieth century, health and medical activities, as reflected in national expenditures, absorbed only 1 to 4 per cent of national wealth (measured by gross national product or GNP). The fraction was greater in the more industrialized countries and less in the less developed countries, where so much had to be spent on food and shelter. As the potentialities of the health sciences expanded after the Second World War (around 1945), the share of GNP devoted to health systems increased almost everywhere – to a level of 6 to 11 per cent in the affluent countries and a level of 2 to 5 per cent in the developing countries.

These higher expenditures were both a cause and a result of collectivized methods of financing, through general taxation and earmarked social insurance funding. They also provoked greater political interest in cost containment through increasing the efficiency of health systems, deliberate planning of the supply of various health resources (personnel and facilities), and controlling the demand for services through different types of cost-sharing by patients. In all but a few industrialized countries, most health expenditures came from government, and therefore served to make health services economically accessible to nearly everyone. In many, if not most, developing countries, governmental programmes were seriously inadequate, and most health expenditures came from the private sector, with great resultant inequities.

Towards the end of the twentieth century, these inequities became a major concern of international health work – a far cry from the original narrow focus on border quarantine. The World Health Organization, the World Bank, UNICEF and other international agencies have become concerned about how each country organizes and operates its own national health system. The horizon of good health is continually expanding, so that national health systems must become broader and stronger to achieve their goal.

One may wonder how this mounting interest in the overall national health system of each country has affected the 'global' role of WHO. Has this focus constituted a departure from the sense of national interdependence that generated, for example, the early conventions to halt the spread of infectious disease? Not at all. In the modern world, the claim that 'disease knows no borders' has become a cliché that no mature health leader repeats. The goal today is now to assure within all countries – rich or poor, large or small – the full health benefits of modern science and civilization. This is not to avert the transmission of cholera from Asia to Europe, but to enrich the lives of Asian people for their own sake. 'One world' should mean not merely to eliminate the need for border quarantine, but to endow each country with the resources and strategies to achieve maximum health for all its people. At this stage in world history, national sovereignty is still respected. Within this reality, the goal of world health means that all the people of every country will have equal opportunity to attain 'the highest possible level of health'.

Bibliography

Aitken, J. T., H. W. C. Fuller and D. Johnson (eds), *The Influence of Christians in Medicine* (London: Christian Medical Fellowship, 1984).

Allan, Ted and Sydney Gordon, *The Scalpel the Sword: The Story of Norman Bethune* (Boston: Little, Brown & Co., 1952).

Arnold, David (ed.), *Imperial Medicine and Indigenous Societies* (Manchester: Manchester University Press, 1988).

Beck, Ann, *A History of the British Medical Administration of East Africa, 1900–1950* (Cambridge, Mass.: Harvard University Press, 1970).

Council for International Organization of the Medical Sciences, *Organization, Activities, Members* (Geneva: CIOMS, 1989).

Dayton, Edward R., *Medicine and Missions: A Survey of Medical Missions* (Wheaton, Illinois: Medical Assistance Program, 1969).

Garrison, Fielding H., *An Introduction to the History of Medicine, Fourth Edition* (Philadelphia: W.B. Saunders & Co., 1966), 789.

Goodman, Neville M., *International Health Organizations and Their Work* (London: Churchill Livingstone, 1971).

Howard, Lee M., 'International Sources of Financial Cooperation for Health in Developing Countries', *Bulletin of the Pan-American Health Organization* 17 (1983), 142–56.

Howard-Jones, Norman, *International Public Health Between the Two World Wars – The Organizational Problems* (Geneva: World Health Organization, 1978).

Idem, The Pan-American Health Organization: Origins and Evolution (Geneva: World Health Organization, 1981).

Idem, The Scientific Background of the International Sanitary Conferences 1851–1938 (Geneva: World Health Organization, 1975).

Hume, Edward H., *Doctors Courageous* (New York: Harper, 1950).

Kohn, R. and S. Radius, 'International Comparison of Health Services Systems: An Annotated Bibliography', *International Journal of Health Services*, 3(2) (1973), 295–309.

Linsenmeyer, William S., 'Foreign Nations, International Organizations, and Their Impact on Health Conditions in Nicaragua since 1979', *International Journal of Health Services*, 19(3) (1989), 509–29.

Macleod, R.M. and Milton Lewis (eds), *Disease, Medicine and Empire: Perspectives on Western Medicine and the Experience of European Expansion* (London: Routledge, 1988).

Musgrove, Philip, 'The Impact of the Economic Crisis on Health and Health Care in Latin America and the Caribbean', *WHO Chronicle*, 40(4) (1986), 132–47.

Roemer, Milton I, *The Organization of Medical Care under Social Security* (Geneva: International Labour Office, 1969).

Turshen, Meredith, 'The Impact of Colonialism on Health and Health Services in Tanzania', *International Journal of Health Services*, 7(1) (1977), 7–35.

World Health Organization, *The First Ten Years of the World Health Organization* (Geneva: 1958).

World Health Organization, *The Second Ten Years of the World Health Organization 1958–1967* (Geneva: 1968).

Index

B

C

D

Index

R

S

X

Y

Z